P9-DUM-808

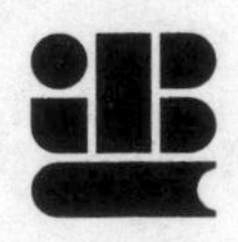

Total Customer Satisfaction

Total Customer Satisfaction

A Comprehensive Approach for Health Care Providers

Stephanie G. Sherman
with
V. Clayton Sherman

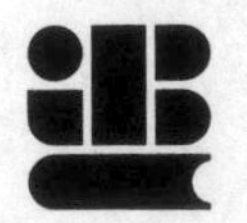

Jossey-Bass Publishers
San Francisco

Quotations in Chapters One and Eight from CEO John Schwartz and data throughout the book from Trinity Hospital are used with permission of John Schwartz and Trinity Hospital.

The quotation in Chapter One from CEO Mark Clement is used with permission of Mark Clement and Holy Cross Hospital.

Jossey-Bass books and products are available through most bookstores. To contact Jossey-Bass directly, call (888) 378–2537, fax to (800) 605–2665, or visit our website at www.josseybass.com.

Substantial discounts on bulk quantities of Jossey-Bass books are available to corporations, professional associations, and other organizations. For details and discount information, contact the special sales department at Jossey-Bass.

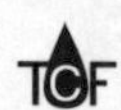
Manufactured in the United States of America using Lyons Falls Turin Book. This paper is acid-free and 100 percent totally chlorine-free.

Library of Congress Cataloging-in-Publication Data

Sherman, Stephanie G.
Total customer satisfaction: a comprehensive approach for health care providers/Stephanie G. Sherman with V. Clayton Sherman.
p. cm.
Includes bibliographical references and index.
ISBN 0-7879-4392-4 (alk. paper)
1. Health services administration. 2. Consumer satisfaction. 3. Patient satisfaction. 4. Medical care—Quality control.
I. Sherman, V. Clayton. II. Title.
RA971.S487 1999
362.1'068—dc21 98-38362
CIP

FIRST EDITION
PB Printing 10 9 8 7 6 5 4 3 2 1

Contents

	Figures, Tables, and Exhibits	ix
	Preface	xiii
	About the Authors	xvii
Chapter 1	Extraordinary Customer Satisfaction: The Facts and the Promise	1
Chapter 2	Eighteen Commandments for Well-Managed Customer Satisfaction Programs	23
Chapter 3	What the Customer Really Wants	87
Chapter 4	Measurement Tools That Work	139
Chapter 5	Calculating the Cost of Dissatisfied Customers	155
Chapter 6	How to Win and Retain Customer Loyalty	181
Chapter 7	The Irrational Nature of Customer Satisfaction: Sweating the Small Stuff	221
Chapter 8	Building the Customer Satisfaction Team	251
Chapter 9	Designing Your Customer Service Strategy	293
Chapter 10	Prescriptions for Sustaining Top Customer Satisfaction Ratings	337
	Recommended Readings	357
	Index	359

Figures, Tables, and Exhibits

CHAPTER 1

Figure	1.1	Satisfaction-Success Cycle	9
Exhibit	1.1	Initiating Total Customer Satisfaction: Task One	20

CHAPTER 2

Figures	2.1	Impacts of Reduced Waiting Times	28
	2.2	Ideation Impacts at Holy Cross Hospital	35
	2.3	Quantifying the Satisfaction-Success Cycle	42
Exhibits	2.1	3C Card	70
	2.2	Sample CEO Welcome Letter	71

CHAPTER 3

Figures	3.1	What Is a Customer?	89
	3.2	The Pareto Principle	91
	3.3	Age Distribution of Patients	113
	3.4	Distribution of Patients by Age and Sex	114
	3.5	Patient Satisfaction by Age and Sex	115
Tables	3.1	Top Ten Issues Most Closely Correlated with the Likelihood of Patients' Recommending a Hospital (Inpatient Services)	93

	3.2	Ten Least Important Factors Correlated with the Likelihood of Patients' Recommending a Hospital (Inpatient Services)	95
	3.3	Forty-Eight Factors Correlated with the Likclihood of Patients' Recommending a Hospital (Inpatient Services)	96
	3.4	Priorities for Customer Satisfaction Improvement (Hospitals)	99
	3.5	Which Aspects of the Emergency Room Experience Correlate with the Likelihood of Patients' Recommending the ER	102
	3.6	Emergency Room Priority Index	104
	3.7	Factors that Influence Recommendations of Medical Practices	108
	3.8	National Priority Index—Medical Practices	110
	3.9	Sample Report—Emergency Department/Room	119
	3.10	Sample Priority Listing	121
	3.11	Holy Cross Sample Customer Satisfaction Report	125
	3.12	Holy Cross Hospital Inpatient Survey Points	127
	3.13	Patient Care by Units	129
	3.14	Call Lights	131

CHAPTER 4

Exhibits	4.1	Vendor Checklist	152
	4.2	Department Survey	154

CHAPTER 5

Figures	5.1	Service Recovery–Time Relationship	165
	5.2	Profitability Components of One Customer	168

CHAPTER 6

Figures	6.1	Customer Feedback Loops	186
	6.2	Customer Loyalty	189
	6.3	Why Loyal Customers Are Profitable	203
Exhibits	6.1	Customer Satisfaction Competencies Checklist	202
	6.2	Sample Internal Customer Satisfaction Survey	215

CHAPTER 8

Figures	8.1	Impacts of Ideation at Holy Cross	253
	8.2	Do-It-Groups and Just-Do-Its: A Flow Chart	276
Exhibit	8.1	Performance Improvement Checklist	258

CHAPTER 9

Exhibit	9.1	Eight Dimensions of Health Care Quality	316

CHAPTER 10

Figure	10.1	The New American Hospital	338
Exhibits	10.1	Self-Audit Test for Work System Effectiveness	342
	10.2	Self-Audit CEO Tips for Sustained Success	355

This book is dedicated to
Jonathan Bently Metzger,
who while living life to its fullest,
has experienced the helpless, vulnerable,
but never hopeless patient experience of
many emergency rooms and too many
hospitals. And to Adam Michael Metzger,
who reminds me daily that love, patience,
and personal support are essential
elements in every healing effort.

This book is also dedicated to all the
mothers of children who will call upon
health care facilities for help, healing,
and hope. We, in turn, hope that this
book will help make every health care
experience during such difficult times
less trying and more satisfying.

Preface

Why are a select few health care organizations better, year in and year out, at delivering extraordinary Customer Satisfaction while others struggle with making progress? What do they know, and what do they do that results in accolades from patients and physicians alike?

About a dozen years ago we began working with health care organizations interested in creating a competitive advantage by boosting organization performance. The idea was to create a New American Health Care Organization—one focused on values and mission while performing exceptionally well in the operational areas of high Customer Satisfaction, low cost, high quality, and employing the best people.

To create the New American Health Care Organization, we borrowed best practices in business and industry in the areas of Customer Satisfaction, cost, quality, and people management, and we adapted them to the health care environment.

The results were favorably astonishing. New American Health Care Organizations are winning in their competitive markets. They are experiencing extraordinary growth in market share even when located in consolidated and shrinking markets, dramatically improved financial results though competitors struggle to survive, exponential increases in employee satisfaction while others experience strikes and layoffs, and national recognition as top-rated health care organizations for Customer Satisfaction. (The philosophy and operating assumption of the concept of the New American Health Care Organization are outlined in the 1993 book, *Creating the New American Hospital: A Time for Greatness* by Dr. Clay Sherman, and will be expanded upon in the 1999 sequel, *Raising Standards in American Health Care: Best People, Best Practices, Best Results.*)

One of the cornerstones for creating a New American Health Care Organization is *Total Customer Satisfaction* as an operational priority. Management and staff must share a common passion for making each health care experience exceptional—a caring, compassionate, healing experience. Providing Total Customer Satisfaction is clearly their reason for being, yet most health care organizations are struggling to boost Customer Satisfaction ratings. It is in their heart to do the right thing, but they simply do not know how to make a difference. This book provides the recipe for success. In a detailed, step-by-step fashion, the "how to's" for boosting Customer Satisfaction are laid out for use by any health care provider, whether hospital, clinic, medical practice, nursing home, home health care agency, or extended care facility. Use the recipe and quickly reap the rewards of success that so many others have experienced.

In the past, cost and quality considerations have driven health care management decisions. New studies indicate that although the majority of Americans believe that the health care industry is changing how it does business in order to better meet consumer demands, the industry still has a long way to go to meet consumer demands. The companies and providers who "put consumers first" are predicted to gain competitive advantage.[1]

For purposes of this book, *Customer* refers primarily to patients but also includes physicians, who play a dual role of Customer of the hospital and partner with the hospital; health plan providers and/or payers, who must be satisfied in order for the health care organization to continue to survive; and employers, who are sourcing health care providers that meet the needs of their employees. In some cases, *Customer* refers to the "internal Customers" of the organization, such as supporting departments, that serve direct patient care-giving departments.

You will notice that throughout the book the word *Customer* begins with a capital letter. Although this usage may not be stylistically correct, it is nonetheless intentional. *Customer* is capitalized out of respect for the people that the word represents, as also is *Associate*, which signifies employees of the organization.

Today's patients, physicians, and payers, who constitute the largest body of health care Customers, are making new and powerful demands on health care providers. These groups are more educated, and are aided by reliable sources of information and the revolution in information technology. In no other industry is the challenge for providing top Customer Satisfaction as complicated as it is in health care.

Our mission in writing this book is to share the philosophy, knowledge, and operational acts that created and sustain the ability of America's top-rated health care organizations to deliver Customer Satisfaction. Our hope is to upgrade the health care experience in all organizations in the years to come.

Thousands of health care leaders have read the forerunner of this book, *Creating the New American Hospital: A Time for Greatness,* and applied the philosophy in their organization. The present book offers you a new level of understanding of how to achieve and effectively manage Customer Satisfaction in health care.

This book presents both fact and anecdote. Without the latter, facts would have little life, and some of the ideas could not be clearly grasped without an example of how to apply them. Further, each idea can be interpreted and applied in a number of different ways. There is no one specific application of each idea that guarantees results. Rather, the value of the book is in the interpretation and application of each idea in a way that fits your organization. The stories demonstrate how each idea can be interpreted and applied in a variety of ways.

In each chapter, concepts are discussed first, then examples provided to illustrate the points, followed by an Action Plan section with specific Tasks to be done in your organization or operation to implement the concepts and achieve the desired results. The approach is "discuss, then do."

Do not take any assignment lightly. For a number of reasons, not all assignments will be possible to implement in your organization. The more assignments that are implemented, however, the greater the results you will see.

Your organization may already have some of the Task work in place. In these situations, evaluate the extent to which your current format is achieving the level of results you desire. If current results are something less than extraordinary, reevaluate what you are doing as compared to what is described in this book, and make modifications. The idea is continuous improvement, not acceptance of whatever is currently provided.

We intend to communicate the mundane but critical aspects that drive Customer Satisfaction ratings, as well as extraordinary actions and accomplishments of top-performing organizations in Customer Satisfaction. After all, patients experience the total package of experiences, which includes more daily, routine health care encounters than exceptional "superservice" events.

Like any good product or service, the *Total Customer Satisfaction Strategy* for health care is an evolving set of ideas and applications. The ideas and applications represented in this book have been successfully implemented in hundreds of organizations in a variety of ways. We are constantly learning of new, no-cost and low-cost ideas that add to Customer Satisfaction and move one organization ahead of others in the competitive pack. This book reflects our most recent thinking and experiences on how to achieve extraordinary patient and physician satisfaction. But the current level of Customer Satisfaction must continue to evolve in order to remain competitive.

Several organizations have worked closely with us in the application and testing of the ideas and action plans presented in this book. Other organizations have been extremely helpful in supplying information and research on measuring Customer Satisfaction in the health care industry. It is not possible to recognize by name all of the organizations and people who have contributed to the *Total Customer Satisfaction* strategy over the years. However, we would like to recognize the following organizations for their continued assistance in this project: Press, Ganey Associates, South Bend, Indiana; Picker Associates, Boston, Massachusetts; Parkside Associates, Park Ridge, Illinois; Trinity Hospital, Chicago, Illinois; and Holy Cross Hospital, Chicago, Illinois.

NOTES

1. Kathryn F. Clark. "Employers Group Ranks Physicians." *Human Resources Executive,* December 1997, p. 18.

About the Authors

Stephanie G. Sherman is a nationally recognized authority on cutting-edge management and one of the most sought after speakers in health care and business today. She has spoken before health care, business, civic, and educational audiences. Her work and writing are changing the way health care conducts business, and continue to break new ground in the ever-changing world of health care. As a keynote speaker and seminar leader for individual organizations, health care systems, associations, and individual executive coaching sessions, Stephanie Sherman delivers simple yet effective approaches to achieve outstanding business and personal results. She is frequently quoted as an expert on personal achievement and business management by radio and print media, including the *Chicago Tribune, Investors Business Daily, USA Today,* and numerous professional journals.

As executive vice president of Management House, Inc., Stephanie Sherman specializes in organization and individual performance improvement seminars and strategy implementation in the areas of customer and employee satisfaction, cost management and quality improvement, business growth, and organization culture development. Stephanie Sherman has completed postgraduate work at the Harvard School of Business and has earned an M.B.A. from Capital University.

V. Clayton Sherman is founder and chairman of Management House, Inc., in Inverness, Illinois. Management House, Inc., provides management and organization development services to a wide range of Fortune 500 companies, hospitals, associations, and emerging growth organizations.

Dr. Sherman's primary consulting experience encompasses wide-scale change processes, organization renewal, and operational excellence. He specializes in hospital revitalization and high-performance management. Clients of Management House, Inc., have been honored with awards such as the Great Comebacks Award, the International Enterprise Award for Customer Satisfaction, the Global Best Practices Award for Customer Satisfaction, the Innovative Practice Award for Human Resources, the Top 100 Best Hospitals Award, and more.

Other books authored by one or both of the Shermans include

Creating the New American Hospital: A Time for Greatness

Make Yourself Memorable: Winning Strategies to Impact Your Boss, Your Coworkers, Your Customers . . . and Everybody Else!

Performance and Promotability: The Making of an Executive

From Losers to Winners

We would like to hear from you. If you are interested in sharing your success stories on how your organization is *Raising Standards in American Health Care* (forthcoming), or if you would like to share your tips and success stories on *Total Customer Satisfaction,* please write, enclosing a self-addressed, stamped envelope, to Stephanie G. Sherman, 1046 Aberdeen Road, Inverness, IL 60067.

Total Customer Satisfaction

Chapter
ONE

Extraordinary Customer Satisfaction

The Facts and the Promise

It is the nature of business today that if you are not getting better, you are getting behind.

The pendulum of Customer influence in health care has significantly shifted in the past few years and continues to shift with gaining momentum in favor of the voice and choice of Customers. In the recent past, health care consumers were at the twin mercies of the physician as to which hospital they would use and of their employers for a limited number of health insurance providers from which to choose. Things have changed.

Government payers and national accreditation organizations are moving to incorporate Customer Satisfaction ratings in their evaluation of health care providers' performance levels. For example, there is a movement under way to incorporate information about Customer Satisfaction into Medicaid reporting, and the Joint Commission on Hospital Accreditation has already mandated measurement of patient satisfaction as a part of their evaluation process. Employers who require employees to pay a substantial share of the cost of health care insurance are under fire to include health care providers that *the employees find satisfactory.*

The health, wealth, and continued existence of health care providers now hinge on the voices of patients, physicians, and insurers. Those who serve Customers well will thrive, and those who serve in a less than acceptable manner will perish.

A recent story in the *Human Resources Executive* cites a San Francisco–based employers group, Pacific Business Group on Health, that published a ranking based on patient surveys of fifty physician groups. The report card that they published focuses on the performance of physician groups rather than on specific health plans. Their goal is to help employees select a service provider that is close to the individual employee's specific needs, then choose a health plan in which that provider participates—an approach contrary to the physician-selection process commonly used elsewhere today. This group rates physician groups on criteria such as patient satisfaction, ease of referrals, and the ability to manage patients' blood pressure and cholesterol clinically.[1]

Surely those bold enough to participate in such an evaluation of their performance levels, if participation is indeed voluntary, would not want to find themselves listed in the lower portion of ratings. Perhaps they wouldn't have participated if they knew where they ranked comparatively.

The race is on to provide exceptional Customer Satisfaction in hospitals, outpatient facilities, emergency rooms, and physician practices. Management of Customer Satisfaction has become a cornerstone to the success of the health care business.

WHAT MAKES CUSTOMER SATISFACTION DIFFERENT?

Customer Satisfaction is different from other health care business indicators because it represents the consumer's *subjective* perception of the quality of the health care experience. In every service business it is the consumer's subjective satisfaction level that determines which organizations get today's and tomorrow's business. The extreme degree of subjectivity in Customer Satisfaction ratings makes consistently high performance levels difficult, but not impossible, to produce. Once an organization has mastered the formula for performing at top levels and has installed the infrastructure necessary to sustain it, the organization will have gained a competitive advantage that other organizations cannot easily reproduce.

A new service or piece of technology that you offer today can be duplicated or purchased by your competitors tomorrow, thus making that particular competitive advantage short-lived. However, your competitors cannot easily replicate the hundreds of small things that you do for patients and physicians to earn extraordinary satisfaction ratings. Nor can they buy or easily duplicate kind, caring, and effective human relations skills that seem so natural for the staff of winning New American Health Care organizations.

Some argue that cost and quality are the driving factors dictating which health care facilities will win the competitive game. They say that those with low cost and high quality will win. All those who hold that philosophy, consider this question: What happens when a low-cost, high-quality health care experience falls short on Customer Satisfaction expectations? The answer is that the consumer, whether patient or physician, will not be back but will find another physician to help them or another hospital to use.

Some leaders call this a "one-time stand." The patient is there for one experience, and the unsatisfactory experience as judged by the Customer is enough to make him change health care providers. Or, the physician practices at an organization for one year, and dissatisfaction with the situation is enough to convince her to change organizations. These one-time Customers seek alternative arrangements where cost and quality are equally good and the total experience is more satisfying.

Health care business cannot be built on a series of one-time visits but it can be destroyed by a series of one-time relationships.

EMERGING POWERS OF EXTRAORDINARY CUSTOMER SATISFACTION

Reports Jerry Seibert, president of Parkside Associates:

> *People like to think that the next field of competition is quality, but quality is hard to measure, and to some degree Customer Satisfaction is a measure of perceived quality. Meanwhile, before and after the quality competition, patient satisfaction will be the final differentiator."*

Why is Customer Satisfaction emerging as a power? What's changed in health care that boosts the power of the Customer? Patients are still patients, and physicians still practice medicine—so what's new? Answer: Everything.

The following nine changes have been highly influential in contributing to the power of the Customer in the health care industry.

More Choices and Raised Voices. Health care consumers have more choices today than they've had in the past. More outpatient facilities, independent clinics, and a variety of alternative health care providers now supply a market that was once dominated by hospitals.

In the past, patients had little or no voice in choosing a health care facility. The patient chose the physician, and the physician dictated which health care facilities would be used based on his or her independent professional opinion or professional relationship with a particular facility. Now health care plans offer a choice of physicians as well as a choice of hospitals. A look through my *PPO Health Care Book of Providers* shows literally hundreds of physicians of various specialties and many local choices of hospitals. As a patient, I can choose my physician, and I can choose the hospital or outpatient facility where I wish to be treated.

In addition to competing among themselves, hospitals must now also compete with various types of outpatient community facilities, such as twenty-four-hour emergency care centers and hospital-managed outpatient specialty centers. Alternatives for where to go for health care assistance are growing in number.

So who's making hospital and outpatient facility choices? Patients are.

Physicians as Business People. Once upon a time the art of medicine was the physician's primary concern. Under the cost reimbursement structure there was little need for physicians to concern themselves with basic business skills because they were paid whatever professional fee they deemed appropriate. Nice work when you could get it.

Enter the changing arena of managed care, slashed reimbursement rates, and the reality that a comfortable livelihood for many physicians has come to depend on their ability to embrace the basics of business, including managing Customer Satisfaction, in concert with their healing skills.

Fundamentals, such as that unsatisfied patients translate into fewer patients and therefore reduced revenue, are being seen and better understood by physicians. Consequently, physicians' sensitivity to patient satisfaction is on the rise. Physicians are seeking simultaneous practice privileges at numerous hospitals to allow them to accommodate patient requests for care at patients' specific hospitals-of-choice. It also provides the physician with an easy and painless way to shift admissions from one organization to the other based on their patients' satisfaction levels with the health care experience.

Physicians as Listeners and Learners. To the extent that physicians have an increased desire to satisfy patients, they want to use hospitals and outpatient facilities known to deliver exceptionally satisfying experiences so as to expand their own, personal reputations.

Through the patient's eyes, the hospital and physician are linked in the overall health care experience. Patients don't necessarily distinguish physician services from hospital services. It's the overall package they remember as an experience. When I had my tonsils removed, I didn't think, "Boy, that doctor was great and the hospital was the pits." I remembered that the overall experience was somewhat less than satisfactory; there were problems that didn't need to be problems.

The adage that "you're known by who you run with" is never more true than in a highly competitive situation in which there will definitely be winners, and there will be definitely be losers. That is why winners want to associate with winners. Winners don't associate with losers. Understanding this phenomenon, smart physicians refer their patients to winning health care facilities where the total health care experience will be as positive as possible.

In the interest of building a medical practice based on repeat business and personal referrals, astute physicians listen for patient feedback on their experience in the hospital or outpatient center. When the patient is happy, everybody is happy. When the patient is unhappy, the doctor hears the complaints, anger, and criticisms. Unhappy physicians mean lost future referrals to your hospital or outpatient business.

So who's listening to Customer Satisfaction ratings? Physicians are, and they are making referral decisions based on patient feedback.

Excess Capacity. It's not new. If you've been keeping up on the health care industry, you know that there are far more hospital beds than needed. The supply of health care providers, such as hospitals, exceeds the demand for such facilities and services, and there is no expectation that the trend will change any time in the near term.

In the healthiest of business situations, when everyone is busy and competition takes the form of who can grow fastest, the battle for market share is keen. But in a consolidating industry such as health care, where the market in total is shrinking and there is not enough business for all operations to continue, competition becomes shark-like.

Health care is competitively shark-like. The loss of one physician practice or one managed care contract can mean the difference between profit and foreclosure for some organizations. That being the case, sharp executives listen carefully to what patients and physicians have to say about Customer Satisfaction in their facility. There is no room for Customer defection.

Obsession with the Right to Satisfaction. Where did all this Customer Satisfaction stuff start anyhow? Who said that people have a right to judge their health care experience or any other experience? What do they know about the technical aspects of health care? How can they possibly judge their experience?

No matter what their level of education or experience, people have an opinion, and they want to share it. With a more intense and vocalized right-to-satisfaction movement under way globally, the voices and choices of patients and physicians have become louder and more clear. They are demanding a satisfactory experience or they won't pay, they won't be back, but they will tell their story of woe to anyone who will listen.

In a 1993 article in *Fortune*, "Meet the New Consumer," the author proclaims that the Customer is not king anymore, "The Customer is dictator." The author pronounces a societal movement toward the "right to satisfaction," a newly proclaimed personal right that supports the drive for greater Customer Satisfaction in health care and in every other aspect of society. And what patients and physicians find to be satisfactory continues to evolve to higher and higher levels. The list of demands is lengthening and patience is shrinking.

Power to Health Plan Providers. "Everybody loves a winner." Winners, for purposes of this discussion, are defined as professionals and organizations whom the Customer deems extraordinary—those who provide a quality service at a competitive price and with a high level of satisfaction.

How do Customers determine who is a winner and who is not? One primary measurement is the collective opinion of the *ultimate Customer*, the patient. The patient is the ultimate Customer because she is the one universal consumer of all segments of the health care business. Patients consume physician services, health care plan provider services, and health care facilities services. As the one universal consumer of all segments of the health care business, patients hold the greatest power, and it is their satisfaction level that a health care business must meet or exceed to survive as a business entity.

Consider the case of health plan providers such as Blue Cross and others who build their business by selling more and more health insurance coverage; the number of covered lives is one indicator of their business performance. In order for Blue Cross to retain current policy holders and recruit new policy holders they must satisfy current and prospective Customers.

Customer satisfaction for health plan providers encompasses important items such as premium costs and coverage, and it also includes heavy-hitting items such as inclusion of the patient's preferred physician and preferred hospital or outpatient clinic as a part of the provider base. When patients are not satisfied with their choice of doctors or health care facilities, they change health insurance plans or companies and move to one that does offer their preferred providers. This means that when patients prefer your hospital or medical practice over others, their preference—the voice of the patient—will be valued by insurance providers, thus making your relationship with insurers potentially more pleasant and definitely more possible.

This all boils down to the single most important factor for winning in the health care provider business: *you* must be the preferred provider—the provider of choice as determined by a large number of patients and physicians.

A Shifting Balance of Power. Exceptional Customer Satisfaction ratings are a strong indicator that an organization is a provider of choice. High Customer Satisfaction ratings typically translate into higher than average Customer loyalty, which in turn better positions the organization to petition for inclusion in the database of premier health plan providers, as well as to negotiate better reimbursement rates for services. A mutually exclusive relationship develops between preferred health care providers and premier health plan providers.

Health plan providers need preferred health care providers in their base of facilities and physicians from which to choose. They don't want to disappoint large populations of Customers who prefer your facility because of highly satisfactory experiences they and other family and friends have had there. In turn, your facility needs to be included in the database of choices that serve a large population represented by premier health plan providers. The power equation between health plan provider and health care facility begins to balance out.

In a summary description of this interactive, interdynamic phenomena, CEO John Schwartz of Trinity Hospitals explains,

> *Customer satisfaction drives organization performance. It's a large circular phenomena beginning with the number of patients that prefer your organization over others.*

The greater the number of patients who prefer your organization over others, the more frequently managed care plans and insurers that feature your organization will be selected. And the more frequently patients request your organization to be part of the insurance package, the greater the level of cooperation you are likely to experience in negotiations with insurers. We call this the Success Cycle. Success in one area, such as Customer Satisfaction management, generates success in another area, and the cycle becomes self-perpetuating. See Figure 1.1 for a visual picture of the Satisfaction-Success Cycle.

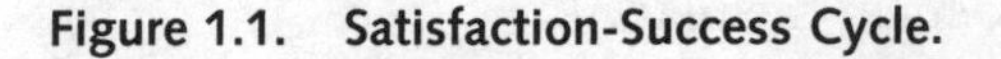

Figure 1.1. Satisfaction-Success Cycle.

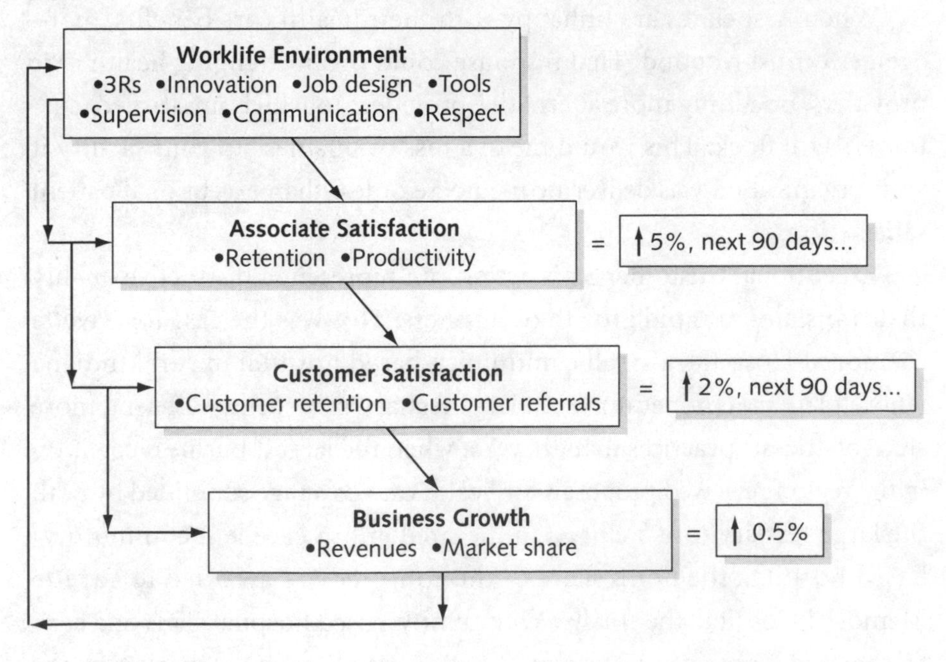

The reverse is also true. If your organization delivers "average" Customer Satisfaction, as measured by reliable firms using comparative national norms for Customer Satisfaction ratings, health insurance organizations are likely to have little or no interest in negotiating better rates with your organization or possibly even in continuing to offer your organization as a part of the package, and your organization will wither.

Employer Obligations. Currently, employers and employer consortiums are conducting formal and informal feedback from Associates regarding their satisfaction with health care providers. Given the high-profile position that health benefits hold in Associates' eyes, the shifting and sharing of health-benefit costs between employer and Associate, and the high proportion of expenses that this benefit represents in the overall benefit package, it is not unreasonable to expect that employers are monitoring satisfaction with the benefit, which translates to monitoring Customer Satisfaction with the health care providers in the plan.

When Associates are unhappy with their health care benefits, management must respond. That response could mean changing health care providers, or adding more alternative providers to which unsatisfied Customers will flock. This would mean a loss of business to your facility if your organization was delivering mediocre or less than exceptional patient satisfaction.

Exceptional Customer Satisfaction can represent a distinctive quality that translates to rapid growth of business. This was the case for Fayette Memorial Hospital, a small·community-based hospital in rural Indiana whose primary competitor was a large tertiary care facility offering more state-of-the-art practices than they. Yet when the largest business coalition in the region reviewed proposals for health care coverage submitted by both the large tertiary care facility and the smaller but excellent community-based hospital, the lion's share of the contract was awarded to Fayette Memorial Hospital, the smaller, community-based hospital. This one contract award represents 70 percent of the covered lives in the market area—

the lion's share of the health care market. The determining factor in awarding the contract, as reported by Fayette Memorial Hospital CEO David Brandon, "was the leadership and management teams' commitment to providing exceptional Customer Satisfaction."

A second example of exceptional Customer Satisfaction serving as the cornerstone for market share growth is that of Holy Cross Hospital in Chicago. With a rapid rise in Customer Satisfaction ratings from the thirteenth percentile to the ninety-ninth and hundredth percentile in the national Press, Ganey Associates database, the organization coincidentally experienced a growth in market share in the range of 3 to 4 percent annually for each of the past four years while competitors experienced a shrinkage in market share to the tune of 1 to 2 percent each year. By building on the Customer Satisfaction cornerstone, combined with an aggressive plan to expand services and the physician base, Holy Cross doubled their outpatient revenues, moving from $9 million of debt in 1991 to more than $5.6 million in profit in 1996.

Holy Cross Hospital CEO Mark Clement reflects on this outstanding performance and explains,

> *Customer Satisfaction alone did not attract all the new patients, but it did allow us to retain each new and existing patient and it made it easier to grow through our external strategies of managed care contracts, new programs, more physicians, and expanded outpatient facilities. If we did not implement the external strategy, we would not grow, and if we did not implement the internal, Customer Satisfaction strategy, we would not be able to retain new physicians and patients.*

New Mandates and the Creation of National Databases.

> *There are real mandates going on regarding Customer Satisfaction. Medicaid will be requiring that Customer Satisfaction surveys be conducted, and employers who are requiring Associates to pay a portion of the health insurance costs are beginning to survey their Associates*

about their opinion of health care providers as well as share Customer Satisfaction information collected by HEDIS [Health Employers Data Information Set] with them.[2]

HEDIS has already begun collecting and making available data on health plans regarding Customer Satisfaction, as member satisfaction is one area of measurement on which health plans are focusing. Measurements in this early stage are a little shaky in that they often cross over from the area of member satisfaction to patient satisfaction. The goal is to measure Customer Satisfaction with the health care plan and how complaints with the plan are handled, rather than focus on complaints with the provider. However, HEDIS often can link the data that they have on health care plans to the providers who cared for the patients.

In short, measurement of Customer Satisfaction with health plans is already under way. And it makes good business sense for executives of health plans to want to know which providers in their plans are contributing to their good name in Customer Satisfaction, and which are tarnishing it.

For those who have nothing positive to contribute in terms of high Customer Satisfaction, the telephone will not be ringing at contract-renewal time. No one will be calling to discuss your role in next year's health plan programs because your organization will have been replaced with one that is more innovative and Customer driven.

UNEXPECTED BENEFITS OF EXCEPTIONAL CUSTOMER SATISFACTION

Providing exceptional Customer Satisfaction is just plain good business, and health care providers who deliver top levels of service do so because it is the right thing to do. However, by doing the "right thing" they coincidentally gain a number of related benefits. The following unexpected benefits have consistently accrued to organizations achieving top customer satisfaction ratings.

Negotiation Power. For the past several years the focus for health plan providers, and consequently for hospitals, has largely been dominated by cost management and driven by reimbursement rates. Predictably, with an initial strong focus on containing cost, the next logical step would be improving quality. In recent years the cost/quality argument has leveled out; providers now realize that both cost and quality thresholds must be met and, in fact, can be met with new management and operating approaches.

Now that the dust surrounding competitive battles over cost and quality is settling, the question is how to distinguish more excellent health care providers from the rest of the mediocre pack. All else being equal (cost and quality), what do winners bring to the negotiating table that others do not? Emerging as the differentiating element between excellent organizations and mediocre ones is exceptional Customer Satisfaction—a representative voice of consumers making the choice of where to spend their health care dollars.

When patient and physician satisfaction ratings indicate that one organization is clearly superior at delivering an exceptional health care experience with a comparable or better level of quality and cost, health care plan providers are more apt to listen intently to what the exceptional provider has to say. Since health care organizations are working to satisfy the same Customers that health plan providers are working to satisfy, the camaraderie between exceptional service-oriented health care organizations and health plan providers strengthens.

To the extent that there is any discretion in establishing reimbursement rates, health plan providers are more likely to use that discretionary decision making to the advantage of health care facilities that are producing highly satisfied patients and physicians. *Result:* better negotiated reimbursement rates, which translate to increased hospital/physician revenues. Teaming up in this way is a win for the health plan provider, who experiences a stabilized and growing base of highly satisfied Customers, and for hospitals and physicians, who receive more revenue for services performed.

Jerry Seibert, President of Parkside Associates, a nationally recognized Customer Satisfaction measurement vendor, succinctly states,

> *The demand for valid Customer satisfaction measurement continues to expand as managed care organizations work to level the field of competition based on pricing. The next field of competition is patient satisfaction.*

Partnership Power. If society has indeed embraced the idea of a "right to Satisfaction," it makes sense to expect that in a fragmented industry such as health care, where each component of an intricate process is delivered by a different organization under different leadership and standards of performance, that Customer Satisfaction ratings for each segment of the business would be critical to identify where unsatisfactory performance is occurring and where immediate changes are required. After all, when one segment of the experience goes sour, an eclipse overshadows all aspects of the experience, and everyone associated suffers to some degree. Consequently, it is essential to know which suppliers are providing less than satisfactory service so that they can be quickly corrected or replaced by others who will deliver desirable Customer satisfaction levels.

"Together we stand, divided we fall" is more true in health care today than it has been in the past. When all components of the delivery process are exceeding Customer Satisfaction thresholds, the system is strong and stands for another day. But if any *one* aspect of the system does not measure up, the system as a whole begins to waver. The more pieces that don't measure up, the more it wavers until Customer opinion becomes decidedly unfavorable, and business ceases to exist. Therefore, it is in the best interest of all providers and vendors working with your organization to measure Customer Satisfaction with their specific piece of the process as well as to measure satisfaction with the overall experience.

Customer Satisfaction measurement becomes the tool by which organizations and systems of organizations identify and fix underperforming subsets of the total system. Subsets of performance that cannot or will not adjust to reflect expected levels of performance should be discarded and a new player or vendor with higher standards recruited to replace it.

In summary, Customer Satisfaction ratings are becoming *the key determinant* of whether or not a business or professional organization continues to exist in the health care business community.

Recruitment of Physicians on Staff. Physicians have two priorities in mind when they select a health care facility at which to base their practice:

1. How well does this facility serve my needs as a physician?
2. How well will my patients like using this facility?

The only indicator of how well an organization meets these requirements is the opinion of its consumers, communicated in Customer Satisfaction ratings provided to the organization.

On the surface, Customer Satisfaction ratings seem to be a simple rating of how people feel about the experience. The reality is that Customer Satisfaction ratings are a measurement of the performance level of the *overall system* supporting the final outcome of a health care experience. To deliver extraordinary Customer satisfaction, numerous components of the system need to work together and work well. For example, staff must be friendly, attentive, and skilled; adequate supplies must be readily available; effective communication systems and equipment need to be in place; and a million other details all have to come together to provide the overall experience that the Customer will rate as excellent. When all components of the organization are operating effectively and at a high standard of performance, this overall quality is reflected in the Customer Satisfaction ratings.

Physicians want to practice in an organization that operates efficiently, and what is even more important, they want to send their patients to an organization that reflects the high level of professional performance that physicians subscribe to themselves. In short, excellent operating systems make it easy for physicians to practice medicine, and keep patients feeling satisfied with the overall health care experience. *Result:* an influx of physicians seeking privileges to practice at the organization that delivers high Customer Satisfaction, as demonstrated at Holy Cross Hospital in Chicago.

Holy Cross Hospital, one of America's top-rated health care organizations in Customer satisfaction (Press Ganey database) for the past several years, was not always the epitome of Customer Satisfaction. At one time, Holy Cross was on the brink of closing its doors. Customer Satisfaction ratings were at the thirteenth percentile nationally, the hospital was financially indebted, and nothing looked promising except the new CEO who had accepted the challenge of saving the organization.

Enter Mark Clement, new CEO. Mark's strategy was to build the infrastructure of the organization as rapidly as possible in order to support the new business that he planned to bring in, and then to build new business. Mark explains:

> *One of the key internal infrastructure components was Customer Satisfaction. We didn't have any money, so we could not compete on technologically advanced services, but we could compete on Customer Satisfaction—build an image of the friendliest, most comfortable and accommodating health care facility. From the image of Customer Satisfaction grew repeat business, and a reputation for serving the Customer well. In turn, this allowed us to recruit more physicians, which means more admissions and services. With our costs under control, more business meant more money to the bottom line, and from the Customer Satisfaction focus we were able to grow the business.*
>
> *Today we are busier than ever with a full census; twenty-seven new community satellite facilities; substantial growth in market share; and money in the bank. We grew out of debt and to a point where it was possible to start rebuilding the technological aspect of our health care business. We could not have done this without the infrastructure support provided by a staff and work systems driven by the desire to provide exceptional Customer Satisfaction.*

John Schwartz, CEO of Trinity Hospital in Chicago, reinforces these sentiments of exceptional Customer Satisfaction in his analysis of the value of Customer satisfaction,

> *Since our Associate Satisfaction and Customer Satisfaction ratings have improved we have seen a significant increase in the number of physicians asking for privileges. The backlog of requests has caused us to streamline the process for credentialing in order to get them on board faster.*

More evidence of the power of providing exceptional Customer Satisfaction.

Public Interest and No-Cost Publicity. Statistical quality and financial measurements for excellence in health care are largely beyond the comprehension of the average health care consumer. Statistics such as cost per adjusted occupied bed mean nothing to the consumer. "How do you adjust the cost of a bed?" is the common question. The notion of mortality rates adjusted for complications elicits, "If it wasn't complicated, they wouldn't be in the hospital!"

The reality is that there are few measurements of excellence in health care that mean anything to the average consumer except the one measurement easily understood and interpreted by the general population—Customer Satisfaction ratings. People know that a facility's high satisfaction ratings mean that they are more likely to have a positive experience at that facility.

Winning awards for Customer Satisfaction brings national publicity and recognition—at no cost—as Holy Cross Hospital happily learned when their organization was named the top-rated health care organization for Customer Satisfaction in 1995. As a result, special news stories were aired on television and full-page reports graced the covers of local and national publications. Again, in 1996, Holy Cross Hospital earned Anderson's "Enterprise Award for Customer Satisfaction," for which a feature story on their success was featured in *Fortune* magazine.

How does this translate to further business results? What is the value of favorable local and national television and newspaper publicity? The argument for inclusion in preferred health plans just became easier, and negotiations for more favorable reimbursement rates just got stronger. Widespread positive publicity elevated the image of the organization, which in turn brought more patients and physicians. And the cost for all this publicity? Nothing more than doing the right thing to start with—providing a health care experience that highly satisfies patients and physicians.

WHAT THE FUTURE WILL BRING

Getting today's health care services in line with Customer expectations is a challenging proposition that will grow ever more challenging as baby boomers grow older and thus become heavier users of the health care system. To get a handle on how boomers and younger people rate satisfaction with health care compared to those who are older, Press, Ganey Associates conducted survey research among 1,007,612 patients from inpatient hospitals around the United States by asking forty-nine standard questions. The results indicate that patients fifty years of age or younger are considerably more dissatisfied with health care services than older generations. Baby boomers had a mean satisfaction of 83.1, a rate significantly lower than that of older folks, categorized as "war babies," "Depressioners," and "GI generation," whose mean scores were 84.5, 85.5, and 85.2, respectively.[3]

Boomers have been raised on the principle of getting what they want when they want it. Movies on demand, money from the ATM, fast food from the drive-through—the fax me, beep me, get me what I need now generation. Their impatience with imperfection and their power as consumers have driven major change in every industry.

Considering that the 1998 U.S. population of baby boomer or younger generations is approximately 77 million, these expectations present a substantial challenge to health care providers in the coming years. Those who master Customer Satisfaction philosophy and practice now will be better positioned to handle the intensified expectations of the aging boomer generation.

ACTION PLAN FOR TOTAL CUSTOMER SATISFACTION

The following is a step-by-step strategy to initiate and implement Total Customer Satisfaction in your organization.

Task 1. Understanding the Impact of Customer Satisfaction. Discuss the nine major changes contributing to the boost in Customer Satisfaction power in the health care industry discussed in this chapter, and add other changes to the list that you see as pertinent to Total Customer Satisfaction management. Discuss why Total Customer Satisfaction management must become a more active initiative within your organization. Use the worksheet provided in Exhibit 1.1 to assist you in this discussion.

Complete your discussion with a prognosis of what will happen to the organization if Total Customer Satisfaction is not brought to the forefront of active and continuous improvement.

Task 2. Gaining Top Executives' Support: Ascertaining to What Extent Customer Satisfaction Management Is a Driver of Organization Performance. To garner the support of top executives for Customer Satisfaction management initiatives, you must first show them that Customer Satisfaction is a driver of overall organization performance. The more executives see Customer Satisfaction as a driver of organization performance, the more importance they will place on efforts to manage and provide extraordinary Customer Service, thus leading to more resources and administrative support for changes needed to enhance satisfaction levels. Winning organizations realize that without exceptional Total Customer Satisfaction they will not and cannot grow as a business. Without it, their very existence in the future is questionable.

Exhibit 1.1. *Initiating Total Customer Satisfaction: Task One.*

Things That Have Changed	Why Action Is Needed
Obsession with right to satisfaction	____________
Physicians as listeners and learners	____________
Physicians as business people	____________
New mandates and creation of national database	____________
Excess capacity	____________
More choices and raised voices	____________
Shifting of the balance of power	____________
Employer obligations	____________

Other:

____________	____________
____________	____________
____________	____________

What is the prognosis for your organization if customer satisfaction is not made an active initiative?

____

____

____

____

If top executives in your organization view Customer Satisfaction management as a simple outcome measurement rather than an executive initiative, your crusade to boost satisfaction levels will be somewhat tougher, but not impossible. To better position Customer Satisfaction management as an executive initiative, begin providing top management staff with information on the quantitative economic and business values of Customer Satisfaction management. (Specific examples are provided throughout this book.) Provide them with readings on the new-found influence of Customer Satisfaction with respect to recruiting physicians, negotiating with insurers, and winning provider agreements with employer coalitions. Then report where your organization's ratings stand compared with regional and national competitors, and accompany this with a plan to make needed changes. Information without a plan to make changes has little impact. Information with a proposal on how to implement improvements has a better chance of gaining approval and winning.

Task 3. Review Physician Relationships. Review trends in admission and patient case loads for each physician for the past three years. Which physicians show a trend of increased admissions and patient utilization of your organization? Which have remained stable, and which show a trend toward a reduced number of patients using your organization? Those with stable or declining patient loads at your facility are probably defecting from your organization and reaching out to another organization. Why?

The reasons for defection are sometimes easily determined when physicians are open and sharing of information. Often that will depend on the relationship that the physician has with the person asking the questions. More mature, trusting relationships between interviewer and physician generally result in a more generous sharing of information. In other cases, deciphering reasons for defection will be more difficult and will require talented conversationalists to help draw out the reasons through easy conversation—a nonthreatening approach. In no case should you count on another paper survey or focus group to provide core information on physician defection.

Physicians who are not building your business through the building of their practice are not loyal and should be your first and foremost targets to correct defection—through improved Customer Satisfaction. In other words, find out why their trend is anything but upward, and make necessary changes to retain these physician groups. Avoid rationalizing any behavior that is not growth-oriented. Make the changes that the doctors reasonably request, and then ask for their business.

Task 4. Analyze Results of Physician Feedback. One area with little or no standardization of information in databases is that of physician satisfaction surveys. Consequently, determining how the level of satisfaction of your particular physician population measures up against that of others is difficult.

If your organization is using a measurement tool for physician satisfaction, audit the contents to assure that the following three points are explicitly covered. If they're there but vaguely addressed, amend the questions in the instrument so that they will address these specific issues directly.

1. How well does your organization serve the needs of each physician?
2. How well does your organization serve the needs of the physician's patients (from which the physician will hear either glowing compliments or raging criticisms)?
3. What improvements in your organization's policies, practices, or work systems would be seen as positive moves by physicians?

We hope that your organization is not using dull and ineffective paper surveys to gather physician information, but rather is investing in the relationship people-to-people. In other words, we hope you are conducting one-on-one interviews with physicians to gather information in a way that nurtures the physician-hospital relationship while gaining a full understanding of where the inadequacies in your organization lie.

NOTES

1. Kathryn F. Clark. "Employers Group Ranks Physicians." *Human Resources Executive,* December 1997, p. 18.
2. Personal interview with Margaret Gerteis, Picker Institute, Boston, Mass., 1998.
3. *The Satisfaction Monitor,* November–December 1997, p. 3.

Chapter
TWO

Eighteen Commandments for Well-Managed Customer Satisfaction Programs

If you only look at customer complaints, you will miss the silent mass of discontent.

The most fascinating aspect of Total Customer Satisfaction management is that most health care providers and leaders seem to understand only narrow segments of what it should encompass, how to achieve it, and how to manage it. The concept of Total Customer Satisfaction has eluded them.

Some health care organizations have garnered successful Customer Satisfaction ratings in spite of themselves. These organizations don't necessarily understand why or how their organization achieved their ranking, or how to sustain it. They tend to have a myopic view of what Customer Satisfaction means. If that view could be widened and shared, they would have the potential to rocket-boost organizational performance to significantly higher levels and to accumulate the rewards and national recognition that accompany such success.

After working with over one hundred health care organizations and talking with and researching hundreds more regarding why they've been successful in attaining high satisfaction ratings, we compiled the following list of Eighteen Commandments of Total Customer Satisfaction. Read through the list and mark those that seem to describe your organization. If you find that your organization is not embracing at least twelve to fifteen of these Commandments, it might be time to reaffirm your organization's commitment to Customer Satisfaction and learn how to better manage this compounding asset.

EIGHTEEN COMMANDMENTS OF TOTAL CUSTOMER SATISFACTION

Only a small portion of health care leaders understand what Total Customer Satisfaction encompasses. Most health care organizations, even top-performing ones, are oblivious to one or more of the following commandments of Total Customer Satisfaction. Organizations operating in the ninetieth-plus percentile in a national comparative database such as Press, Ganey Associates or Parkside Associates are probably missing at least four or five of these commandments with some frequency. Organizations rated in less than the ninetieth percentile are delivering a lackluster performance and falling short on most of the Eighteen Commandments for Total Customer Satisfaction. The description *lackluster* may seem somewhat tough or critical at first glance, but it's not. Although noble efforts have been offered by most health care organizations in the name of Customer Satisfaction, their efforts typically fall far short of what is needed.

This situation is not entirely the fault of the individual health care organization; after all, it serves a challenging and difficult customer base, while providing complicated services requiring simultaneous delivery of extraordinary technical, scientific, and artistic skills, often in critical, life-and-death situations. Let's face it, health care is unlike any other business. Customers are more sensitive, particular, and demanding—and rightfully so. After all, they have entrusted their health and life to you.

Use the following list of Eighteen Commandments of Total Customer Satisfaction to audit your organization's performance level and awareness of Customer Satisfaction needs. Omission of any one Commandment in daily operations can have a significantly adverse impact on an otherwise excellent Customer Satisfaction initiative.

Commandment 1. Constantly Measure, Monitor, and Share Customer Feedback

Customer Satisfaction feedback and informal measurement should occur minute by minute, hour by hour, and day by day. With each encounter with patients, Associates should be able to uncover opportunities for Customer satisfaction that are germinating or that have already occurred, and at that moment correct the situation, and thus salvage or improve the patient/provider relationship.

With respect to formal, survey-style Customer Satisfaction measurements, most organizations choose to receive feedback quarterly. More aggressive organizations request it monthly. Those that truly understand the dynamics and power of Customer Satisfaction collect it daily and report it weekly. The more frequently information is monitored, the more likely you are to correct a souring situation before it does great damage.

Example. The attitude of staff on a particular nursing unit sours. Patient Satisfaction assuredly will be poor until the attitude problem is discovered and corrected. There are fifteen beds on the unit. They are filled to capacity, and the length of stay for each patient is about five days. Calculating mathematically, we know that about 270 patients would rotate through that unit in a three-month period (quarterly basis). That means that at least 270 patients plus their family and friends would be subjected to an unpleasant and unsatisfactory experience before management received a Customer Satisfaction report highlighting this problem. It seems a little late at that point. Major damage has already been done.

If, on the other hand, data were collected weekly, management would know at the end of the first week that there appeared to be a problem, and that would be confirmed at the end of the second week and corrected before the end of the third week. Damage would have been contained to about sixty-three patients rather than 270 patients.

Commandment 2. Accept No Customer Defection as Inevitable or Negligible

It continues to amaze us to see the number of patients who get up and walk out of hospitals, clinics, emergency rooms (ERs), and physician offices never to return simply because they had to wait too long. Waits of one, two, and sometimes three hours plague organizations and cause the irreplaceable loss of Customers.

Patients and physicians "defect" or leave an organization, never to return, for four primary reasons:

1. The waiting time is too long. They need faster service.
2. The cost is more than they can afford.
3. They are concerned that the quality of service is not satisfactory.
4. The overall experience is unsatisfactory for a number of reasons.

Waiting time is the easiest cause of Customer defection to detect and correct before it occurs. *Waiting time* is the length of time a patient waits to have their needs addressed efficiently. Some call this Customer *sacrifice*, meaning that the Customer must sacrifice their time and other opportunities in order to obtain your services. How much are you asking your Customers to sacrifice?

Waiting consistently occurs in the admissions office, registration office, physician's or department's waiting room (appropriately named), and examination and testing rooms. Patients and physicians are waiting to get test results, waiting to be told what to do next, waiting to go home. It is almost as though waiting time is an expected part of the service process in health care. To be served on time is a rarity.

Waiting time in a typical ER can often be one hour or more. I've watched people in need of medical assistance get up, hobbling and bleeding, to leave the ER because they don't feel that they can *wait* any longer.

Customer defection is an outcome of this kind of unsatisfactory health care experience.

Customer Defection. Each time a patient defects, revenue is lost to the organization. What is more important, with each patient defection, you have probably lost that patient and the health care business that he represents for a lifetime as well as the lifetime health care needs of others whom he influences.

Skills for detecting incipient patient defections and recovering services should be taught to managers and staff in all departments, particularly those serving external Customers. To identify points of defection look for

- Waiting times in excess of fifteen minutes
- Uncomfortable waiting areas
- Patient anxiousness

Waiting Times in Excess of Fifteen Minutes. Do not be surprised if the list of patient/customer services with typical waiting times in excess of fifteen minutes is very long. The length of the list might suggest that excessive waiting time is more the norm than the exception at your organization, and therefore staff feel that it should be tolerated, or even expected. After all, that's the way it is everywhere in your organization.

To correct unacceptable waiting times, look first to the work-system flow chart. When you fix the waiting-time problem, the cycle time for the work process will be shortened; this translates to increased productivity as well as increased Customer Satisfaction—a winning combination for the organization, physician, and patient. (See Figure 2.1.)

Uncomfortable Waiting Areas. Uncomfortable waiting areas can be remedied with different furniture and by adding entertainment such as television, reading materials, aquariums, and toys to distract patients. If

Figure 2.1. Impacts of Reduced Waiting Times.

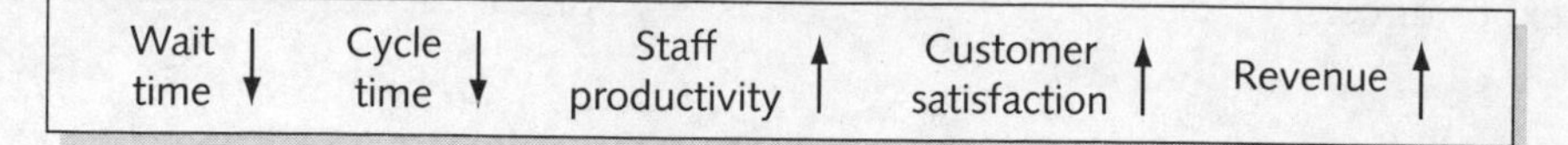

your organization is still using industrial-strength plastic chairs connected to one another with a steal rod and designed with a hard bucket seat, the kind one sees in a bus station, think again. There's no need to invest in plush recliners, but something with a little padding, an attractive design, and room to sit without feeling that you're imposing on the person in the next seat makes a world of difference. These alternatives are not much more costly than the "bus station" seats, and they go a long way toward creating a more positive experience and retaining potential defector patients.

As for distractions and entertainment, think of adult patients as children in grown-up bodies. When kids are distracted with something entertaining or interesting to them, they settle down for longer periods. The same is true for adults. Provide adult-type distractions and entertainment, and be creative about it. TV and newspapers are good, but you can do more. Crossword puzzle books, computer games, aquariums, or fish bowls are novel. Do not limit your thinking to traditional paths.

Patient Anxiousness. Patient anxiousness is a condition that escalates one unsatisfactory patient situation, which otherwise might have been salvaged, into a complete catastrophe. Calm the anxious patient with frequent staff visits, reassuring messages, and updates on the situation. Inform patients and visitors on the expected arrival time of the doctor or status of other sources of delay as well as sequential steps in their health care experience. Information makes people feel less out of control and more involved in what is happening. It builds an understanding and prevents small irritations from becoming all-consuming problems.

Comprehensive Nature of Customer Satisfaction. Organizations interested in obtaining results in key business areas such as increased revenue and profitability need to get a handle on Customer defection. Hundreds of Customer defections are occurring in average and small-sized hospitals each year. Thousands occur in larger health care organizations. This represents a loss of tens of thousands and conceivably millions of dollars of revenue to any one organization.

Commandment 3. Evangelize Customer Satisfaction at Every Level in the Organization

If managers and staff don't know what their level of performance in Customer Satisfaction is, they cannot make changes to improve upon it. If you cannot measure it, you cannot manage it. Without concrete data to the contrary, most Associates and managers are likely to be of the opinion that they are performing at a satisfactory level and doing well in meeting the needs of patients because it is in their hearts to want to do well for patients. However, good intentions frequently do not translate to high Customer Satisfaction.

Managers and staff need frequent communication on measurable activities that correlate to Customer Satisfaction in order to maintain it as a priority in what is routinely a crisis management environment with more demands on people than is reasonable. Frequency of communication must be high and channels of communication varied to gain and retain Associates' attention. For example, some New American Health Care Organizations require department managers to conduct weekly departmental team meetings on Customer Satisfaction. The structure of the meetings is predetermined, and managers are expected to follow a prescribed agenda, which looks like the following:

Standard Agenda

1. Review the most recent feedback on Customer Satisfaction measurement.
2. Identify the top three irritations or issues for the week.

3. Establish problem-solving groups around the top three issues.
4. Determine the status of solutions to previous unresolved problems.
5. Devise additional ideas for improving Customer Satisfaction.

Customer Satisfaction is thus prominently kept in front of executives, managers, and Associates.

In addition to the structured departmental meetings, the CEO holds monthly meetings on Customer Satisfaction with the management team. And every executive conference contains at least one agenda item on Customer Satisfaction. Patients' letters of commendation, as well as letters of complaint, are shared with management and staff. Weekly internal newsletters include information on performance, tips, anecdotal stories of exceptional Customer Satisfaction, and targets for additional attention.

Notice that the communication of ideas, performance reports, tales of jobs well done, and suggestions for specific improvement needs sets up a constant drumbeat for Customer Satisfaction, and it is being generated mostly from the top of the organization down to Associates, thus sending the added message, "This is important information. This is a priority for the CEO." Also note that the media for communication are varied and include all of the following:

- Printed newsletters and meeting agenda
- Graphic reports displaying performance levels
- Verbal messages from the CEO, VPs, and department managers
- Verbal and videotaped stories of heroic achievements in Customer Satisfaction as told by real patients and physicians and replayed for staff
- Symbols of goals and achievements in the form of rewards and recognition awarded by the CEO
- Considerable time in new Associate orientation dedicated to Customer Satisfaction
- On-going training and coaching by managers and staff who are deemed exceptionally skilled in managing Customer Satisfaction.

If managers and staff do not see evidence that the organization places a high priority and importance on Customer Satisfaction ratings, they will not naturally and consistently place a priority on the innovation needed to improve performance levels.

Amazingly enough, many executives believe that a single report on Customer Satisfaction distributed once each quarter is adequate to motivate staff to make necessary changes. One message per day may be adequate, but one message per week or per month or per quarter will bring little or no improvement.

Commandment 4. Every Customer Contact Is an Opportunity to Measure, Manage, and Master Customer Satisfaction

Often the formal source of data collection and reports on Customer satisfaction—most frequently the postdischarge survey process—becomes the only source of data collection. Organizations come to rely on their paper survey responses almost entirely for feedback information. What this means is that only a portion of the picture on Customer Satisfaction is presented. What are not gathered in the paper survey are information and ideas from the patient's perspective on how the service may have been better performed. The basis of Customer comparison remains unknown, and an important source for ideas on how to improve performance is blocked.

Although open-end comments are provided for in the paper survey format, the likelihood of patients condensing the description of an idea for improvement or comparison of your services to those that are superior into a few short lines that are meaningful to you is small. A means for collecting this valuable information is needed.

The easiest and most natural way of collecting this information is through caring conversation with patients and family, and empathetic listening on the part of staff. When two people are in close proximity, such as in a patient room or exam room, it is only appropriate that there be some communication between them. Communication is a sign of caring, a sign of a relationship. It is also a technique for reducing anxiety and stress.

Often staff enter a patient's room, conduct the clinical tests or processes required, and leave with little or no communication other than "primal grumbling" of fragmented sentences, such as "just taking your vital signs" or "we need to do. . . ." Opening a channel of communication takes little time and brings great rewards in terms of improved Customer Satisfaction for that particular patient, valuable ideas for improvement for future patients, and greater staff satisfaction.

Nursing and patient care staff routinely complain that they would like to have more time to spend with each patient, but the workload is such that they just can't. This type of situation leaves both the patient and health care provider unsatisfied. And to some degree, it is a cop-out—an excuse for not developing a relationship and doing the hard work of listening.

To overcome this situation, alternative channels of communication need to be created to meet the differing needs of patients, family, and visitors. Processes such as the "Three-C Card: Complaints, Criticisms, and Compliments," a Customer Hotline, and Adopt-a-Patient programs provide these channels of communication. (Each is discussed in detail later in this book.) Effective, active listening and questioning techniques go a long way toward identifying potential patient and physician problems before they emerge and transforming potential unhappiness into opportunities for greater satisfaction.

Customer satisfaction feedback generally comes in the form of survey ratings, Customers' ideas for improvements to the current process, and complaints. Whereas in the old, worn-out, conventional thinking Customer complaints were viewed as burdens, new Total Customer Satisfaction thinking sees Customer complaints as opportunities to recover from an unsatisfactory experience and salvage what otherwise might become a lost Customer. Customer complaints pose a learning opportunity that points out changes needed in the system.

Satisfaction survey responses provide only a part of the picture. Organizations striving for excellence in Customer Satisfaction use multiple communication channels, formal and informal, to gain a truer picture of Customer Satisfaction and to better influence ratings in the future.

Commandment 5. Use Big D to Drive Improvements in Customer Satisfaction

D stands for *dissatisfaction. Big D* represents *major dissatisfaction.* To effect change in any type of organization, Big D with the status quo is a given. Complacent organizations within which there is no dissatisfaction with present performance will not change until someone in authority becomes significantly dissatisfied with the current state of affairs and makes their major dissatisfaction known.

Executives often come to understand the value of a major Customer Satisfaction initiative but are frustrated with their inability to make a difference in performance levels. Although money, resources, and ideas are poured into the initiative, nothing seems to result from it. Ratings may rise a little, then fall or stabilize at a level less than the goal.

Executives cannot motivate people to change unless the people who deliver the service see a need to make the change. Nonetheless, the singular most important ingredient in creating Big D within the organization is the appearance of major dissatisfaction on the part of the CEO. The blood-boiling variety of dissatisfaction that the CEO feels must be transformed and effectively communicated to management and staff. It is the display of CEO dissatisfaction that grabs staff attention.

As CEO, you can choose any number of reasons to create Big D and exploit those reasons to strike awe into staff. For example, the reason could be that a VIP is not highly satisfied with the health care experience that occurred at your organization, or that Customer Satisfaction ratings from the last period are not at the targeted goal. Maybe you receive a critical letter from a prominent business person, or perhaps you lose an important contract (any contract is an important contract). The reason could be that *service just is not good enough for the people you are serving!* As CEO, you have the liberty of choosing the object of your dissatisfaction, and if Big D is big enough and widely communicated to Associates, it will act as a catalyst to motivate people to want to make changes. Until Big D is apparent and frequently referred to, change will not occur, no matter how badly you need it or want it to happen.

To gauge the current level of Big D in your organization, order a complimentary copy of the *Organization Performance and Readiness Assessment* instrument available from Management House, Inc.

Commandment 6. Commit to Customer Satisfaction BHAGs

BHAGs are *B*ig, *H*airy, *A*udacious *G*oals, often referred to as *stretch goals,* or goals that are attainable but only with extraordinary effort and work. Executives wanting to achieve top Customer Satisfaction ratings need to take an aggressive approach to establishing goals. People (staff) are moved by dreams to achieve. As the wise man said, "If you can dream it, you can achieve it. Believe it." Staff believe it.

One organization reported, when asked about their Customer Satisfaction BHAG, that they wanted to move from the eighty-sixth percentile to the eighty-ninth percentile in Customer Satisfaction. A goal of three percentage points increase in Customer Satisfaction ratings is *not* a BHAG.

To want to be number one in Customer Satisfaction is a BHAG. A goal to move into the ninetieth-plus percentile on Customer Satisfaction ratings within a national database of like health care organizations is a BHAG. But to aspire to small, incremental shifts in Customer Satisfaction ratings is not a BHAG.

The beauty of Customer Satisfaction BHAGs is that they are entirely achievable. It is possible to go from the thirteenth to the hundredth percentile or to number one nationally in seven months, as you can see from the success story of Holy Cross Hospital shown in Figure 2.2.

Notice in Figure 2.2 that once a strategy for Total Customer Satisfaction was operationalized (around August 1993), satisfaction ratings quickly responded. For a closer look at how the strategy for Total Customer Satisfaction was constructed at Holy Cross Hospital—and ideas about how to construct one at your organization see Chapter Nine.

Figure 2.2. Ideation Impacts at Holy Cross Hospital.

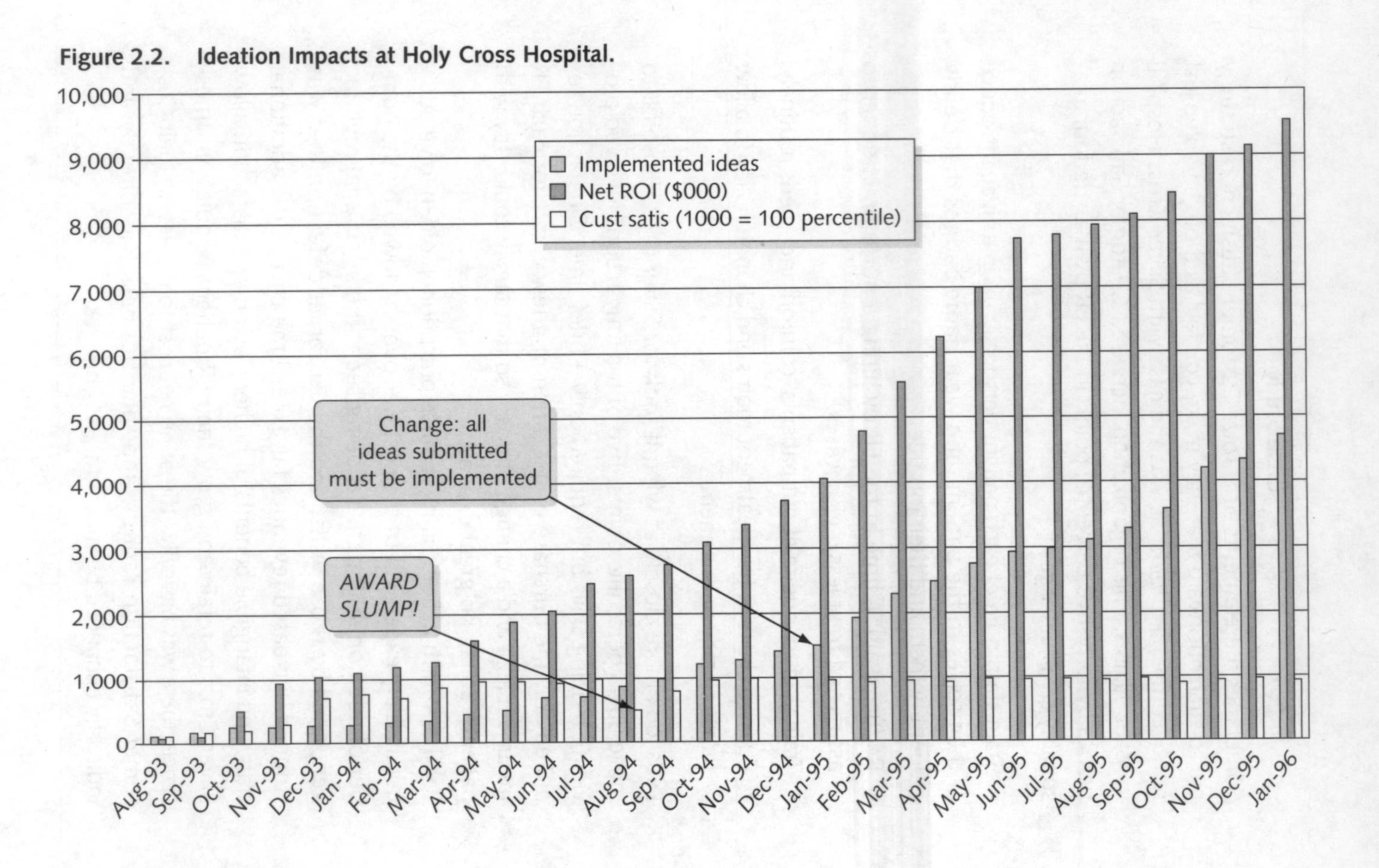

Case Study

Sometimes the elements of a Total Customer Satisfaction strategy are so straightforward that they make you feel as though you've just removed the blindfolds, as was the case with Silver Cross Hospital in Joliet, Illinois. This organization increased Customer Satisfaction ratings by forty-five percentile points in the ER by making four, reasonably small, changes:

- Train staff to greet each patient personally upon arrival, introduce themselves to the patient, and wear name badges that clearly identify them and their job title.
- Reduce waiting time in the ER by hiring a nurse practitioner to assess and treat less critical cases.
- Train staff to inquire about patients' comfort and needs routinely.
- Put two chairs in the treatment rooms and change policy to allow family to stay with patients.

Let's look more closely at what it took for Silver Cross Hospital to move up 45 percentile points. Two of the four actions involved providing training skills but required only a brief time. One action required only the purchase or relocation of a few chairs for each ER treatment area and a change of policy so that family could stay with patients. So far, no great expense.

The fourth action, hiring a nurse practitioner, did involve additional salary expense, but the cost was overshadowed by the number of additional ER patients being seen, the additional revenue generated by those visits, and the Customer defection that was stopped. Increased revenues far exceed the cost of the additional staff, and intangible benefits of higher Customer Satisfaction allow Silver Cross to retain and grow their ER patient population. In essence, there was basically little or no net cost to increasing their Customer Satisfaction ratings, and their business was directly and indirectly enhanced by making these changes.

Now, don't run out and make the same changes in your ER and look for the very same results. That may or may not happen. Certainly implementation of these changes will enhance your ER service, but the extent of the improvement will depend on what your Customers see as a deficit in your ER operations. No one formula represents the entire story for every ER.

Commandment 7. Be Critical in Your Interpretation of Customer Satisfaction Ratings

Four- or five-point rating scales are common; typical satisfaction rating categories are *excellent, above average, average, poor,* and *very poor.* Ratings of *above average* and *excellent* are generally interpreted by health care management to mean that the experience was at least better than the average experience. Consequently, there is a common sense of relief when Customer Satisfaction ratings rank in the *above average* and *excellent* categories. The sense of relief is related to a false sense of security in thinking that *above average* ratings translate into loyal Customers.

The reality is that only a portion of those patients or physicians who rated your organization as *excellent* will be loyal to your organization. Those who rated your organization *above average* or lower, and even a portion of those who rated the experience as *excellent,* are no more loyal to your organization than they are to any other organization. They are as likely to use another facility the next time they need health care services as they are to use your facility.

Excellent ratings are the only ratings that should give you some sense of having provided a superior experience and thus *some sense* of Customer loyalty among those who grant it. *Excellent* as a rating is defined as "the very best experience known by the rater."

The subjective, relative nature of *average* and *above average* ratings make them almost meaningless. *Average* ratings depend on the patient's comparative base. *Average* compared to what? The same is true for *above average.* Compared to what? How much better than *average* do you have to be in order to be *above average*? Keep this perspective in mind, the mean or average performance level represents the best of the worst, or the worst of the best.

Proper interpretation of Customer Satisfaction ratings rarely leads executives to feel a sense of relief or satisfaction in ratings that are *above average* or less. Rather, it moves them to greater anxiety, at least until they see the greatest proportion of Customer Satisfaction ratings move into the *excellent* category.

Commandment 8. Listen to the Special Needs of Every Customer

Listen. Can you hear them? Patients, physicians, and staff are telling you what they are thinking and feeling every day. They are sending you clues, but management typically turns a deaf ear on the messages, too busy to listen and consider what the messages mean.

Nurses say, "I want to spend more time with patients. Patients need me to spend more time with them. Quality is declining. It takes too long to do anything. Patients need. . . ." Physicians are saying, "My patients are unhappy because . . ." and "I can't bring more patients here because. . . ." Staff are saying, "If only we could do it this way it would be so much better. The patients would like it better if. . . ." Patients are saying, "Please, I need to do it this way. It would be so much better for me if. . . ." Yet few of these comments translate into immediate actions for improvement.

Two Ways To Compete. There are two ways to compete in a mass-market service business like health care. One is to think that the business is merely about performing a function, delivering a set of medical skills, performing a test, and reading the results. This is known as the *commodity mind set.*

The other way to compete is to go beyond the function and compete on the basis of *providing an experience.* In New American Health Care Organizations, services are delivered as comfortably and conveniently for each patient as possible. That means that each Customer is considered special and unique, and that the hospital is a special place where it is expected that each customer will have individual needs unlike any others.

To learn what these special needs are, Associates must learn to listen actively and empathetically to what the patient/Customer is trying to communicate. Until staff are trained to listen and respond, and management is comfortable trusting and valuing the legitimacy of requests for improvements and changes made by patients, physicians, and staff, an organization will never reach the ranks of excellence in health care.

Commandment 9. Associate Satisfaction = Customer Satisfaction = Success

Intuitively we have always believed that satisfied Associates deliver services that generate greater Customer Satisfaction, which in turn is good business practice, but there is little statistical evidence to support this belief until just recently. Now researchers can put trust into what previously was an intuitive feeling because the cause-and-effect relationship between satisfied Associates and high Customer satisfaction has been statistically proven and documented.

Clas Forney International Group, an econometric statistician group from the University of Michigan, has statistically validated and proven the undisputable relationship between Associate Satisfaction levels and Customer Satisfaction levels, and to some degree can quantify the financial impact of this relationship for the Sears Corporation, which funded this original research.

Associate Satisfaction Drives Customer Satisfaction. In the Sears research project, a direct relationship between organization work life and Associate Satisfaction was found. Associate Satisfaction generates Associate retention, which in turn provides greater productivity levels for the organization.

Associate retention represents knowledge and expertise in the Associates' particular job function that directly impacts Customer relationships and overall organization productivity. After all, tenured Associates are typically more knowledgeable about the products and services they supply, how the organization functions, and how to work around barriers to get results. In the end, they deliver more services in an excellent manner and in a shorter period of time, thus achieving both Customer and management Satisfaction.

To test this thinking, consider your personal reaction when seeking advice from a service provider. Do you want to talk to the new trainee that has been on the job a couple of weeks, or do you want to talk to the guy who has been there ten years and knows what's happening? That's why organizations put the words *trainee* on name badges to warn Customers that this person might not have all the answers at the tips of their fingers, and to ask Customers to be patient with the training time needed for this new Associate. Associate retention drives productivity and Customer satisfaction.

Research at Sears quantified the linkage between Associate and Customer satisfaction. When Associate Satisfaction went up 5 percent, ninety days later Customer Satisfaction would rise 2 percent, and ninety days after that profits would increase 0.5 percent. The obvious question is this: If this happens at Sears, would it also happen in health care?

At this point, the statistical relationship has not been proven in a health care organization. However, the same people who shop at Sears use health care facilities, and to the extent that satisfied Associates in any job function provide the same benefits of employment retention and increased productivity to their organization, it would seem logical that the Associate-Customer satisfaction relationship would hold true in health care as well as in any business where the majority of Associates are working directly with the Customer.

The questionable factor would be the degree to which Associate Satisfaction correlates to Customer Satisfaction in health care. Would health care providers need to experience the same 5 percent increase in Associate Satisfaction in order to generate a 2 percent increase in Customer Satisfaction, or would something greater or lesser be needed? The point is that an increase in Customer Satisfaction is directly correlated to an increase of some value in profits.

Customer Satisfaction and Profitability. Intuitively, it has been thought that increased Customer Satisfaction leads to increased revenues or profitability. As noted above, in quantifying the relationship of Customer Satisfaction, employment retention, and increased productivity to profitability for Sears, Clas Forney International Group found that a 2 percent increase in Customer Satisfaction generated a 0.5 percent increase in profits ninety days later.

The question is, *why* does increased Customer Satisfaction generate greater profits? The answer is that high Customer Satisfaction creates Customer loyalty, which translates to repeat business from current customers and Customer referrals for new business.

Clearly, Sears customers are personally in control of their discretionary spending decisions and can choose to buy more services and products from Sears; therefore, the impact of Customer loyalty for Sears is easy to understand. Happy Sears Customers will tell friends and neighbors about their good fortune at Sears, and these referrals translate into new, additional sales for them. Do these same dynamics apply in a health care situation? At first blush, one might say that the two situations, Sears versus health care, are entirely different and therefore not comparable at all. But a closer look reveals numerous similarities.

For example, health care Customers include patients, physicians, and insurers. Each of the Customer groups has a choice of where to receive health care services. Just as shoppers have a choice of retailers, patients, physicians, and insurers have a choice of health care providers. Therefore, providing extraordinary Customer Satisfaction to health care Customers could generate a dynamic somewhat similar to that generated by a loyal retail Customer: repeat business and new referrals. Satisfied Customers, whether in a retail or health care business, talk about their experiences and refer others to suppliers who satisfy the Customer.

The next question is the extent of the relationship between high Customer Satisfaction and increased business success. For Sears, the relationship is a 2 percent increase in Customer Satisfaction yields a 0.5 percent increase in profits ninety days later. For health care organizations, the exact figures will certainly be different because the financial structure and requirements are different. However, the relationship of increased Customer Satisfaction to increased business success is undisputable. (See Figure 2.3.)

Research on the Associate-Customer satisfaction relationship goes back to 1985 with research by Benjamin Schneider and David Bowen. Following their research, Leon Schlesinger conducted further studies on the Associate-Customer relationship and established close links between Customer and Associate satisfaction in organizations such as MCI, Merry Maids, Xerox, Major U.S. Travel Service, and others. In all cases in which data allowed statistical analysis, the relationships between high Associate Satisfaction and high Customer Satisfaction were statistically significant but never exact.

In cases in which data analysis was less precise, the results nevertheless supported the same general conclusion: There is a relationship between Associate and Customer Satisfaction. These and other experiences have led us to conclude that in the absence of data regarding either Customer or Associate Satisfaction, one can be predicted from the other.

Figure 2.3. Quantifying the Satisfaction-Success Cycle.

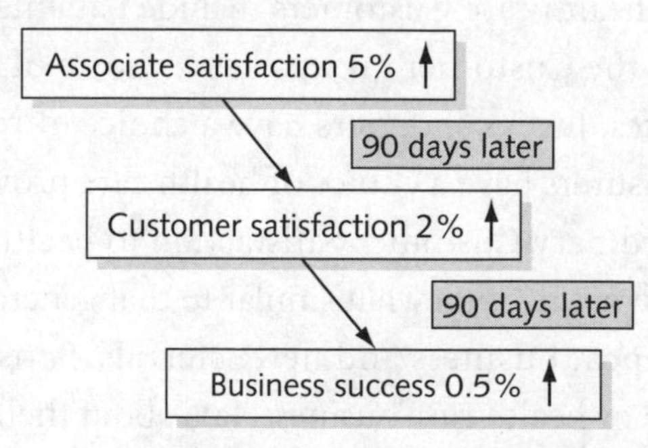

A Reflective Relationship. The *Satisfaction mirror*, as Schlesinger calls it, is the mirror effect between Associate and Customer Satisfaction whereby satisfied Associates serve Customers in ways that create happier, more satisfied Customers.

You can see a Satisfaction mirror in its simplest form in a restaurant where waiters and waitresses enthusiastic about their jobs not only communicate their enthusiasm to Customers but also go out of their way to make the Customers' dining experience pleasant. Customer satisfaction is expressed through positive comments and a larger-then-usual tip that reinforces the relationship and increases the employee's enthusiasm for the next Customer.

Health care is unlike the restaurant business except that it is a service business, and its ability to be successful is directly linked to each Associate's desire to serve. Therefore, hiring happy Associates and keeping them satisfied is an essential part of the formula for creating satisfied Customers. Happy nurses, certified nursing assistants (CNAs), housekeepers, clerks, and therapists provide a more pleasant and cheerful healing environment for patients. The personal happiness of staff is directly translated to a better, more positive and caring health care environment for patients.

Unfortunately a significant number of health care CEOs do not recognize the value of a healthy quality of work life and satisfied Associates. They speculate that if union organizers are not knocking on their door, or if letters of complaints and grievances from Associates do not number more than one or two a month, things are good enough; if they are compensating Associates at a competitive rate, that is all that matters. *Wrong.*

Monetary compensation alone is not enough to overcome dissatisfaction with the quality of work life and other concerns, such as lack of personal concern, inappropriate or inadequate supervision, poor communication, and lack of work tools. Schlesinger's research predicts that to know your Associate Satisfaction level is to predict your Customer Satisfaction level.

Protecting Associate Satisfaction. If the goal is to improve Customer Satisfaction, first look at Associate Satisfaction. Jerry Seibert, president of Parkside Associates, Inc., a national health care Customer Satisfaction measurement firm, has reviewed Customer Satisfaction trends in hundreds of cases. We are particularly interested in Jerry's experience with Customer Satisfaction ratings following the merger of two organizations.

Jerry explains that when two organizations with equally healthy Customer Satisfaction ratings merge, statistical trends show that there will be a significant dip in ratings beginning about the time that merger information is known by Associates, and continuing until some time after the merger is complete and shakeout from job changes and employment insecurity settles down. Why? Because prior to the merger announcement, happy Associates focus on their job of delivering excellent health care, and Customer Satisfaction runs high. When the future of employment turns questionable in terms of what will happen to jobs in the wake of the merger, *specifically what will happen to my job,* staff become distracted from the focus of providing health care. Distraction, or preoccupation with what will happen to job security, is conveyed to the patient through Associate-Customer interactions and subsequently is reflected in Customer Satisfaction ratings. As soon as merger mania settles down, and job security is reestablished, Customer satisfaction ratings typically resume their higher levels.

When management makes it easy for Associates to do their job right by providing them with necessary tools, policies, and support, they find Associates who are happier and not distracted from their primary function of delivering care. Nordstrom's retail store management clearly believes that the goal of complete Customer Satisfaction is achieved through satisfied Associates. Nordstrom's Associates are backed up with operating systems and policies that make it easy to serve the Customer and resolve Customer needs. In turn, Nordstrom's Associates cite their positive interactions with Customers and freedom in exercising their own judgment in their relationships with Customers as important qualities in their work environment—the "reflective relationship" in action. It has no beginning and no end.

Commandment 10. Manage Associate Turnover to Manage Customer Satisfaction

Regardless of the reason for Associate turnover, it is an unfortunate phenomena for the organization. There are two primary types of turnover. The first is turnover due to natural causes, and the second is turnover due to dissatisfaction among Associates.

Natural Causes. Turnover resulting from a spouse's transfer, a return to school for further personal development, or other reason outside the employment relationship is a called *natural cause of termination.* There is no relationship between the action of terminating employment and the work environment. It is a "no-fault" situation.

Nonetheless, natural-cause terminations have a direct impact on patients and physicians because of the break in patient-staff relationships. This is particularly disruptive for patients and physicians who have routine encounters with the same staff repeatedly, such as patients who are regularly scheduled for testing, treatments, or checkups.

Through routine visits, patients come to know what to expect in terms of the staff's personalities. They can count on the responsiveness of staff and the organization, have confidence in staff's professional skills and knowledge, and have trust in staff's personal judgment. In short, a relationship has been established between patient and staff. When that relationship is disrupted, Customer Satisfaction is also disrupted until a new, acceptable relationship develops with the replacement staff, at which time Customer Satisfaction should rebound to prior levels.

Dissatisfied Associates. The second type of Associate turnover has its roots in an unhappy work environment. All other things being equal, why would someone leave employment if it is as good as, or better than, what other employers provide?

The root cause of Associate dissatisfaction is unique to each individual. Granted, some people are naturally unhappy (and therefore should not be selected for employment in a health care organization), but they represent a small minority of dissatisfied Associates. Aside from the issue of selection, Associate dissatisfaction is most frequently generated in one or more of the following situations:

1. Associates perceive inequity or unfairness in the workplace.
2. Associates experience conflicts between personal values and organizational demands.
3. Constant irritations that are brought to the attention of management are not resolved.

Given that Associate turnover is a true indicator of the extent of Associate Satisfaction, and unhappy or dissatisfied Associates correlate to lower levels of Customer Satisfaction, proactive management of the causes of Associate turnover will directly and positively affect Customer Satisfaction ratings.

Commandment 11. Accept No Excuses for Poor Customer Satisfaction

When initiatives to boost Customer satisfaction do not provide the expected substantial results, there often is a tendency to justify lower-than-desired ratings or to rationalize why better Customer Satisfaction ratings were not achieved. The following are common justifications:

- "Oh, it's the construction project. No one can get excellent ratings in the midst of a major construction project."
- "If we weren't doing such a good job, we wouldn't be so busy, and people wouldn't have to wait, so these ratings must be wrong."
- "People with this kind of diagnosis are bound to be cranky. No one could satisfy all their needs."
- "We have limited resources and you can't make everybody happy."

Justifications are excuses for nonperformance. Excellent Customer Satisfaction is manageable in any situation, given some consideration and preplanning. For example, during a major construction project at Trinity Hospital, the following proactive management actions were undertaken:

- Nursing units were shuffled to temporary locations in the facility farthest from the construction site in order to minimize the volume of noise to patients. This action was taken at the expense of temporarily reducing maximum census for the construction period, which constituted a reduced cap on possible revenue. The payoff was higher Customer Satisfaction ratings and greater overall revenues in the long term.
- The noisiest construction work was scheduled during standard work hours of 9 to 3 P.M. daily, thus making it easier to manage patient expectations regarding the noisiest period.
- Patients were advised that construction noise would end at 3:00 P.M.
- As many patient tests and treatments as possible were scheduled at testing sites away from the patient rooms and construction noise during the 9 to 3 P.M. period.
- Patients were advised of the construction noise prior to admission and reminded of the situation again at the time of admission, thus creating awareness in advance and a familiarity with the idea that there will be some construction noise during the visit.
- Necessary sleep aids were readily available from patient care staff.
- Reassuring, positive comments from staff regarding the benefits of the new building were made continuously in the presence of patients to help create an appreciation for the temporary inconvenience. Staff were trained to make comments along the lines of, "The results of this construction project will make it much more convenient for patients to. . . . I realize that it's a little noisier now than usual, but they will be done at 3:00 P.M. so you can rest better this afternoon. Is there anything I can do to make you more comfortable? Would you like a set of headphones with music?"

It has been said that every man is rational in his own mind. Rationalization and justification of less-than-excellent Customer Satisfaction ratings is simply an excuse for weak performance.

Commandment 12. Reward, Recognize, and Reinforce Excellent Associate Performance for Customer Satisfaction

At one level it is appropriate to count on the intrinsic values of health care delivery to motivate people to do good work. On another level, people are asking themselves, "But, what is in it for me? Why should I do more? Give more?"

Behavioral science research teaches us that people respond favorably to reward, recognition, and reinforcement. Behavior that is reinforced will be repeated. If top Customer Satisfaction ratings are the goal, there must be some reward, recognition, and reinforcement for achieving that goal—a prize for performing well. Unfortunately, some organizations still depend solely on the strength of each individual Associate's internal value system to make a difference in Customer Satisfaction performance. These organizations are routinely disappointed with small, periodic increases in Customer Satisfaction at best.

New American Health Care Organizations, however, now include Customer Satisfaction ratings as part of management's performance review process and compensation package and as an incentive for staff performance. Although we would like to think that Customer Satisfaction is something everyone should concern themselves with for its own sake, unfortunately that is not the case. However, Associates will concern themselves with an initiative when there is a payoff for performance.

When the BHAG for outstanding Customer Satisfaction ratings at Hays Medical Center was reached within the prescribed period, all Associates received a $100 bonus to reinforce specific behaviors that brought about specific results. The organization could afford to make this payout because patient referrals were on the rise, thanks in great part to extraordinary Customer Satisfaction performance in a short time.

Reward, Recognition, and Reinforcement. Not all rewards and recognition need to be in the form of cash compensation. Frequent, inexpensive, but meaningful recognition goes a long way to keeping people interested in doing just a little more, going that extra, special mile to make a difference. New American Health Care Organizations use daily, spontaneous recognition to put life into the work environment and communicate a sense of appreciation for work well done.

Trinity Hospital awards Associates the Fireball Award, a jaw-breaker candy too big to put into your mouth and too hot to keep there long anyway, along with a Fireball Certificate handed out by the CEO, for exceptional Customer Satisfaction–promoting behaviors. Departmental staff gather around, and public relations staff are on hand with a camera when the award is given. The photo is posted in the department, and mention is made in the hospital newsletter. Associates are proud to receive the Fireball Award. Co-workers get in on the fun, and it keeps everyone talking about what behavior was good enough to get an award. Reward, recognition, and reinforcement for desirable or improved behavior keeps Associates motivated to do more and makes the work environment more pleasant.

Commandment 13. Balance the Seven Areas of Key Business Results

A myopic focusing of attention on one or two business initiatives at the cost of overall organizational performance management is a dangerous approach that tilts organizational performance out of balance. The other five or six key results areas require equal executive attention.

This happened with the "quality improvement" craze of the early 1990s. Organizations rushed in with fists of money for consulting fees and training, thus feeding an obsession with improving quality at the expense of time, attention, and resources for people, Customer Satisfaction, and other fundamental business management needs.

Case in point: Florida Power and Light, a prior Malcolm Baldrige Award winner for quality, was obsessed with quality improvement and the goal of winning the Baldrige Award in 1993, but at the expense of total organization performance. Yes, they won the award, but at the expense of losing sight of the primary mission of the organization to provide power to consumers. Today, just a few years after winning the Baldrige Award for quality, local newspapers jokingly call Florida Power and Light "Failing Power and Light" as they publicly discuss the astounding Customer dissatisfaction rate, which has recently risen to 36 percent.[1]

The Seven Key Areas of Business Results. Top Customer satisfaction ratings come as a result of managing all seven Key Result Areas (KRAs) of business correctly and in a balanced way. The seven KRAs are

- Customer Satisfaction
- Productivity
- Economics
- Quality
- Organization Climate
- People Growth
- Innovation

A balanced business focus is required at all times. A myopic focus on Customer Satisfaction can generate extraordinary ratings for a time. However, high Customer Satisfaction ratings in a myopically focused setting are likely to be inflated and temporary, gained at the expense of one or more of the other key business result areas. The result will be a rough, splintered organization trying to manage in a constant state of chaos rather than a smoothly running machine that moves with ease from one initiative to another, each of which interlocks easily and without conflict.

Commandment 14. Establish Uniform Standards of Performance for Customer Satisfaction—Accept Nothing Less

Sustainable high Customer Satisfaction performance requires a universal application of standards of performance for all staff and departments. Standards of performance that are currently in place in most health care facilities are frequently not universally applied or enforced. One department will have strong Customer Satisfaction standards, but another department will have no specific standards. Consequently, overall organizational satisfaction ratings will never reach top levels. To create an organization capable of delivering a consistently extraordinary level of Customer Satisfaction, uniform performance standards must be put into place for all Associates. Areas to be managed by uniform standards of performance include personal appearance, personal hygiene, and manners.

Personal Appearance. High standards of personal appearance for all staff creates a sense of unity and greater professionalism within the organization. Without standardization, variances in personal appearance are dramatic and distracting. A sense of professionalism is missing. One must look the part of a professional as well as act the part.

Housekeeping staff in health care facilities have typically worn uniforms and consequently have portrayed a more professional appearance. Appropriate uniforms should be determined for the business office staff, registration and admitting staff, and others in administrative, non-patient-care roles. Benchmarking top-rated hospitality service organizations such as Marriott Hotels and Suites, Four Seasons Hotels, or major airline carriers renowned for excellent Customer Satisfaction such as British Air is a good place to start. Notice that all uniform selections are coordinated in color and style, yet allow for personal selection of sweater, skirts, slacks, blouses, and jackets. Some degree of personal choice is provided but the overall impression is uniformly planned.

Patient care uniforms should be given equal thought and planning. Rather than adopting a rainbow of colored smocks of pinks and greens, some tie-died, some with teddy bears, some with flowers, establish a consistent style, color, and design line for patient care provider uniforms. In no case should jeans, colored tennis shoes, excessive jewelry, make-up, or cologne be permitted. Men's hair length and earrings should be regulated. The objective is to eliminate the variation from Associates' appearance. You should be able to line up all Associates from patient care departments and see that they are dressed alike, identifiable by appearance, and all portraying a professional image.

When you move to greater structure and more requirements in professional appearance, there will probably be some upheaval from a small group of Associates. The kind of objections you will receive are typically short-lived. The greater population of staff find a uniform standard for dress at work a relief, and the uniform sense of professionalism in the organization has a positive impact on Associate pride. Soon thereafter the raised standards of professionalism will become a part of the culture of your organization, and dissatisfied parties will quiet down or disappear. Remember the short-lived controversy that developed when you moved to become a smoke-free environment? The same dynamics will play out when raising dress code standards.

Personal Hygiene. It is almost embarrassing to think that this topic has to be addressed. Unfortunately, common standards of personal hygiene do not exist. Specific standards for personal hygiene should include items such as facial hair for men and women (preferably not), colognes, breath and body odor, fingernails, and general overall tidiness in personal appearance. Some might want to argue that items such as length of hair are personal decisions. The point is, when a positive impression on the Customer is the goal, all variables that can affect the Customer's perception must be controlled and standardized, including individual decisions with a wide range of results, not all of which are acceptable. A specific list of requirements should be developed at your organization. Be specific, leaving no opportunity for individual variance.

One obvious item for inclusion on your list of "Don't Do's" is gum chewing. A recent visit to a hospital revealed three out of four Associates in the preoperative department chewing gum. Whether people chew gum to ease the stress of the work or to counteract boredom matters not, gum chewing presents an annoying, unprofessional appearance, not to mention maintenance requirements caused by used gum stuck on anything from the underside of a table top to the bottom of a trash can or floor and the offensive odor of chewed gum. Remember the gum stuck under the desk top in high school? Well, these are the same gum-chewing people, only they are twenty years older. Gum snapping, jaw wrenching maneuvers of gum chewers take the professional polish off an otherwise highly skilled Associate.

At one point, IBM marketing staff were known for a particular image that included gender, height, hair style, general physique, wardrobe design, shirt color and design, shoe design, and more. All components of appearance as well as behavior were standardized. Some people want to call this rigidity. Others see it as standardization at a higher, more professional level. Health care organizations that impose higher standards of professional image upon Associates set the stage for higher Customer satisfaction ratings.

Manners. Ritz Carlton staff are trained to use a standardized greeting as they encounter Customers. It is "Good morning, Sir," "Good afternoon, Madam," or "Good evening, Sir." It is not "Hi, how are ya?" from one Associate, and "Good to see you!" from another Associate. It is a standardized, mannerly, professional yet personal exchange from all Associates, all the time. The Ritz Carlton attitude is that they are "Ladies and Gentlemen serving Ladies and Gentlemen." Health care professionals are also "Ladies and Gentlemen serving Ladies and Gentlemen."

If we were to take this concept of standardized greetings from the Ritz Carlton and adapt it to health care, scripts would be created for staff to use in the following situations:

- Greetings for patients, visitors, and one another while in public areas
- Self-introductions for staff and others entering a patient room or greeting visitors
- Responses to common questions such as "How do I get to . . . ?"
- Apologies for what appears to be a Customer inconvenience
- Responses to angry patients or visitors
- Responses to patient requests that you can fulfill
- Responses to patient requests that you can't fulfill
- Departures from patient rooms or testing areas
- Who goes through the doorway first
- How to interrupt politely, when interruption is necessary
- How to ask questions that will be viewed by the patient as demonstrating care and concern
- How to clean up when you see something out of place
- How to give corrective guidance and direction to guests in a kindly, professional manner

One of the strengths of the Disney Corporation is standardization of Associate performance levels. Disney Associates are expected to behave as though they are "on stage" or in character while in public areas. Only in restricted "Associate only" areas are Associates permitted out of character.

Disney embraces specific performance behaviors for everyone. For example, if you are lost and need directions, Disney staff know that they are expected to walk Customers to their destination—something that top-performing New American Health Care organizations have adopted from Disney. If Customers appear to need something special, Disney staff are expected to offer to try to get it for you—another standard that health care staff can adapt. Standardization of Associate behaviors creates a pleasant, managed environment with a positive managed outcome for all Customer groups.

Commandment 15. Benchmark Against Only the Most Excellent Companies and Don't Limit Your Options to the Health Care Industry

It is time to break away from the "me-too" mentality that health care organizations have traditionally had. Benchmarking against yourself to see how much you've changed or improved has some merit in that it provides one small piece of information—how much your performance has changed compared to prior performance. It does not, however, tell how your performance compares to competitors', which is what the real ball game is all about. Keeping score with competition is how winners and losers are named. Regardless of what you deem your performance level to be, self-comparison to the performance of others determines your level of excellence.

Benchmarking your organizational performance against others in the health care industry, however, is akin to copying the best of the worst in Customer Satisfaction practices. The results are minimal, if any, improvement for you. There is some value in the effort to learn what other, better-performing health care providers are about. But learning about what competitors are doing can hardly be called benchmarking, as most health care competitors are not benchmark organizations.

Making Benchmarking Pay Off. The process of benchmarking in its truest sense involves selecting a performance leader, researching how they do what they do, and making adaptions of their process, or components of it, to be used to improve your organization's performance. To achieve distinguished Customer satisfaction ratings, look outside of health care to organizations with a record of exceptional organization performance in other industries.

Benchmarking efforts should not be myopically focused on Customer Satisfaction practices only. Benchmark the most excellent operating components of each organization, adapting them to health care and your organization. These operating systems are the subsystems within your organization that make it possible to deliver exceptional Customer Satisfaction.

For example, if the distribution process in your organization is faulty, getting needed supplies to manage patient care will be difficult and time consuming, thus affecting Customer Satisfaction. Benchmarking Federal Express or UPS distribution systems provides insight on how to transport goods quickly and cheaply through the organization. If these companies can move a letter from Boston to Los Angeles in two days, health care organizations can learn to move a bandage from central supply to the ER in ten minutes or less.

Other organizations to consider benchmarking include Southwest Airlines for how to handle difficult Customer relations, Marriott Hotels for admissions, discharge, food service and hospitality functions, and Hewlett-Packard for Associate training and selection processes. The list does not stop there. Consider local service providers that you find exceptional, and ask to visit their operation for ideas that you can adapt to your business. Community businesses are proud to share what they can with their health care providers.

Commandment 16. Free Associates to Problem Solve and Create Customer Satisfaction

Top Customer Satisfaction can only be delivered in an organization in which management trusts Associates with spontaneous decision making (within well-defined financial limits and organizational values) in Customer-centered problematic situations. If all problems must be referred up the bureaucratic ladder from Customer through Associate, supervisor, department manager, to vice president and possibly to CEO and then back down the chain in reverse order before a problem is solved, extraordinary Customer Satisfaction will never be attained. There's not enough time, and Customer frustration becomes the dominant and destructive force.

Many leaders pay great lip service to goals of superior Customer Satisfaction. Priorities for Customer Satisfaction are pronounced by leaders in marketing campaigns, community presentations, and Associate meetings.

The reality is that the organization lacks the infrastructure, staff training, and value-centered empowerment and management style necessary to support rapid and appropriate Customer-driven problem-solving. Bureaucracy in the problem-solving process remains, and Customer problem-solving situations continue to be lengthy. With the passing of time also passes the possibility of excellent Customer Satisfaction.

Organizations that are top-performing in Customer Satisfaction have Associates that are trained in a standardized behavior format and ready to solve Customer problems on the spot at the moment they arise. They have been trained in exactly what to say to defuse an unhappy situation, how to handle Customer complaints, and what to say to reduce Customer anxiety. Research shows that when a Customer problem is quickly resolved (that means immediately following the incident), the likelihood of retaining the Customer is nearly 100 percent. Conversely, the longer it takes to solve the problem, the more likely it is that you will lose the Customer for life and not even know it until they never return!

Those of you who wish to learn how to transform your organizational culture into one that supports exceptional Customer Satisfaction, read the book *Creating the New American Hospital: A Time for Greatness* (Jossey-Bass), and call Management House, Inc., for a copy of the *Do-It-Group (DIG) Guide* for rapid problem solving.

Commandment 17. Link Up with Physicians

Without the support and integration of physicians and physician office staffs into the Customer Satisfaction initiative, the best-laid plans for Customer Satisfaction improvement fall flat at the implementation stage through opposing or apathetic physician behaviors and practices.

Executives talk freely about significant initiatives such as Customer Satisfaction improvement without planning for the participation of the medical staff. Early rationalization is that Customer Satisfaction is something that the health care facility must provide, but little consideration is given to how to integrate participation from the medical staff. *As a point of guidance: Anything that involves a patient or what is being done to a patient also must actively involve the patient's physician.*

Failure to involve medical staff in a participatory manner compromises efforts and results. In the words of CEO John Schwartz of Trinity Hospital,

> *If you don't involve your medical staff early, you're dead in the water.*

Commandment 18. Value and Measure Customer Share First, Market Share Second

Customer share represents a measure of the amount of business that your organization is getting within the framework of the total amount of business that each Customer could possibly represent to you. For example, when a physician (who is also a Customer to a hospital) brings half of her patients to your hospital for admission, the customer share that is presented is 50 percent, or half of what the potential business represented by this physician actually is. Perhaps your organization's statistics show that you have 70 percent of the new birth market, but you have only half of this doctor's admissions. There is obviously a substantial amount of customer share yet to be gained that will in turn contribute to the market share calculation.

Look first at Customer share measures in order to determine what additional, specific actions need to be taken to boost Customer Satisfaction for a specific Customer base. These are the actions that will consequently build specific business success for your organization.

Review: Eighteen Commandments of Total Customer Satisfaction

1. Constantly measure, monitor, and share Customer feedback.
2. Accept no Customer defection as inevitable or negligible.
3. Evangelize Customer Satisfaction at every level in the organization.
4. Every Customer contact is an opportunity to measure, manage, and master Customer Satisfaction.

5. Use Big D (major dissatisfaction) to drive satisfaction improvements.
6. Commit to Customer Satisfaction BHAGs.
7. Be critical in your interpretation of Customer Satisfaction ratings.
8. Listen to the special needs of every Customer.
9. Associate Satisfaction = Customer Satisfaction = Success.
10. Manage Associate turnover to manage Customer Satisfaction.
11. Accept no excuse for poor Customer Satisfaction ratings.
12. Reward, recognize, and reinforce excellent Associate performance for Customer Satisfaction.
13. Balance the seven areas of key business results.
14. Establish uniform standards of performance for Customer Satisfaction—accept nothing less.
15. Benchmark against only the most excellent companies and don't limit yourself to the health care industry.
16. Free Associates to problem solve and create satisfaction.
17. Link up to physicians.
18. Value and measure Customer share first, market share second.

NINE REALITIES OF TOTAL CUSTOMER SATISFACTION

Realities are rules, maxims, facts, and teachings that are positioned to be factual and undisputable. In the previous section, Eighteen Commandments of Total Customer Satisfaction, we identify the cardinal rules of the game. The rules emerged over a period of years of studying, discussing, and observing behaviors and decisions of hundreds of health care executives. In each case, when a rule or practice seemed to be coming into belief, we asked what kind of thinking the executive or team had undertaken in order to get to their specific action point. Why did they make the decisions that they made? From those answers we identified Nine Realities of

Customer Satisfaction that are widely operating in the health care industry. You will probably identify with most of them to some degree.

Read through the following list of realities and assess how many, if any, of them are operating in your organization. Although each of these realities can be debated endlessly, we will explain why we stand behind them and what we have found to be the truth about Customer Satisfaction.

Reality 1. Staff Training Is a Crucial But Not Exclusive Solution to Gaining Customer Satisfaction Ratings

Staff training is certainly one part of the solution to boosting Customer Satisfaction ratings. It is not, however, adequate on its own merit to make a significant or lasting improvement in Customer Satisfaction. To the extent that staff training provides greater understanding of what is needed by patients, physicians, and other Customers, it is helpful. To augment and support a good training effort, however, a system is needed for generating and rapidly processing new ideas for continuous improvement in work systems that support Associate's efforts to serve the Customer. Such a system has been designed and successfully implemented in hundreds of health care organizations via implementation of ideas through the DIG or Do-It-Group process.

In short, the DIG process calls for a small group of four or five Associates coming together to solve a work-related problem quickly. DIG processes operate under specific rules and timeframes, and each member of the DIG has a specific role to play in the process. DIGs are not committees and should not exist any longer than it takes to solve the problem (usually four or five weeks). Once the solution to a problem has been identified and approval for implementation given, DIG members implement the solution and disband. The process is expeditious and allows Associates to participate in solving many of their work-related problems.

Most work-related problems can be broken down into "bite-sized" issues that can be resolved in thirty to forty days. (See the *DIG Guide,* available through Management House, for details on how to manage the DIG process in your organization.)

Reality 2. You Can Control Customer Defections

Nearly every day patients walk out of the Emergency Room without receiving the service for which they came. They walk out of testing and treatment waiting rooms routinely without receiving their tests; and they walk out of your organization unsatisfied more often than you know.

The greatest cause of Customer defection is dissatisfaction that is not addressed quickly enough. By reducing waiting times prior to service, managing waiting times through providing routine updates, distraction, and entertainment to help pass the time, and providing a caring, compassionate staff to assist with paperwork and process details, walk-out Customer defections can be dramatically reduced or eliminated. Patients don't want to have to go to another provider, but there is a point at which they have an overwhelming feeling that they must walk out of your door rather than wait another minute.

Patients and physicians who are unhappy about any portion of their health care experience are potential defectors. They can be salvaged if the situation is handled correctly at the point of dissatisfaction. *Timing* is the key element in managing defections. The more quickly problematic situations are corrected, the more likely you are to salvage the Customer relationship for the long term.

Quickly is a relative term. Problematic situations that are resolved on the spot or within twenty-four hours are problems from which the organization has a high probability of recovering the Customer relationship. The longer the time between the point of incidence and the point of resolution, the more likely you are to lose that Customer forever.

Reality 3. You Only Think You Have a Lock on Your Market

Once upon a time rural hospitals in particular had a lock on regional health care because physician coverage was not as fluid as it is today. There was only one hospital that served a market, so patients and physicians had little or no choice of where to go. However, state-of-the-art communication systems and an evolution in health care management by health plan providers makes it increasingly easy for patients in rural areas to be cared for by urban physicians. Telemedicine is one possibility. Remote clinics operated by large urban medical centers constitute a second alternative. Transportation to predetermined health care providers, paid for by the health plan, is a third possibility. Creative solutions to what was once a hostage health care situation continue to evolve.

Where there is a market, there is a way. Greater populations of people have alternative health care providers available to them. No one has a lock on any market. If you think you have a lock on any particular market, you will be at a major disadvantage when the competition unexpectedly arrives with heavy armor ready to do battle over the market you thought you had a lock on. All markets are fair game. Be prepared to defend your market with a Total Customer Satisfaction strategy.

Reality 4. Patients Have Choices of Which Health Care Providers They Use

As mentioned earlier, physicians control where some of their patients are admitted, but a growing number of patients have control over where their physicians admit them. Most health plans provide for a selection of facilities that enrollees can use for health care services. Based on either past experience with a particular facility or the reputation of a particular facility, patients determine where they definitely do not want to go and where they would prefer to go for health care treatment. Physicians, in turn, are attempting to accommodate patient requests. Therefore Total Customer Satisfaction is the competitive advantage used to help assure that patients choose your facility for health care services.

Reality 5. You Can Please Just About Everyone

There will be a few patients who, regardless of the mountains moved for them, will not be entirely pleased with their health care experience. However, the majority of patients and physicians can be pleased within reasonable limits. There will be patient requests that for medical reasons cannot be accommodated, but given a proper explanation of why the request cannot medically be provided and the option of a substitute for the request, patients generally find the overall situation to be acceptable.

Total Customer Satisfaction is an attitude. It requires a commitment to going beyond the obvious. It requires a commitment to creativity in patient problem-solving and a relentless pursuit of Satisfaction.

Reality 6. A Sampling of Appropriately Constructed Customer Satisfaction Tools Does Represent the Opinion of the Majority of Customers

In some cases, when the Customer Satisfaction survey instrument has not been validated or when the number of returned surveys is less than that required to be statistically validated, a sampling of opinions will not represent the majority of opinions. This is part of the case made for utilizing a professional, credible vendor for Customer Satisfaction measurement.

There is a specific volume of survey returns necessary to assure statistically that the responses of the completed surveys represent the majority opinion of those who experienced your organization. Surprisingly, it is not a particularly large number. The number of returns needed to be assured that summary ratings are representative of the general population of those who used the service is directly related to the volume of patients served. When the number of completed surveys reaches the designated threshold, you can feel confident that the summary opinion does represent the general opinion of those using the service during that period.

Think of it in terms of a grade school report card on your child's learning. If the teacher gave only one test and the child failed that test, would you believe that the one test was a representative picture of the child's knowledge on that topic? Of course not. However, if the teacher gave nine tests and the child did poorly on each test, would you feel more confident that the final grade, although it is a poor one, is more reflective of the child's knowledge on this topic? Of course. Does the teacher need to give a very large number of tests to judge a student's knowledge level? No. They need to give only a sufficient number of exams to demonstrate the overall knowledge level.

The same is true for Customer Satisfaction feedback results. An organization does not need excessive numbers of feedback results to gauge the overall performance level of the organization properly. The key is in the quality and validity of the survey instrument. Therefore, it behooves each organization interested in Customer Satisfaction management to subscribe to the services and database of a quality provider of Customer satisfaction measurements and discontinue do-it-yourself efforts.

Reality 7. Managed Care Contracts Are Awarded on the Basis of Cost, Quality, and Customer Satisfaction Ratings

In the early phases of managed care, contracts were awarded largely on the basis of cost of services. As the cost debate heated up and quality of care appeared to be sacrificed in the effort to reduce costs, the quality of care factor was added to the selection formula. Now the third element of Customer Satisfaction is being added to the formula, and when all else is equal, meaning cost and quality considerations are equally strong, Customer Satisfaction ratings make the difference between being named a preferred provider or not.

Reality 8. Only Those Who Rate Your Organization as **Excellent** Have Any Loyalty to You

Although *above average* Customer Satisfaction ratings are definitely worthy of pride, they are not good enough to assure patient and physician loyalty. As discussed in Chapter Six, the Xerox Corporation conducted extensive studies on Customer loyalty relative to Customer Satisfaction ratings. They found that only a portion of those who rate their experience with the company as *excellent* are loyal to the organization. This is also true of the health care experience. The balance of Customers, some of whom rate the experience as *excellent* and others as less than *excellent*, are just as likely to go to another organization as to return to your organization.

The best strategy for building patient and physician loyalty, and the business, is to increase the percentage of *excellent* Customer Satisfaction experiences.

Reality 9. Total Customer Satisfaction Is the Number One Goal of Every Successful Organization

When everything else is changing in and around the organization, attention to the way Customer Satisfaction is managed is imperative. A change in one aspect of the work process may mean that other changes are required to sustain top Customer Satisfaction in the overall health care experience.

One hospital was seeking advice and a process for making improvements in what was then a mediocre level of Customer Satisfaction. When they learned how much work was required to acquire top Customer Satisfaction ratings, they decided that they had too many other major initiatives, such as reengineering the admission process and revamping the information system, to handle a significant Customer Satisfaction initiative.

Fast-forward twelve months: Now this very same organization has a new and expensive admission process that as a patient I have experienced and see no improvement in. Behind the scenes they have installed a larger, more powerful computer, they have redesigned the admissions forms, they have built new admission desks and enhanced the waiting rooms. They have enhanced elements of the process, but what they improved did not have any impact upon the Customer. When I arrived in the admissions department to be processed for my X-ray, I still had to wait. I still had to provide the same old personal contact information, insurance information, and all the details that I had provided just one month previously. The system might have been improved, but it had no impact on me as the Customer.

Question: Was their investment in the reengineering process worth it, or might patients and physicians have been better served with a Customer

Satisfaction process that identifies which components of the admission process and information system were in need of improvement?

Review: Nine Realities of Total Customer Satisfaction

1. Staff training is a crucial but not exclusive solution to gaining Customer Satisfaction ratings.
2. You can control Customer defections.
3. You only think you have a lock on your market.
4. Patients have choices of which health care providers they use.
5. You can please just about everyone.
6. A sampling of appropriately constructed Customer Satisfaction tools does represent the opinion of the majority of Customers.
7. Managed care contracts are awarded on the basis of cost, quality, and Customer Satisfaction ratings.
8. Only those who rate your organization as *excellent* have any loyalty to you.
9. Total Customer Satisfaction is the number one goal of every successful organization.

ACTION PLAN FOR TOTAL CUSTOMER SATISFACTION

What makes the difference between dreaming and achieving is an action plan. The following action plan will help you make Total Customer Satisfaction a reality.

Task 1. Provide Training on Customer Defection Detection. Defection detection is a skill used to recognize when a Customer is ready to leave your organization for the services of another. All departments that serve patients and physicians should be trained in Customer defection detection and how to remedy potential Customer defection situations quickly. Some of the content of the training would include identification of defection points and behaviors, methods to calm an anxious patient, and a process for quickly solving unhappy patient situations.

Identification of Defection Points and Behaviors. Typical defection points are waiting times in excess of fifteen minutes, uncomfortable waiting areas, and unresolved anxiety in patients or physicians.

Waiting times often seem longer than they are, particularly for health care services. To better manage waiting time defections, update patients on the length of the waiting time at least every fifteen minutes. Knowing how long the wait will be provides some sense of relief to the patient and keeps the waiting time in perspective. Frequent updates make the patient feel that they are informed.

When advising patients of the revised waiting time, explain briefly why the delay is occurring, a tactic that often makes acceptance of the delayed situation less irritating. A sample update might sound like this: "Mr. Jones, we apologize for the delay in getting your X-ray taken. An unexpected emergency case arrived and a child involved in a sporting incident needed an emergency X-ray. We should be able to do your X-ray in about 20 minutes."

Methods to Calm an Anxious Patient. Patients' anxiousness is usually relieved with frequent communication about the status of their case combined with distractions of entertainment.

Establish a standard procedure for communication to anyone waiting for anything. Fifteen-minute intervals are recommended. This means that patients or visitors who are waiting would receive an update on the status of their situation from a staff person every fifteen minutes. Even if the updated information is not entirely positive (the doctor has been delayed another thirty minutes), the courtesy of providing the information and keeping the patient informed is of greater comfort than no information at all.

The type of communication is just as important as the frequency of communication. A standardized content for messages should be learned by all staff. Each message would include the following components:

- A kind, caring inquiry as to how the patient or visitor is doing.
- An inquiry as to whether anything more can be done for that patient at the moment.
- An update on the waiting situation and what specifically can be expected next.
- Reassurance that it is of personal importance that the patient be cared for quickly.

A Process for Quickly Solving Unhappy Patient Situations. There are many problem-solving approaches taught throughout the industry. The best ones are those that have only a few steps (three to four) within short times and that provide Associates with the freedom to take corrective measures on the spot. Whichever problem-solving approach you choose to use, be sure it includes the following training components:

- Techniques and speech patterns to use for calming upset people.
- Techniques for empathetic listening to identify patients' needs; that is, sorting through the patient's words to find the meaning.
- Skills for finding full or partial solutions, even if they are not in response to the exact Customer request that was made.

Basic Needs for a Comfortable Waiting Area. Uncomfortable waiting areas can be remedied by providing comfortable furniture and adding entertaining distractions such as a television, reading materials, aquariums, toys, and refreshments. Be sure that there is enough seating for everyone. Personally test the waiting room furniture for comfort. Be objective. Could you sit comfortably in the chairs for up to an hour?

Task 2. Revisit Your Customer Satisfaction Communication Activities. How frequently do the CEO and vice presidents communicate in person, writing, or symbolically on the topic of Customer Satisfaction? How frequently do managers and staff see messages about Customer Satisfaction? How many media are being used to send Customer Satisfaction messages to staff, patients, physicians, and others?

Whatever the level of current communication is, it may be insufficient or inadequate to make a substantial change in performance results for Customer Satisfaction. *More* communication from the top of the organization is needed, more frequently, and via more channels of communication to make the message have an impact on Associates. Create an action plan to augment what is presently being done in Customer Satisfaction communication by using the ideas described below as a starter.

3C Card—Complaints, Compliments, and Comments. The objective of the 3C Card is to collect feedback from patients and visitors. Each piece of feedback, whether it is a complaint, compliment, or comment, is something the organization can learn from. It tells us what we're doing right, and therefore should be doing more of, and it tells us where improvements are needed, and perhaps even how to make the improvements.

3C Cards should be readily available throughout the organization, primarily in waiting or resting areas with a corresponding drop box nearby or via postage-paid mail-in form. Drop boxes generally are more successful because the card can be completed and mailed all at the same time and location. When the card has to go from the health care facility to a mailbox, the probability that it will not get mailed is higher. See Exhibit 2.1 for an example of a 3C Card.

CEO Welcome Letter and Customer Satisfaction Pledge. The model welcome letter shown in Exhibit 2.2 comes to us from Holy Cross Hospital. Notice that it includes a message about Customer Satisfaction at Holy Cross Hospital, personal peace and satisfaction, information about how the patient will be cared for, information on changes occurring at the hospital, and an open invitation to contact the president's office for problem-solving needs.

Exhibit 2.1. *3C Card.*

Welcome to Hope Springs Eternal Hospital.
You are more than a patient or visitor—you are our guest.
We are dedicated to serving you with dignity, kindness, and courtesy.
Your satisfaction is our primary concern.
We appreciate the opportunity to be of service to you.

(Chief Executive Officer's Name)

Hope Springs Eternal Hospital is dedicated to listening and responding to your needs. At Hope Springs Eternal Hospital we are interested in your comments, concerns, compliments.

Please complete this form and return it at any nurses station drop box. Or simply detach this postage-paid card and drop into any U.S. mailbox.

Comments: __________

Complaints: __________

Compliments: __________

OPTIONAL

NAME: __________
ADDRESS: __________
CITY: __________ STATE: ______ ZIP: ______
PHONE: __________
ROOM # __________ DATE: ______

Date pt. response received: ____ Date forwarded to mgr. ____ Date action taken: ____

Exhibit 2.2. *Sample CEO Welcome Letter.*

Dear ________,

Welcome to Holy Cross Hospital. Although a hospital stay can sometimes be difficult, I want to give you my personal commitment that our doctors, staff, and volunteers will do everything possible to exceed your expectations for quality medical care, comfort, and peace of mind.

Whether your visit lasts for one day or many, I trust that you will leave our hospital with firsthand knowledge of why Holy Cross is consistently ranked among the top 1% of hospitals nationwide for patient satisfaction. In the meantime, I want you to know about some changes underway that are designed to improve the care that we provide to our patients and their families.

You may have already noticed that Holy Cross is in the midst of a complete renovation that will make our hospital more welcoming. Our lobbies, for example, are being renovated to provide a more attractive, comfortable setting for our visitors. On patient floors, the single, centralized nursing stations are being replaced by multiple, smaller stations located closer to the patient rooms. This new design enables our nurses and other caregivers to spend more time in your room and respond to your questions and requests more quickly.

Another improvement is the way that our staff provide care. During your stay at Holy Cross, most of your medical care will be provided by a "Care Pair" that includes a registered nurse and a patient care technician. Meanwhile a customer service technician will make sure your room is tidy, your meals are tasty, and you have everything you need to be comfortable. Moreover, all of these professionals will be assigned to you on a consistent basis, enabling you and your family to grow familiar with each of them.

Throughout your stay, please don't hesitate to let any of these individuals know how Holy Cross can do a better job meeting your needs. If there is anything I can personally do to make your visit more comfortable, please don't hesitate to call me at ________. Even during evening and weekend hours, you can reach me or someone else on the Holy Cross' senior leadership team by dialing this number.

Thank you in advance for giving Holy Cross Hospital an opportunity to help you enjoy better health. My best personal wishes to you for a speedy recovery.

Sincerely,

Mark C. Clement
President

This approach accomplishes the following objectives:

- Advises patients how to contact the president, should they need or want to, thus providing a problem-solving approach that also makes each patient feel that they have access to someone in authority.
- Provides information on how patient care is provided and what to expect from various types of staff members. This avoids misunderstandings and sets the stage for the patient to expect service that he will find highly ratable.
- Advises patients of the priority of Customer satisfaction at your facility. This breaks down barriers or reservations that patients sometimes feel, and opens up the communication channel from patient to Associate as to what is needed to better serve the patient's needs.
- Keeps staff alerted to the high priority of delivering Customer Satisfaction; they will not want to be reported to the CEO as a problem.

Use your welcome letter as a quasi-marketing piece. Communicate information about your organization that makes it an exceptional place to come for health care needs. If changes are occurring in or around the facility that are visible to the patient, point them out and explain how the changes will positively affect patients and health care delivery. It is a means of establishing expectations early in the patient-provider relationship.

Another Approach. I came across the following message in a hotel which, in the simplest of interpretations, provides a small measure of the type of hospitality required of a hospital. Nonetheless, the message is appropriate for any organization in which people are overnight guests, not necessarily of their own free will. You may want to use portions of this message as a part of your organization's welcome message. An adaptation of this message for hospital use might be as follows:

> *Because this hospital is a human institution to serve people, we hope that God will grant you peace and rest while you are under our roof.*

May this room and hospital be your second home. May those you love be near you in thoughts and dreams. As we get to know you, we hope that you will be comfortable and happy as if you were in your own house.

May the reason that brought you our way be healed. May every effort you make and every message you receive move you closer to peace. When you leave, may your journey be safe.

We are all travelers. From "birth 'til death" we travel between the eternities. May those days be pleasant for you, and a joy to those you know and love you best.

These messages could be reproduced in colorful, artistic posters as inspirational quotations reminding staff of the importance of Customer Satisfaction and posted in locker rooms and staff lounges. They would serve as a message from management and a pleasant reminder and attitude adjuster. Integrate organization values into all messages and highlight them on banners.

Table Tents. Table tents in the cafeteria with Customer Satisfaction tips from your own staff are fun topics for lunchtime conversation while serving as reminders of Customer Satisfaction priorities and providing visibility and recognition to Associates offering the tips.

"Customer Satisfaction Corner" in Your Weekly Newsletter. Within each internal news publication a column could be dedicated to Customer Satisfaction topics. Content ideas may include anecdotal Customer Satisfaction stories, copies or excerpts from favorable letters written by patients and physicians about staff performance, tips on delivering Customer satisfaction, recognition of those receiving Customer satisfaction awards, updates on how the organization as a whole is performing in Customer Satisfaction, which departments have exceeded performance standards, which departments are sorely lacking in performance, and other related topics.

Television Remote Reporting. There should be a television in every patient room. In the Marriott Hotel there is a television in every room. At the Marriott, guests can use the television to enter a complaint about their room or service, and an appropriate person from the Marriott follows up to correct the situation. In-house television systems can be used for remote reporting in hospitals as well.

Patient Hotline. At Trinity Hospital in Chicago, patients can dial the "hotline" and reach a manager or appointed staff person to handle any kind of problem at any hour of the day, any day of the week. When they dial the hotline number, the first message they receive is from the CEO of the hospital thanking them for taking the time to use the hotline and allowing staff the opportunity to serve patients.

Following the CEO's instructions for how to use the hotline, there is a menu of possible types of problems for the patient to choose from; for instance, housekeeping, food service, maintenance, nursing. If a menu item is selected, the patient is immediately connected with a trained staff person from that specific department who can solve the patient's problem quickly. If a menu item is not selected, the patient reaches a hotline operator who takes the message and forwards it to the appropriate staff person for immediate follow-up.

A period of one hour is established as the standard of performance for resolving the problem. If it cannot be immediately resolved, the patient is advised about what action will be taken to resolve the problem, and when to expect this action will be taken.

Where there are multilingual patient populations, the menu and instructions should be provided in the most frequently used languages. The name of the game is to communicate.

Task 3. Assess How Customer Satisfaction Data Collection Is Managed in Your Organization. Look at both formal and informal processes of collecting Customer feedback. Top-performing organizations do not rely solely on printed postdischarge satisfaction surveys for feedback but seek out as many sources of feedback as possible. If your organization is not employing at least three means to collect Customer feedback, you are probably not collecting enough valuable information to significantly affect satisfaction ratings.

The following list of methods to collect Customer feedback should start you thinking:

- Focus groups
- Empathetic staff listening with a system to process what is learned
- Postdischarge surveys
- Interviews
- Adopt-a-Patient process
- Effective patient advocacy
- Hotline for Customer problem-solving
- Television remote reporting
- 3C Card: Compliments, Criticisms, and Comments

Select at least one or two additional methods of data collection and begin collecting the information that will make a difference.

Task 4. Evaluate Your Organization's Systems for Rapid Processing and Implementation of Ideas for Improving Customer Satisfaction. Can your organization take Customer feedback and quickly implement improvements in the way work is done? Or is the bureaucracy and process bogged down? If you have a system that allows managers and staff to process ideas for improvements easily and quickly, your assignment is to review the process and streamline it further to make it even better.

If your process is bureaucratic and cumbersome, order the *DIG Guide* from Management House, Inc. for instructions on how to process hundreds of ideas simultaneously, efficiently, and rapidly.

Task 5. Assess the Degree to Which Managers and Staff Are Aware of Big D (Major Dissatisfaction) in Your Organization. Are there real or created crises around which the CEO can express Big D? If not, Big D must be created in order to make change happen. Big D can exist in the heart and mind of the CEO. "Yes, I want more from this organization. This community deserves the best health care available," is a common CEO chant. But until the passion for improvement is translated and communicated to management and staff, the desire for change has no impact. At the moment that the CEO's desire for improvement, or her dissatisfaction with the status quo, is translated and communicated in a passionate way to Associates, it takes on new power—the power to motivate change. If there is no Big D in your organization, work with your CEO to identify issues that can be exploited with Big D energy and serve as the driver to change.

Organizations that are highly sensitive to criticism, such as those located in small communities where the slightest criticism can be misconstrued or twisted, are advised to base their Big D on "righteous" issues, such as "the community's right to the most excellent health care services," as the medium through which Big D is expressed. This helps frame the community's perception of the CEO's expressed dissatisfaction and avoids twisted, unfavorable, and unfair interpretations.

Task 6. Evaluate Customer Satisfaction Ratings for Your Organization. What percentage of patients rate your organization as *excellent*? What percentage rate it as *above average*? The goal is to have all ratings in the *excellent* category. If the majority of Customer Satisfaction ratings are in the *above average* or lower performance categories, your organization is at risk for Customer defection.

Customer loyalty is gauged by a percentage of the responses rating the organization as *excellent*. Further, if less than 92 percent of all Customer Satisfaction ratings are in the *above average* or higher performance categories, there is more negative news than positive news about your organization being spread in the community via word of mouth.

To move Customer satisfaction ratings up, begin focusing on those patient populations and situations earning *above average* performance levels first. What is needed to move them from *above average* to *excellent?* Look at the data you have collected. What does it tell you? If it does not present possible answers to the situation, then go directly to the patient population that rated you *above average;* probe and listen until you've identified possible solutions to the dilemma.

Example: British Airways found itself in a comparable situation. Customer satisfaction on routes to and from Japan seemed to be stuck in an *above average* satisfaction rating. One of the problem areas was food service. This was puzzling to British Airways, and their management could not figure out what the problem could be. They were serving first-quality, authentic Japanese meals, yet Customer Satisfaction was at a standstill. It was not until British Air staff talked with in-flight Customers further did they realize that the evaluation of the authentic Japanese meals served on the flights was evaluated by Japanese Customers as "good for a western effort." Notice that they did not say "good," but qualified the statement.

In these same exploratory discussions, British Air learned that Japanese people prefer to eat smaller portions of food but more frequently, and that their food is typically served in a particular style of Japanese bowl or plate. Further, they learned that a particular meal is enjoyed at the midnight hour by a large population of Japanese people. These are details that otherwise would have totally eluded British Air staff had they not talked directly with Customers. After British Air made these changes, the Customer satisfaction ratings from Japanese fliers immediately moved up.

Perhaps you should spend time talking with the patients and physicians that rate your hospital *above average.* If you listen, they will tell you what you need to do to move into the *excellent* category.

Task 7. Provide Listening Skills and Anxiety-Relief Training for Staff and Managers. Start with those involved most directly with patients and physicians, and then work to include all Associates. Training content should include the following:

- How to read body language to determine what a patient, physician, or visitor is actually communicating.
- How to ask concise, probing questions that make patients respond with specific opinions.
- How to indicate that you are empathetically listening, and what is being said is important to you.
- How to calm apparently anxious patients, visitors, and staff members.

Then put listening and anxiety relief skills into action. Establish listening standards of performance for staff. For example, each staff member is to actively listen and submit two new ideas for Customer Satisfaction improvements each week. Standards of performance push "desired" performance behaviors, such as active listening, into "required" performance behaviors, such as problem-solving groups, and change begins to happen.

Task 8. Review Associate Attitude Survey Results. The results of Associate attitude surveys for your organization should be current, within the past six months at least, to be of value. If results are older than six months it is time to arrange for an update. If results are within twelve months, compare the results of the Associate satisfaction survey with those for Customer Satisfaction for the same period. There will be a correlation. This is the satisfaction-mirror dynamic, as previously discussed. In departments where Associates are satisfied and happy with overall work life, where they rate supervision as *above average* or *excellent,* and there is an overall good feeling about work, Customer Satisfaction ratings should be correspondingly high.

Departments with poor Associate attitude ratings will probably have correspondingly low Customer Satisfaction ratings. Or it may be that a number of policies or protocols need to be modified to relieve irritating circumstances. Whatever the cause, it's important that it be identified and resolved for Customer Satisfaction efforts to be realized.

Ferret out reasons for low Associate satisfaction, and work with the Human Resources Department to make changes that are needed. Perhaps leadership in a particular department is inadequate, and a change in leadership would make the difference in Associate performance and Customer Satisfaction levels. Attitude flows from the top down, and it is essential that Associate Satisfaction be high if the goal is to achieve extraordinary Customer Satisfaction.

Task 9. Study Associate Turnover Rates. Compare turnover rates at your organization to other excellent service organizations to determine what a normal turnover rate is. Avoid comparing your turnover rates exclusively with other hospitals. Consider comparisons with regional health care statistics, and more appropriately, with other industries of similar profile.

Typical rationales for comparing regional turnover are the commonality of business in the same region and challenges within the same set of circumstances. The thinking is that comparison of turnover rates among like organizations in the same region should represent a good comparison. Although this thinking is somewhat logical and makes sense in some special situations where unique regional influences are a driving factor of turnover—for example, a shortage of skilled staff—for most health care organizations, most of the time, it is an inadequate comparison.

New American Health Care Organizations identify current and projected employment challenges, such as projected shortages of skilled staff, and move preemptively to make changes to neutralize the problem before it becomes an emergency. In dealing with staff shortages, such organizations quickly put in place extraordinary initiatives for staff recruitment and retention because they realize that the many costs of staff turnover will far exceed the costs of aggressive practices for staff recruitment and retention.

A more productive line of thinking is to compare your organization's performance with the best performers in the industry. Look to the *Top 100 Hospitals* list published by *Modern Health Care* for contacts with which to benchmark. Although qualifications for *Top 100 Hospitals* recognition do not include Associate turnover rates, the eight quality indicators upon which they are measured are achieved via outstanding Associate performances. Top organization performance is not achieved without a positive staff of Associates. Other industries with which to conduct turnover comparisons are high-quality, high-tech organizations such as Hewlett-Packard where the competition for the best performers is keen and the organizational culture is very close to that of a New American Health Care Organization. Beware of comparisons to other electronic industry organizations, where chaotic entrepreneurial states of organization leadership are in place and proper benchmarking is not available.

You can easily see when a person, whether patient or Associate, is satisfied and happy, just as you can easily see when they are unhappy. There is no hiding an unhappy person. Associates who deliver great Customer service transmit a pleasant, serving attitude. Unhappy Associates cannot deliver consistently excellent Customer service. Their unhappiness is transparent, easy for patients and everyone else to see. Sometimes we become so accustomed to the unhappiness transmitted by some people that it becomes gauged as "normal" and therefore acceptable.

It is now time to get a complete reading on the satisfaction level of the Associate population in your organization. Fix the things that need fixing to increase satisfaction, change or adjust attitudes where they need it, and change or adjust staffing and job assignments if individuals can't or won't make their own internal, peaceful adjustments. The commitment must be to Total Customer Satisfaction, which cannot occur with people who are fundamentally unhappy at work.

Task 10. Evaluate Reward, Recognition, and Reinforcement (3Rs) in Your Organization as They Relate to Customer Satisfaction Initiatives. What new programs can be created to build motivation for achieving the Total Customer Satisfaction goal and also add fun to the work environment? Work with your Human Resources Department to modify managerial and Associate compensation programs, and support and incentivize achievement of BHAG Customer Satisfaction goals.

Two, equally important, types of recognition, reward, and reinforcement programs are needed. One is formal and the other is informal. *Formally,* a manager's compensation for any given period should be directly related to both the individual department's and the overall organization's Customer Satisfaction ratings. This requires managers to achieve goals in areas where they have direct responsibility and accountability, and at the same time to play as team members by helping other managers who are having difficulty meeting their goals. When an organization's payout schedule is based on the performance of the sum of the parts of the organization, it creates an incentive for all management to work together. Organizationwide Customer Satisfaction goals cannot be achieved unless all managers achieve their individual departmental goals. It is an all-or-none game. Everybody wins, or nobody wins.

Frequent *informal* recognition and reinforcement keeps the initiative of high Customer Satisfaction in view as a priority for staff, reinforces the types of behaviors required to achieve the goal, and lightens up what otherwise might become an undesirable work environment. This approach may include no-cost and low-cost recognition from the CEO, department manager, and VPs, recognition at a meeting or in a newsletter, a Million Dollar candy bar and personal thank you, tickets to the movies, a special lapel pin, a photograph and announcement in the local newspaper—the list goes on and on!

Your job is to create a Recognition Action Council, as described in the book, *Creating the New American Hospital: A Time for Greatness,* and get the wheels of recognition spinning on all levels, formally and informally within the organization. If your organization is undertaking less than four or five specific recognition programs simultaneously within each fiscal quarter, then you are reward-starving Associates. There is no threat or harm in overrecognizing the good work or changed behaviors of people. It costs next to nothing and brings you many good results in the future.

Task 11. Evaluate Whether Leadership Balances the Seven Key Result Areas. In any business there are seven Key Result Areas (KRAs) that require expert management attention, as discussed earlier in this chapter. If the executives balance their attention among the seven KRAs well, emphasis on Customer Satisfaction will probably produce good results. Your responsibility is to assess whether the seven KRAs are receiving an appropriate balance of executive attention, resources, and priority. If the balance of attention is out of kilter, identify which KRAs are being neglected, and make plans to bring them back into balance as quickly as possible. It is also valuable to assess how or why they originally went out of balance in order to avoid making the same mistake twice.

Neglected KRAs will show as poorly performing components of the organization in the near term, and will distract management from long-term commitment to top Customer Satisfaction ratings. A balanced interest in managing each Key Result Area is imperative. No one KRA is any more important than the others. However, when ineffective management or attention to a KRA occurs, performance in that KRA will fall so dramatically as to cause a near-crisis situation to which we must respond—again distracting management and perpetuating an unbalanced approach to KRA management. Balanced KRA management is required before top Customer Satisfaction ratings can be achieved.

Task 12. Identify Where Uniform Customer Satisfaction Standards of Performance Should Be Developed. Earlier in this chapter we discussed standardized performance levels for every Associate and every patient-physician-visitor interaction. For example, greetings would be standardized, personal hygiene would be standardized, and frequency of patient visits by staff would be standardized. What performance standards are your organization willing to adopt and uniformly enforce? Work with the management team to establish uniform standards of behavior and work performance for all staff, including uniform standards of performance for situations specifically unique to particular staff. Standardize performance behaviors, time tables, and expected results in every possible area of operation within the organization.

Create an internal training program for standardized skills and expected behaviors for all Associates. Support this initiative with modifications in Human Resources policies to reflect the use of standardized practices as part of every job description, for which disciplinary action can be levied if these standards are not met.

Task 13. Evaluate Management Development and Staff Training Needs in the Areas of Customer Satisfaction Management, Problem-Solving Skills, and Relationship Management. Meet with the department responsible for training and education to review topics and content of management development and training programs provided to managers in the past twelve months. What managerial level training and development has occurred to enhance management's understanding of and ability to deliver Customer Satisfaction?

Building managerial muscle and skill is one way of protecting your investment in departmental leaders who already house the greatest percentage of intellectual capital that your organization possesses. Give them the skills to better handle individual situations, and train and coach other Associates in areas that have immediate Customer Satisfaction payoffs. Do not stop with basic, superficial training delivered by an outside training organization. Get into the details of advanced Customer Satisfaction management at your organization. For instance, what types of patient profiles have what types of preferences? What differences and preferences are presented by the various age categories of patients?

The more management understands the dynamics of Total Customer Satisfaction management, the more they can make adaptations in practice that will boost and sustain top Customer Satisfaction performance. The goal is to bring the knowledge level of members of management to a common point of understanding on Customer Satisfaction management and then to raise the standard of that understanding to a new and higher level.

If no such training has occurred, discuss the option of creating an internally delivered training program for Customer Satisfaction management and additional staff training needs, as referenced above, by using the information provided in this book as an outline and the tasks in the book as assignments. Beware of purchasing commercial Customer Satisfaction program offerings, as they are typically "light weight," and what you are after is a *Total Customer Satisfaction* training curriculum. If your organization has already invested in a one-day Customer Satisfaction seminar, use that as a base upon which to build and expand your knowledge to the more advanced concepts brought forth in this book.

For training references on Total Customer Satisfaction, contact Management House, Inc., Inverness, Illinois.

Task 14. With the CEO, Review Plans to Involve Medical Staff in Customer Satisfaction Initiatives. There is only so much that an organization can do solo before it must have the coordination and support of physicians and vendors in order to continue to improve the level of patient satisfaction. If physicians' office staffs have not undergone Customer Satisfaction training, will the hospital provide that for them? If physician practices are not participating in Customer Satisfaction measurement systems of some significance, how can they actively engage in a system that will have a payoff for the physician as well as the hospital? How will physicians with less than desirable patient satisfaction levels be managed? These are topics for decision making with the executive team.

When your organization undergoes internal radical improvements in Customer Satisfaction management, it is also a naturally good time to assist physicians with a value-added service of training their staff. A by-product of this training is a stronger bond and greater unity of thinking between physician office staff and your staff in the area of Customer Satisfaction management. The objective is to develop and implement an action plan that actively involves physicians and physician practices in Customer Satisfaction management—for their benefit and yours.

Task 15. With the Marketing and Business Development Staff Analyze Your Organization's Customer Share. Begin with the demographics for your market. Identify the profile(s) that represent 90 percent of the people in your market area. Notice that we did not say 90 percent of the market share, but 90 percent of the people within your service area. Profile by profile, starting with those that represent the greatest percentage of people in your service area, identify the various types of health services that each profile of Customer would typically need or make health care choices about. For example, if your demographic profile indicates that there is a large percentage of twenty- or thirty-something females in your service area, what percentage of these potential Customers do you currently serve (market share), and to what extent are these Customers coming to your organization for all their health care needs (Customer share)?

The extent of Customer share that remains potential new business is the easiest target to scope-in first, as that Customer is already familiar with your organization and will have less resistance to expanding the services they acquire from you than a new Customer might have to become initiated to the organization. Build your business by building Customer share first, as it is an easier mark if Customer satisfaction ratings are high. Then move to increase market share targets.

If Customer Satisfaction ratings are not high, the argument is even stronger for working toward building Customer Satisfaction with the Customers you already have before working to attract new Customers who, by virtue of your present, less than satisfactory delivery and ratings, may quickly become one-time Customers.

NOTE

1. Vincent Mallardi. "FP&L, Failing Power & Light." *Business Plus!*, February–March 1998, p. 7.

Chapter THREE

What the Customer Really Wants

Some consumer expectations should be treated as absolute performance standards.

A few years ago, when hospitals first were starting to think in terms of Customer and marketing, you couldn't utter the words *Customer* or *market* without people being very critical of you. People would have amateur-type discussions regarding who the Customer really is. Is it the patient, physician, or insurer? What's the answer to that question? All are Customers. Who else is a Customer? Family, friends, payers, vendors, and other departments are also Customers.

Why are we helping these various types of people? The answer: because they are our Customers. If you're in a patient care area, who's your Customer? In central supply, who's your Customer? The answer is sometimes the same and sometimes different.

For political reasons we often choose to pay more attention to physicians as Customers, but they are really only agents chosen by the ultimate Customer, the patient.

WHAT'S A CUSTOMER?

The word *Customer* comes to us from medieval French. The Customs officer was the person who stood at the border of France, and if the pot-and-pan manufacturer wanted to sell wares in France, he would go to the Customs officer and pay to cross the border. Now, however, the *Customer* gives the money instead of receiving the money.

The idea of a Customer is a person who is granting you a privilege. I cannot think of any higher privilege that any person or Customer can give to an organization than what patients give to a hospital and physician—the privilege of serving health, the quintessential element of life.

If I go to McDonald's, as a Customer I give them the privilege of giving me a meal for which I am willing to pay. But how big a privilege is that? If I bring you my son, I am bringing you the most precious thing I have. It is a great privilege to serve that precious person.

Each time the patient rings the call light or the bell on the desk, it is a privilege for you to serve that patient. Without that attitude, one should not be employed in a health care organization. It is time to do a gut check. Do you feel a deep privilege to serve?

Other meanings attached to *Customer* from the dictionary include "a person that you have to deal with," as in "tough Customer." Let's face it, some Customers are not nice. Some are nasty. Some are downright rude. Wouldn't it be nice if we could have the slogan that we only provide services to pleasant, placid patients? So a person comes in and is not nice. Do you say, "I'm sorry, you'll have to go over to this other hospital, because we only deal with pleasant Customers"?

Another concept is that of being *custom-made.* No organization can do everything that everybody wants exactly the way they want, when they want it. That would be total customization. But all of us know that we have to respond a little differently in each case. So how can we provide a standard service with standard costs, and at the same time apply some details that will fit the needs of a particular person?

The concept of a *Customer* also includes someone who purchases as a patron—a habitual Customer. (See Figure 3.1.) The term *patron* comes to us from the ancient Romans. A *patron* was a person who did favors for another, without whom that person might be lost. An unpleasant picture from Roman times is that slavery was part of their society. If a patron or owner of a slave freed that slave, as was sometimes done, the person who had done the freeing still retained certain legal rights.

Figure 3.1. What Is a Customer?

Customer: n, mef, a collector of customs and duties

1. One who purchases goods from another, a buyer, a patron
2. A person one has to deal with: a tough or cool customer
3. A habitual patron of a particular shop
4. Something "custom made" for individual customers

Patron: n, rom, a protector of a dependent

1. A person who is a customer, client or paying guest
2. A person who supports with money . . . an institution

—The Random House Unabridged Dictionary

In management, a customer is:
1. A person of power and the definer of success
2. The primary focus and purpose of the enterprise
3. A participant in and beneficiary of what we do
4. A giver of meaning to our lives

A customer is NOT:
1. A piece of meat on a gurney or a diagnostic label
2. A person deserving anything less than respect or dignity

A more pleasant picture of *patron* can be found in the concept of guardianship in our society. In addition to being the parent of your children, you are also their legal guardian. You look out for them, are responsible for them, guard them. And when a teacher or other community resident can't deal with the child, she goes to you, the guardian, and you tell them what can be done with the child, or what the child should do.

Guardians have power over their wards. Customers are our guardians. They have power over us. If many of your guardians decide to go somewhere else, will you feel the impact of their power? When you walk past patient rooms and the beds are empty, do you feel the impact of their power?

We live in a competitive society. People who think of their Customers as people of power are motivated to give outstanding value. If you can satisfy a tough Customer, you must be doing a good job. In management, the Customer is the definer of our success.

A Customer is the beneficiary of the work you do. Whoever is, or whatever groups of people are beneficiaries of your work, these people are your Customers.

WHAT THE CUSTOMER REALLY WANTS

What the Customer wants is what the Customer wants. Nothing different. It's a simple concept but one that people seem to have trouble grasping. If you give Customers what they want, they will be satisfied. If you give them more than they thought they would get, they will be ecstatic. It's that simple. The magic, however, is in knowing what Customers want.

Some management teams make a strategic error. They think they know what Customers want. This error is further exasperated when management comes to believe that all Customers want the same things. It is a big, fat error to think that all patients want the same things, or that management knows what most Customers think and want.

All patients and physicians are individuals with unique quirks and idiosyncrasies, specific opinions they are predisposed to hold (some of which are formidable), and specific requests that will make their encounter with you more pleasant for them. To the extent that the goal is to create health care experiences that exceed patients' expectations and satisfy patients' needs at a memorable level, the health care experience must be somewhat customized for each patient. In an industry in which standardization of best practices is rapidly homogenizing clinical protocols, customization of service on a grand scale does not seem possible at first thought. That is not to say, however, that at some level customization is not only possible but required to earn high Customer Satisfaction ratings and create greater Customer loyalty.

If all aspects of the health care experience cannot be customized, we need to ask the following questions: Which aspects of the health care experience are most important to patients, and can those aspects be managed in a way that will make patients feel that you are doing something special for them? What accommodations can you make for them that they did not expect? These are manageable aspects of a health care experience that organizations seeking high Customer Satisfaction ratings must focus on and master first. Excellent performance in these areas will serve as the greatest influence on the overall health care experience for the greater population.

Pareto's 80/20 management principle, illustrated in Figure 3.2, states that 80 percent of the results in most situations are produced by 20 percent of the variables. This principle is applicable in the study of Customer Satisfaction. If 80 percent of the patient's satisfaction rating is influenced by 20 percent of the work or care that is done for them, it follows that patients judge the overall health care experience by 20 percent of the work or care that they see and directly experience. The all-important 20 percent includes basics such as friendliness of staff, attention paid to patients' personal concerns, degree to which staff take patients' health problems seriously, and so on.

Figure 3.2. The Pareto Principle.

It is not enough to be busy—so, too, are the ants.
The question is, what are we busy about? —Thoreau

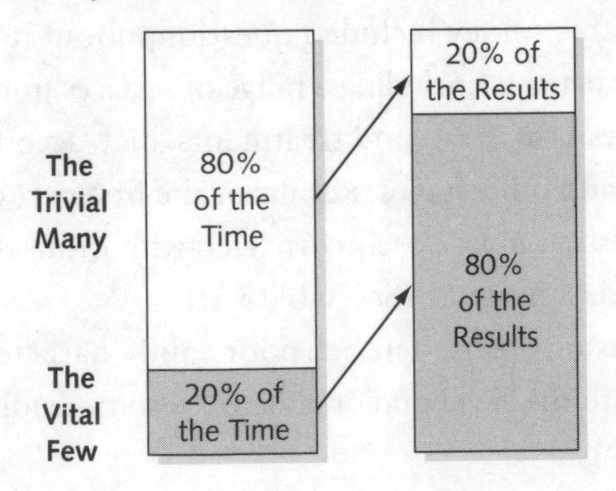

Case in point, of the forty-eight measured aspects accountable for the likelihood of a patient to recommend a hospital, as measured by Press, Ganey Associates, the top ten items, or 20 percent of the forty-eight total aspects, are significantly more closely correlated to the likelihood to recommend than the remaining thirty-eight.

TEN ISSUES MOST CLOSELY CORRELATED WITH THE LIKELIHOOD OF PATIENTS' RECOMMENDING A HOSPITAL

If you could know with some degree of certainty what the top ten patient issues most closely correlated with the likelihood of patients' recommending your hospital are, what would you do with that information? The answer should be to focus on that information as a priority, and test your hospital's ability to consistently meet or exceed expectations on those top ten issues. Thanks to the research work of Press, Ganey Associates, a leading Customer Satisfaction measurement firm, this information is available.

According to Press, Ganey Co-director Rodney F. Ganey, the firm recently compiled data from 545 hospitals in forty-four states. The study included responses from 1,007,612 patient surveys analyzed during the twelve-month period extending from December 1995 to November 1996. An average of 1850 patients per hospital completed the surveys, which included forty-nine standard questions.

The tested, reliable survey included questions about topics deemed most meaningful by patients, including a range of services from admissions to nursing staff, physicians, tests and treatments, diet, accommodations, family and friends, and other issues. Results of the first part of the survey identify the top ten issues most closely correlated with the likelihood of patients' recommending a hospital. (See Table 3.1.)

A quick analysis of the top ten behaviors and characteristics most closely correlated with the likelihood of patients' recommending a hospital indicate the following:

Table 3.1. *Top Ten Issues Most Closely Correlated with the Likelihood of Patients' Recommending a Hospital (Inpatient Services).*

	Correlation Coefficient
1. Staff sensitivity to the inconvenience that health problems and hospitalization can cause	.71
2. Overall cheerfulness of the hospital	.70
3. Staff concern for your privacy	.65
4. Amount of attention paid to your special or personal needs	.63
5. Degree to which nurses took your health problems seriously	.63
6. Technical skill of nurses	.61
7. Nurses' attitude toward your calling them	.60
8. Degree to which the nurses kept you adequately informed about tests, treatment, equipment	.60
9. Friendliness of nurses	.60
10. Promptness in responding to the call button	.55

Source: Press, Ganey Associates news release, January 10, 1997. Used with permission of Press, Ganey Associates.

- Nine out of the top ten qualities have to do with the nursing staff. Eight of these nine qualities address intangible areas of measurement such as attitude, sensitivity, and attentiveness—qualities that might be characterized as "caring," that people delivering health care should consistently be concerned with displaying, and that are determined by behaviors that can be developed through training.
- Three of the top ten qualities have to do with friendliness, attitude, and cheerfulness of the staff and hospital.

Clearly, when your organization standardizes staff behaviors and responses in a manner that assures that nursing staff and others express basic friendliness, concern, and empathy in every patient encounter, you will have mastered the top ten qualities that affect a patient's likelihood of recommending your hospital.

TEN LEAST IMPORTANT ISSUES CORRELATED TO LIKELIHOOD OF PATIENTS' RECOMMENDING A HOSPITAL

To the extent that the top ten qualities are important as a place to focus initial Customer Satisfaction initiatives, the bottom ten, or ten least important issues, should also be understood. In a business environment where resources of time and financial support are routinely rationed, the ten least important issues listed in Table 3.2 should be lower on your list of priorities for resource support when striving to make a rapid and significant improvement in the likelihood that patients will recommend your hospital. This is not to say that these functions are not important, or that they do not have an impact on overall Customer Satisfaction ratings, because they do. However, the degree to which excellence in performance will influence the patient's likelihood of recommending your hospital is somewhat less for these qualities than for the top ten qualities listed above.

This lower correlation to the likelihood of a patient to recommend a hospital should not be used to diminish the goal of providing excellence in each of these areas. Overall Customer Satisfaction ratings are still influenced by all forty-eight factors, and it is the orchestrated or synchronized application of excellence in all forty-eight areas that creates top-rated organizations.

A quick analysis of the ten least important behaviors and characteristics indicate that six fall into the hospitality category. Attention to issues such as room temperature, quality and temperature of food, and likelihood of receiving the food you ordered are not high on the priority list for recommending a hospital. Certainly attention to such details adds some degree of comfort to the patient's experience, yet these amenities are not enough to change a person's mind about recommending a hospital facility. As Rodney Ganey states in his summary analysis of the data,

> *Patients expect less of hospital food and accommodations and do not allow dissatisfaction with these areas (should that occur) to mask the importance of other issues.*

Table 3.2. *Ten Least Important Factors Correlated with the Likelihood of Patients' Recommending a Hospital (Inpatient Services).*

	Correlation Coefficient
1. Room temperature	.35
2. Likelihood of getting food you checked off on the menu	.34
3. Quality of the food	.36
4. Noise level in and around the room	.36
5. Speed of admission process	.36
6. Temperature of the food	.37
7. How well your blood was taken	.37
8. How well IVs were started	.38
9. How well things worked (TV, lights)	.39
10. Length of time you had to wait in the X-ray department	.39

Source: Press, Ganey Associates news release, January 10, 1997. Used with permission of Press, Ganey Associates.

The factors deemed most important by patients in their consideration of whether to recommend a hospital are listed in Table 3.3.

An assessment of all forty-eight factors and their correlations indicates that the role physicians play in the patient's overall likelihood to recommend a hospital is reasonably small. The correlation factor of physician-related concerns is in the range of .44 to .41 compared with the top ten factors, which had correlation factors in the range of .71 to .55 with nine of the top ten factors falling in the .71 to .60 range. This would mean that if your organization is experiencing poor Customer Satisfaction ratings, the reason probably does not stem from physician relations with patients but is related to hospital controlled operations.

Remember, this is the rank ordering of forty-eight key aspects of an inpatient health care experience with respect to how important each item is in the patient's view regarding whether to recommend a hospital. It is not a report on your specific hospital's performance. However, that information is available as a custom report from Press, Ganey Associates if you are one of their clients in Customer Satisfaction measurement.

Table 3.3. *Forty-Eight Factors Correlated with the Likelihood of Patients' Recommending a Hospital (Inpatient Services).*

	Correlation Coefficient
1. Sensitivity to the inconvenience that health problems and hospitalization can cause	.71
2. Overall cheerfulness of the hospital	.70
3. Staff concern for your privacy	.65
4. Amount of attention paid to your special or personal needs	.63
5. Degree to which nurses took your health problems seriously	.63
6. Technical skill of nurses	.61
7. Nurses' attitude toward your calling them	.60
8. Degree to which nurses kept you adequately informed about tests, treatment, equipment	.60
9. Friendliness of nurses	.60
10. Promptness in responding to the call button	.55
11. Information given you or your family regarding your condition/treatment	.55
12. Nurses' attitude toward your visitors	.55
13. Courtesy and attentiveness you received from the business office	.54
14. Advice given about how to care for yourself at home	.51
15. Adequacy of explanation of tests and treatments	.50
16. Hospital's concern not to discharge too soon	.49
17. Cheerfulness	.48
18. Respiratory care	.48
19. Physical therapy	.47
20. Social services	.46
21. Courtesy of staff who started the TV	.46
22. Accommodations and comfort for visitors	.46
23. Courtesy of people	.44
24. Daily cleaning	.44
25. Staff who transported you to and from your room	.44
26. How well the physician kept you informed about treatments	.44

Table 3.3. *Forty-Eight Factors Correlated with the Likelihood of Patients' Recommending a Hospital (Inpatient Services), cont'd.*

	Correlation Coefficient
27. Courtesy of the person who took your blood	.43
28. Physician's concern for your questions and worries	.43
29. X-ray technicians' concern for your comfort	.43
30. How informative the physician was in dealing with your family	.43
31. When you were told you could go home, the time you had to wait before you could leave the hospital	.42
32. Adequacy of visiting hours	.42
33. Courtesy of person who cleaned your room	.42
34. Explanations you were given about your diet if you were on a special diet	.41
35. Amount of time your physician spent with you	.41
36. Visitors rating of the hospital's cafeteria/coffee shop	.41
37. Courtesy of admissions personnel	.41
38. Volunteers	.40
39. Length of time you had to wait in the X-ray dept.	.39
40. How well things worked (TV, call button, lights)	.39
41. How well IVs were started (quick, little pain)	.38
42. How well your blood was taken (quick, painless)	.37
43. Temperature of the food (cold food cold, hot food hot)	.37
44. Speed of admissions process	.36
45. Noise level in and around the room	.36
46. Quality of food	.36
47. Likelihood of getting the food you checked on the menu	.36
48. Room temperature	.35

Source: Press, Ganey Associates news release, January 10, 1997. Used with permission of Press, Ganey Associates.

PRIORITIZING EFFORTS TO ACHIEVE CUSTOMER SATISFACTION

In the role of CEO or organizational leader for Customer Satisfaction initiatives, you have to make important decisions regarding where to focus leadership and staff time, energy, and problem-solving efforts to change the status quo. Your choice of targets and your effectiveness in making change will determine whether your organization's Customer Satisfaction ratings improve.

The first step to improving Customer Satisfaction performance is to identify the priorities for improvement that will make a difference in *your* organization's Customer Satisfaction ratings. These priorities are likely to be different from those at your competitors' organization. Your priorities are based on the level of performance of *your* staff and supporting systems as perceived by *your* patients, a perception that is unique to *your* organization.

If we were to compare all hospitals nationally (545 hospitals), looking at the patient's ratings of the hospitals' level of performance for each of the forty-eight measured Customer Satisfaction qualities in the database and correlating these performance levels to the question "How likely the patient is to recommend the hospital?", your report, or *priority index*, would show which measured qualities need to be improved first in order to have the greatest impact on the likelihood to recommend the hospital. The formula for prioritization is based on a combination of two factors:

1. How highly correlated each performance factor is to likelihood to recommend your organization
2. How poor the average level of performance is for each of the highest correlated qualities

Performance qualities that have a high degree of correlation with the patient's likelihood to recommend the hospital *and* have the poorest average performance rate as determined by patients are given the highest priority for attention. In other words, the *priority index* is the statistically validated list of where to place your efforts to improve Customer Satisfaction in order to reap the greatest payoff to the hospital in terms of greater likelihood to recommend your organization for services. The survey data compiled by Press, Ganey Associates yields the top ten *priorities* for performance improvement shown in Table 3.4 for hospitals overall.

Comparing the top ten qualities most highly correlated with recommending a hospital to the priority index shown in Table 3.4, we can draw the following conclusions:

Staff sensitivity is a top-priority area. Staff sensitivity to the inconvenience that health problems and hospitalization can cause is the quality most highly related to the likelihood of recommending the hospital. It is also the area of performance that patients perceive as the organization's worst!

Table 3.4. *Priorities for Customer Satisfaction Improvement (Hospitals).*

	Priority Index
1. Staff sensitivity to the inconvenience that health problems and hospitalization can cause	.79
2. Staff concern for your privacy	.74
3. Degree to which nurses keep you adequately informed about tests, treatment, and equipment	.73
4. Overall cheerfulness of hospital	.71
5. Adequacy of explanations of tests and treatments	.69
6. Hospital's concern not to discharge you too soon	.67
7. Information given your family about your condition and treament	.67
8. Courtesy and assistance you received from the business office	.67
9. Cheerfulness	.66
10. Explanation you were given about your diet if you were on a special diet	.64

Source: Press, Ganey Associates. Used with permission of Press, Ganey Associates.

Likelihood-to-recommend items equals priority items. Seven of the top-ten qualities for the likelihood to recommend are also in the top ten of the priority index for Customer Satisfaction ratings. This means that seven of the ten most important performance areas in terms of Customer Satisfaction as rated by patients are also areas in which hospitals are performing poorest as rated by their patients.

Top-priority items are mostly intangible. Six of the top-ten priority areas for performance improvement are related to intangible needs that should be conveyed by staff (see Table 3.4, items 1, 2, 4, 6, 8, and 9).

The correlation rating and the priority index provide a focus for your Customer Satisfaction initiatives. Given effective change-management skills and organization leadership, this focus should increase the likelihood of patients' recommending your hospital and produce immediate and significant improvements in overall Customer Satisfaction ratings.

This type of planning can be customized for your particular organization by ordering a custom report. Of course, your Customer Satisfaction data must be in the database, meaning that you must be a Press, Ganey Associates client, in order to conduct the statistical correlations and determine your organization's particular priority index. If you are participating in that database or plan to begin participating in it, the value of the custom report is that it will more sharply focus your efforts to improve Customer satisfaction, thus providing greater return on your investment of time, talent, and dollars.

FACTORS THAT INFLUENCE PATIENT SATISFACTION WITH THE EMERGENCY ROOM

The emergency room is often called the front door to the hospital, as many inpatient admissions come through the emergency room (ER) first. For many organizations the ER is consistently the busiest department, serving as much as 70 percent of the total patient volume in any one year. Whether ER patients become inpatients, outpatients, or simply remain ER patients, Customer Satisfaction with the ER visit is critical to the continued existence of the organization. An unsatisfactory ER visit can translate to lost future ER visits and lost inpatient/outpatient business. At the other end of the spectrum, a patient's positive ER experience may enhance the possibility of that patient selecting your hospital for future inpatient or outpatient services.

With a database of 302 hospitals and 124,627 patient responses, Press, Ganey Associates conducted research to determine which aspects of the ER experience were most highly correlated with the likelihood of the patient's recommending the ER. Twenty-seven aspects specific to the ER experience were rated. The results are listed in Table 3.5.

From this data we can draw the following conclusions:

The top items relating to ER recommendation are subjective. Six of the top ten aspects of the ER experience (see Table 3.5, items 1, 3, and 6 through 9) address subjective, intangible, attitudinal, relationship qualities. Two of the six most highly correlated aspects of the ER have to do with ER staff and physicians "taking the patient's problem seriously." This means that physicians and staff who demonstrate and share a sense of concern and seriousness about the patient's condition will rate significantly better than those who do not.

Relationship items dominate the list of factors contributing to the likelihood of patients' recommending an ER. Of the fifteen aspects of the ER most highly correlated with the likelihood of patients' recommending it (which represent the top one-half of the twenty-seven measured qualities), nine, or more than half, deal with intangible, personal perceptions of relationships to doctors, nurses, and other staff. The patient's desire is to feel attended to, taken seriously, comforted, and treated courteously.

Table 3.5. *Which Aspects of the Emergency Room Experience Correlate with the Likelihood of Patients' Recommending the ER.*

	(124,827 patients) (302 hospitals) Correlation with Likelihood to Recommend
1. Staff cared about you as a person	.80
2. Informed about delays	.73
3. Nurses' attention to you	.69
4. Nurse informative re treatments	.69
5. Adequacy of info to family/friends	.68
6. Courtesy shown family/friends	.68
7. Nurses took problems seriously	.68
8. Doctor's concern for comfort	.66
9. Doctor took problem seriously	.66
10. Doctor's information re treatment	.65
11. Waiting time to see doctor	.65
12. Technical skill of nurses	.64
13. Nurses' concern for privacy	.63
14. Doctor's courtesy	.63
15. Nurses' courtesy	.63
16. Doctors informative re home care	.63
17. Waiting time to treatment area	.59
18. Let family/friends be with patient	.58
19. Comfort of waiting room	.56
20. Courtesy of blood technician	.51
21. Helpfulness of registration	.51
22. Privacy during registration	.48
23. Insurance-billing process	.48
24. Skill in taking blood	.48
25. Waiting time in X-ray	.48
26. Courtesy of X-ray tech	.45
27. Convenience of parking	.37

Source: Press, Ganey Associates, February–April 1997, research and development report, ER Department. Used with permission of Press, Ganey Associates.

"Staff cared" is the hottest item for patients in ER recommendation. By far the most important aspect of the ER experience from the patient's point of view is "staff cared about you as a person," with a correlation factor of .8 compared to the next greatest correlation factor of .69. What the patient expresses greatest value for is a caring, sensitive staff. This does not discount the unspoken expectation and trust that patients have for the clinical component of care. There is an unspoken expectation that each professional will provide the best possible clinical care.

EMERGENCY ROOM PRIORITY INDEX

How does each factor that is correlated with recommendation fit with the patient's perceived performance of that factor? It is not only the patient's perception of how important each aspect of the ER experience is in recommending the ER, but also the patient's perception of how well the organization fulfilled those needs that determines the overall satisfaction rating and likelihood to recommend. This is called the *priority index for likelihood to recommend the ER.*

The priority index for the ER is calculated in the same way that the priority index for inpatient services is calculated, discussed earlier in this chapter: by combining the rank order of the highest correlation score for each aspect of the ER experience with the rank order of the lowest average performance score for each aspect. *Result:* a prioritized list of specific aspects of the ER experience on which to focus in order to make the most significant impact on Customer Satisfaction ratings as quickly as possible. Table 3.6 shows the ER priority index.

Reports of this nature are available for physician practices, outpatient services, and other specific standardized departments in a hospital such as obstetrics and pediatrics. To acquire specific data for your organization, contact Press, Ganey Associates in South Bend, Indiana.[1]

Table 3.6. *Emergency Room Priority Index.*

	r rank	m rank	Priority Index
1. Informed about delays	1	8	9
2. Staff cared about you as a person	1	11	12
3. Adequacy of info to family/friends	4	10	14
4. Nurses informative re treatments	7	9	16
5. Nurses attentive to you	6	12	18
6. Waiting time to see doctor	17	3	20
7. Comfort of waiting room	21	4	25
8. Waiting time to treatment area	22	5	27
9. Doctors informative re treatment	14	13	27
10. Courtesy shown family/friends	5	22	27
11. Nurses' concern for privacy	10	18	28
12. Doctor's concern for comfort	12	17	29
13. Nurses took problems seriously	9	23	32
14. Privacy during registration	26	7	33
15. Doctors informative re home care	19	14	33
16. Convenience of parking	29	6	35
17. Doctor took problem seriously	15	20	35
18. Technical skill of nurses	11	26	37
19. Waiting time in X-ray	24	15	39
20. Skill in taking blood	23	16	39
21. Nurses' courtesy	13	27	40
22. Let family/friends be with patient	16	25	41
23. Doctors' courtesy	18	24	42
24. Helpfulness of registration	25	21	46
25. Insurance-billing process	28	19	47
26. Courtesy of blood technician	20	28	48
27. Courtesy of X-ray technician	27	29	58

r = total correlation factor
m = average performance level, rank ordered
Source: Press, Ganey Associates, *National Priority Index—Emergency Department,* June 1997. Used with permission of Press, Ganey Associates.

THE MOST IMPORTANT CUSTOMER SATISFACTION QUESTION FOR ORGANIZATIONS

The single most important factor in measuring Customer Satisfaction is *how likely the Customer is to recommend your organization to others. Likelihood to recommend* translates to *likelihood for repeat business.* Systems for measuring Customer Satisfaction prepare a report card on how well the organization is meeting the expectations of its Customers. It is the overall Customer Satisfaction level that determines whether the patient's experiences contribute to that patient recommending your services to friends and family and the likelihood of that patient returning to your facility should they need health care services. *Repeat business* from current Customers and *new business* referred from current Customers are the lifeblood of thriving organizations in any industry.

One of the complicating factors in deciphering the value of Customer Satisfaction ratings is the inherent subjective nature of personal evaluations. For example, two people sitting in the ER waiting to be seen by the physician are subjected to the same environmental circumstances, yet they will have two very different ratings of the ER experience based on their personal values. Patient A is a busy executive, father, and all-around good guy. He has twice as many things to do as there is time to do them in. A long wait in the ER is a major annoyance for him. If there is a waiting time, the rating of his likelihood to recommend the ER may be very low. Patient B is a college student on spring break. He doesn't seem to mind waiting in the ER as long as he is made somewhat comfortable. The waiting time is not a highly valued item for him; all other things being equal, he may have a higher likelihood of recommending the ER than Patient A.

Two different people experiencing the same circumstantial situation will have two different experiences. Hence, the importance of "satisfying" each patient based on the special set of needs that a particular patient has. For Patient A, a decidedly more difficult patient to satisfy, waiting time is a major dissatisfier. A trained staff person would have identified this patient's special situation and made as many accommodations or exceptions to the system as possible to build greater Customer Satisfaction and payoff for the organization as well as for the patient. Because of the subjective nature of evaluating an experience, the ratings for each aspect of the health care experience are important in that they represent the degree of excellence with which that piece of work was conducted. The goal is to accommodate each patient's needs to the greatest degree possible. The accommodation that is required is likely to be somewhat different for each patient.

At this point you might be asking, "How is it possible to accommodate all the special needs and requests with slim staffing and other rationed resources?" It is possible and it is simpler than you might think. Refer to the Tasks in the Action Plan section at the end of this chapter to help you create an environment and develop staff able to meet and exceed Customer expectations with no additional staff and a higher level of Associate morale.

Regardless of how patients or physicians view various aspects of the health care experience, the ultimate question is, "Would you recommend this facility to your friends and family?" It is around this core question that decisions regarding improvements and changes should be made.

THE MOST IMPORTANT SATISFACTION FACTOR FOR PATIENTS

Whether you look at the ten most highly correlated inpatient needs for likelihood to recommend your organization, or at the ER's most highly correlated needs for likelihood to recommend, there is a consistent pattern of patient voices that shouts aloud what they want and value most in their health care experiences. Patients want staff that are concerned, courteous, caring, and comforting.

- Concerned. Staff cares about the patient's well-being—all aspects of it, including the patient's feelings, the inconvenience that hospitalization and health problems present, the ability of friends and family to be comfortable and visit.

- Courteous. Displays proper manners, holds polite conversation, acknowledges the patient's situation, has pleasant, positive, cheerful attitude and demeanor.
- Caring. Looks after the details of the patient's stay, inquires as to patient's status, is attentive to patient's needs and those of visiting family and friends, is sensitive to uncomfortable clinical care needs.
- Comforting. Reassuring, supportive, encouraging, soothing. Gives proper pain management, etc.

WHAT PATIENTS WANT FROM MEDICAL PRACTICES

The objective of the 1997 Press, Ganey Associates study was to determine which of the twenty-eight qualities associated with the likelihood to recommend a clinic or private medical practice are in greatest need of improvement and which are being performed reasonably well, as judged by 67,088 patients in ninety-two facilities or medical practices. The combined input from the organizations gives a composite profile of the ninety-two operations.

This study distinguishes between health care clinics and physician offices. As in the previous studies, the primary question is what characteristics or qualities influence a patient's likelihood of recommending your clinic or medical practice to family members and friends. The results are shown in Table 3.7.

Notice that the top four factors most highly correlated with the likelihood of recommending either the clinic or private physician's office are based on the patient-physician relationship. They are not related to medical or clinical skills but to how the patient perceives the physician. Is the doctor concerned for the patient's comfort? Is she or he showing respect for the patient's questions and providing clear explanations? Was the amount of time spent with the patient appropriate, as judged by the patient? Each of these four areas are easily managed by employing fundamental interpersonal skills and techniques.

Six of the top ten qualities fall into the category of patient/medical staff (doctors *and* nurses) relationship. In addition to the top four qualities,

Table 3.7. *Factors that Influence Recommendations of Medical Practices.*

	Likelihood of Recommending Clinic	Likelihood of Recommending Doctor
1. Doctor's concern for your comfort	.60	.70
2. Doctor's respect for your questions	.59	.72
3. Clarity of doctor's explanation	.59	.69
4. Length of time doctor spent with you	.56	.65
5. Nurses' concern for your problem	.56	.51
6. Convenience of office hours	.55	.50
7. Ease of obtaining test results	.54	.58
8. Courtesy of nurses	.54	.49
9. How promptly was call returned	.52	.52
10. Availability of doctor on phone	.51	.52
11. Waiting time to see doctor	.50	.47
12. Friendliness of person who took call	.49	.44
13. Comfort of waiting area	.49	.44
14. Ease of phone access to service	.48	.43
15. Courtesy of receptionist	.47	.44
16. Helpfulness of info/reg desk	.47	.42
17. Ease of obtaining desired date/time	.47	.42
18. Length of wait in reception area	.46	.42
19. Speed of registration process	.46	.45
20. X-ray staff concern for comfort	.46	.43
21. Comfort of registration wait area	.45	.43
22. How well bill handled and explained	.45	.44
23. Courtesy of radiology technician	.45	.45
24. Skill with which tests were taken	.45	.43
25. Courtesy of lab technician	.44	.45
26. Waiting time in lab	.41	.41
27. Waiting time in X-ray	.40	.39
28. Parking convenience	.37	.33

Source: Press, Ganey Associates, March/April 1997. Used with permission of Press, Ganey Associates.

which involve physicians' interactions with patients, two qualities involve patients' interaction with nurses: specifically, courtesy of nurses and nurses' concern for patient's problem. In contrast to the patients' emphasis on the importance of interpersonal relationships with physicians and nurses, the lab technicians' courtesy and the X-ray staff's concern for patient comfort are in the bottom ten qualities correlated with the likelihood to recommend a clinic or physician practice.

This brings up the question of whether or not patients clearly and consistently distinguish between nurses and other health care providers wearing white clinical lab coats or nursing whites. Do they realize that the person taking their X-ray or drawing their blood is not a nurse? To be on the safe side, we consider the politeness and caring qualities of X-ray staff and lab technicians to be equally important as for nursing staff. Then it doesn't matter whether patients distinguish between health care professionals or not. They'll all be rated as winners.

COMPARISON OF HIGHLY CORRELATED QUALITIES TO ACTUAL PERFORMANCE

The priority index for the likelihood to recommend a clinic or physician's practice indicates which of the twenty-eight most important qualities are presently being performed well and which need improvement. A look at the general profile of all clinics and physician practices participating in the survey shows that four of the six top ten qualities most highly correlated with the likelihood to recommend are indeed being performed quite well by both physician practices and clinics (see Table 3.7, items 1 through 4). Patients also rate the actual courtesy of nurses in clinics and physician practices as positive (Table 3.7, items 5 and 8).

Table 3.8 prioritizes the twenty-eight qualities in terms of where improvement in performance is needed. Five of the top ten qualities calling for improvement are in the area of time and availability (see Table 3.8, items 1, 2, 4, 7, and 8).

Table 3.8. *National Priority Index—Medical Practices.*

67,088 patients, 92 facilities
1. Availability of doctor on phone
2. How promptly was call returned
3. Ease of phone access to service
4. Speed of registration process
5. Helpfulness of info/reg desk
6. Ease of obtaining desired date/time
7. Length of wait in reception area
8. Waiting time to see doctor
9. Comfort of registration area
10. Convenience of office hours
11. Friendliness of person who took call
12. Comfort of waiting area
13. How well bill handled and explained
14. Courtesy of receptionist
15. Ease of obtaining test results
16. Nurses' concern for your problem
17. Waiting time in lab
18. Parking convenience
19. Waiting time in X-ray
20. Courtesy of nurses
21. X-ray staff concern for comfort
22. Length of time doctor spent with patient
23. Courtesy of lab technician
24. Doctor's concern for your comfort
25. Clarity of doctor's explanation
26. Skill with which tests were taken
27. Courtesy of radiology technician
28. Doctor's respect for your questions

Source: Press, Ganey Associates. Used with permission of Press, Ganey Associates.

Four of these five areas of performance can be improved with better patient management and higher standards of staff performance. For example, the standard of performance for returning telephone calls should be twenty minutes for office staff and no more than one hour for physicians. Adopting this standard means that other work systems will also need adjustment and a priority system for returning telephone calls will have to be established. Physicians involved in surgery or an emergency case may not always be able to return the call within an hour, but designated office staff can return the call for the physician to keep the communication channel to the patient open and relieve patient anxiety. Currently available telecommunications tools make this standard of performance for returned calls reasonably easy to master.

Speed of registration is a work process noted as needing improvement. Perceptions that the registration process is too slow may have as much to do with the preliminary organization of the paperwork and ease or fluidity with which office staff administer the process as it does with the actual length of the process. An efficiently operating registration process requires only three to five minutes of patient time and can be conducted upon arrival of each patient, with no waiting.

Performance improvement in the "waiting" areas listed above can be improved with modifications to the scheduling process. Batching patient treatments together is one technique. This would mean scheduling patients with common treatment needs on the same day or in the same half of the day. For example, Ob/Gyn physicians might schedule all annual or routine gynecological exams on the same day of the week or all in the morning. By batching like work together as much as possible, time allocations per patient become more predictable and routine, thus making it more likely that office staff and physicians can keep to prescribed patient schedules. A second example of batching patient work might be to schedule patients with emergency pleas such as, "I have to see the doctor today!" at the end of the day, when the appointment will not interfere with routine work.

Numerous variables account for delays and waiting times in reception and treatment areas. Office staff know why delays are occurring better than anyone else. Convene the staff and ask them to identify why delays are occurring and to make recommendations about how work and patient schedules can be better managed to at least reduce, if not altogether avoid, delays.

Parkside Associates conducted a research project comparable to that of Press, Ganey Associates. Their objective was to identify what factors or qualities of the medical practice experience are more powerful in predicting the likelihood of patients' recommending a medical practice. Their research involved 178 medical practices and 30,575 patients. The results can be analyzed according to numerous variables, such as patient age, insurance type, and size of medical practice.[2]

ANALYSIS OF PATIENT SATISFACTION SCORES

When all variables are held constant, and two people are subjected to the same set of factors and experiences, it would seem logical to assume that the overall experience would be reasonably similar for both parties. But the complexity of people and their perceptions voids the logic of that assumption. Consequently, managing top Customer Satisfaction scores in health care can be more art than science in some respects.

To help understand what some of the trends in Customer Satisfaction ratings are, Press, Ganey Associates conducted research on patient satisfaction scores by age and gender. A patient population of 264,132 were included from 464 hospitals. Figures 3.3, 3.4, and 3.5 show patient satisfaction results by patient age and gender. First, let's look at the distribution of patients by age (see Figure 3.3). We see that the majority of patients fall into the age group of eighteen to seventy-nine. The heaviest concentration is in the fifty to seventy-nine year range. This information tells us where to focus first, as this age group represents the majority of patients, yet the information is still inadequate. Further detail is needed.

Figure 3.3. Age Distribution of Patients.

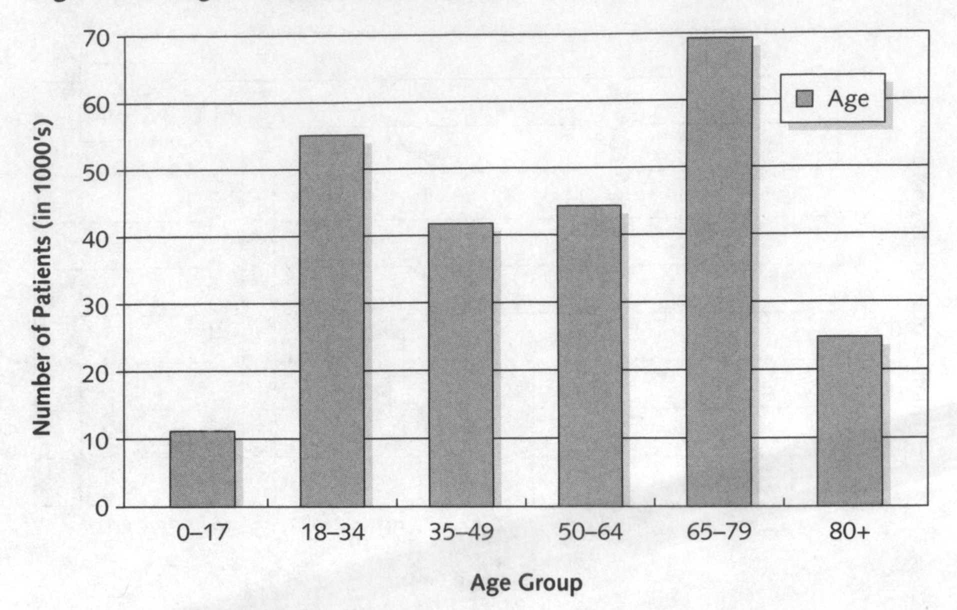

Note: 464 hospitals; 264,132 patients.

Source: Press, Ganey Associates, 1997. Used with permission of Press, Ganey Associates.

Let's look at Figure 3.4 for a distribution of patients by age and sex. This information provides a better focus on male and female responses within each age group. Gender information is important because it may lead to greater specificity about how to better satisfy the total population.

Could it be that female patients have priorities different from those of male patients? A partial answer to that question is found in a further breakdown of information in Figure 3.5. This level of data breakdown is where we begin to get a profile of the differing satisfaction levels of various genders and ages of patients.

Satisfaction Scores by Age

Notice that the highest satisfaction scores are given by patients between the ages of fifty and eighty and older, a population constituting more than half of all patients. This could lead one to think that older patients are more

Figure 3.4. Distribution of Patients by Age and Sex.

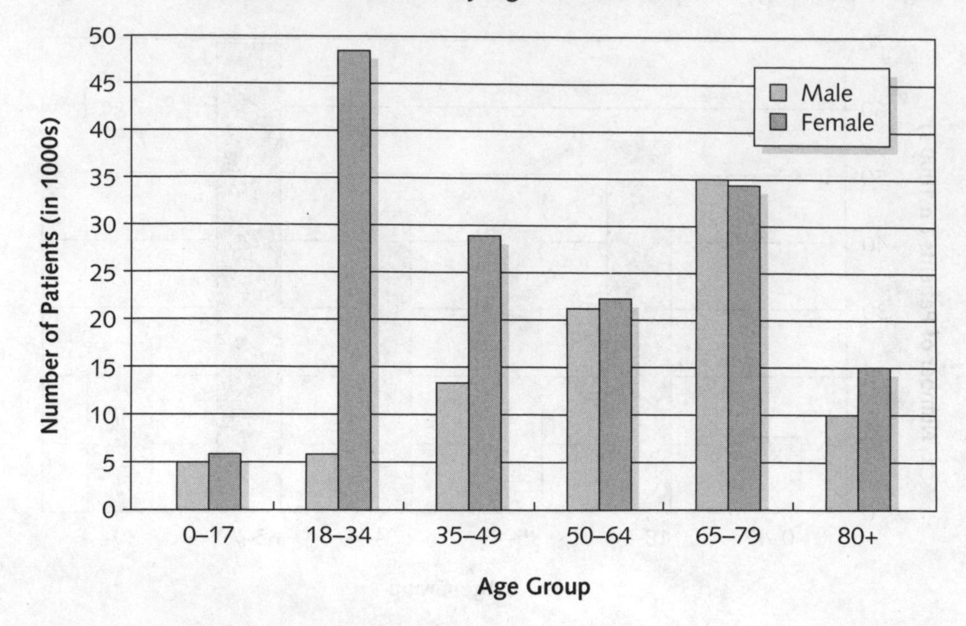

Note: 464 hospitals; 264,132 patients.

Source: Press, Ganey Associates, 1997. Used with permission of Press, Ganey Associates.

gracious and appreciative of health care providers, or that younger patients are more critical. In either case, additional feedback from patients under the age of fifty could help identify what specific changes are needed to increase satisfaction levels for this population.

Among the fifty to eighty-plus patient group (Figure 3.5), the men are clearly more generous in their Customer Satisfaction ratings than the women. In the age groups eighteen to forty-nine, the women are more highly satisfied than the men. The reasons for the disparity in satisfaction are not clear from this research. However, these findings beg for additional feedback from the younger male group as to what is needed to improve their Customer Satisfaction ratings. These data can then be compared with what older male patients find satisfying in the health care experience to see whether there is a relationship.

In general, research findings present the notion that patients of different genders and ages need to be treated differently in order to stabilize Cus-

Figure 3.5. Patient Satisfaction by Age and Sex.

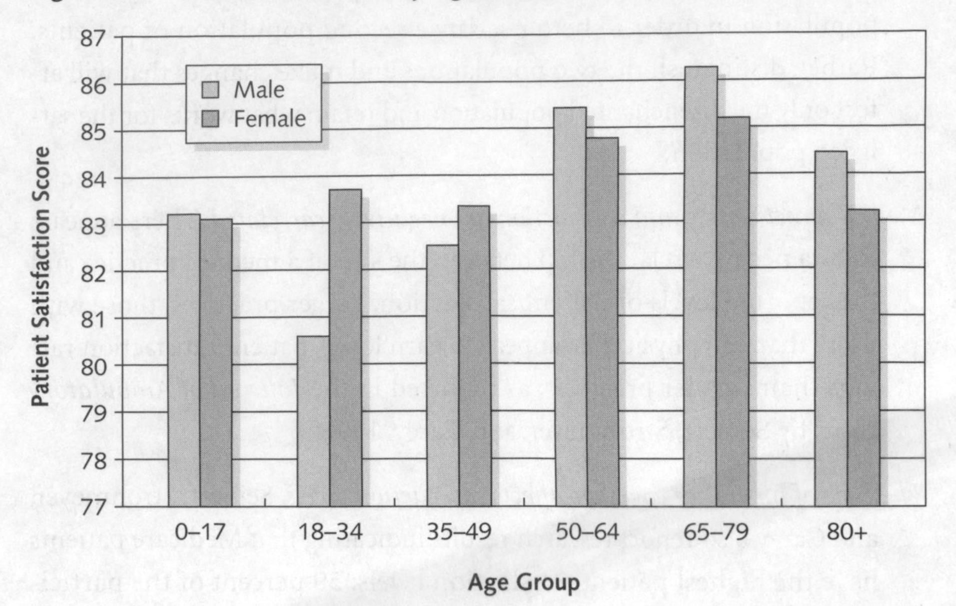

Note: 464 hospitals; 264,132 patients.

Source: Press, Ganey Associates, 1997. Used with permission of Press, Ganey Associates.

tomer Satisfaction uniformly at top levels for all patients. What other factors are known to influence patient satisfaction?

Age and customer satisfaction are positively correlated. In the research of Parkside Associates and Press, Ganey Associates, the conclusions are fairly the same with respect to patient age. Patients who are in their mid-forties or older have a substantially higher level of satisfaction with their health care services in both the physician's office, as documented by Parkside Associates, and in the hospital, as documented by Press, Ganey Associates. The flip side of this discovery is that patients younger than mid-forties are significantly less satisfied with their health care experience in both the physician's office and inpatient hospital setting. This would direct our initial Customer Satisfaction efforts to exploring what needs must be addressed in younger patients, and what needs are already well met in the older patients. Don't change what is working for one population in order to better satisfy a second population of patients. Rather, distinguish the two populations and make changes that will affect only the disenchanted population and retain what works for the satisfied population.

Medical practice size and satisfaction are negatively correlated. There appears to be a negative relationship between the size of a medical practice and the reported levels of patient satisfaction. Larger practices, those with more than ten physicians, appear to earn lower patient satisfaction ratings than smaller practices, as reported in the *Journal of Ambulatory Care,* by Seibert, Strohmeyer, and Carey, 1996.

The type of insurance coverage affects satisfaction levels. Seibert, Strohmeyer, and Carey also report research results indicating that Medicare patients have the highest patient satisfaction levels: 59 percent of the participants rate the medical practice experience as *excellent.* Health Maintenance Organization (HMO) and Preferred Provider Organization (PPO) patients have the lowest patient satisfaction ratings: only 44 percent rate the overall medical practice experience as *excellent.*

Given these research findings, it would seem appropriate to organize large medical practices of more than ten physicians in such a way as to make the work processes and patient interaction feel more like a smaller medical practice. This could be done by devoting administrative and clinical staff specifically to a physician and grouping physicians with relatively like practices together for on-call coverage, and by creating mini or subphysician practices within the scope of a larger medical practice. This may even mean having different waiting rooms for patients of various physician subgroupings, and a mini-team of clinicians and support staff assigned to the patients of particular physicians. The goal is to personalize the physician-patient relationship and reduce bureaucracy and the feeling of insignificance.

ACTION PLAN FOR TOTAL CUSTOMER SATISFACTION

Task 1. Review Output Results from Your Customer Satisfaction Measurement System. Preceding sections of this chapter show that some aspects of the health care experience are more important to patients than others. To find a starting place for improving Customer Satisfaction management, we recommend that you look at the output available from your current Customer Satisfaction measurement system.

Measured data should be in distinct databases: one for inpatients, one for outpatients, one for ER patients, one for community clinics or free-standing practices, and one for each physician's practice. If your data are not available in these distinct patient populations, change your collection and reporting methods as soon as possible. Forgo the value of historical data, as they are of little value to you if they are not collected according to distinct populations.

Task 2. Verify Correlation Factors Between Satisfaction Survey Questions and Likelihood to Recommend. Can statistically sound correlations be drawn between the various aspects of the health care experience that you are measuring (questions on your Customer Satisfaction survey instrument) and the likelihood of the patients' or physicians' recommending your organization, or to use the facility again should the need arise? In other words, is there a statistical correlation between each question on your Customer Satisfaction survey and the likelihood to recommend your facility? This question should be answered by your Customer Satisfaction measurement vendor.

If you can draw these correlations, rank the measured aspects of the satisfaction survey results in ascending numerical order according to each item's correlation factor to the likelihood to recommend your facility. The largest or greatest correlation factor should be first on the list, the second largest correlation factor would be second on the list, continuing until all correlated factors are numbered in descending order, with the smallest correlation factor having the largest and last ranking number. This represents the rank order of measured aspects of the health care experience (items on the Customer Satisfaction survey) from most important to least important (if there is such a thing as least important), as reported by your particular patient population. Rank ordering gives some indication of where you should invest immediate and particular attention. A sample report would look like the ones prepared by Press, Ganey Associates and presented in this chapter.

Table 3.9 provides a sample section of a report for easy reference. Your report should have the same format. The only difference will be that the correlation number and specific measured activities will be different, based on your patient satisfaction feedback.

Task 3. Create a Priority Index for Your Organization. Assess your organization's average response to each correlated satisfaction question and create a priority index for your organization. Will your Customer Satisfaction measurement vendor supply you with a custom report for your organization that calculates and displays the mathematical average or mean responses from your patients to each of the questions on your survey tool? In other words, what is the average patient rating for each of the measured activities? Average patient responses are called the *mean.*

If your Customer Satisfaction measurement vendor cannot provide this information, you might want to reassess the value of the information that they can provide. There are two options at this point: Change providers and let the measurement organization do the work, or stick it out and shoulder more of the administrative burden within your organization by conducting the calculations yourself. In the latter case, you will still require the cooperation of the measurement vendor to provide you with the data from which to collect, calculate, and summarize the findings.

When the data are available, report the mean responses to each of the survey questions next to the correlation factor for each question. In Table 3.10,

Table 3.9. *Sample Report—Emergency Department/Room.*

	Correlation with Likely to Recommend	r rank
1. Staff cared about you as a person	.80	1
2. Informed about delays	.73	2
3. Nurses' attention to you	.69	3
4. Nurse informative re treatments	.69	4
5. Adequacy of info to family/friends	.68	5
6. Courtesy shown family/friends	.68	6
7. Nurses took problems seriously	.68	7
8. Doctor's concern for comfort	.66	8
9. Doctor took problem seriously	.66	9
10. Doctor's information re treatment	.65	10
11. Waiting time to see doctor	.65	11
12. Technical skills of nurses	.64	12
13. Nurses' concern for privacy	.63	13
14. Doctor's courtesy	.63	14
15. Nurses' courtesy	.63	15
16. Waiting time to treatment area	.59	17
17. Let family/friends be with patient	.58	18
19. Comfort of waiting room	.56	19
20. Courtesy of blood technician	.51	20
21. Helpfulness of registration	.51	21
22. Privacy during registration	.48	22
23. Insurance-billing process	.48	23
24. Skill in taking blood	.48	24
25. Waiting time in X-ray	.48	25
26. Courtesy of X-ray tech	.45	26
27. Convenience of parking	.37	27

the average patient response is the *m ranking*. Add the mean score *(m ranking)*, and the correlation factor *(r ranking)* together to arrive at the priority index number. Finally, order the questions on the survey according to the priority index figure, starting with the smallest index figure at the top in the number one spot, the next smallest priority index figure in the second position, etc. The largest priority index figure should be last on the list. A sample of the final priority index report that you generate should look something like that found in Table 3.10.

At this point you have generated the priority index for your organization—a listing in priority order of the areas of service that need improvement—by combining the highest correlation factor and the lowest average performance score as determined by your patient population. The obvious places to begin making improvements, as viewed by patients, are in the measured activities with the smallest priority index figure assigned to them. The smaller the priority index number, the greater the impact will be when you improve performance in that area. Changes in these areas will afford your organization the greatest impact on likelihood of patients' recommending your facilities to friends and family.

If you cannot draw these correlations, or cannot gather the average performance levels for each of the survey questions, the usefulness of your Customer Satisfaction survey data is limited at best, and we recommend that you consider engaging a professional Customer Satisfaction measurement vendor to assist in future measurements. Three credible firms to contact are Press, Ganey Associates, Parkside Associates, and the Picker Institute (see Note 1 at the end of the chapter for addresses).

Task 4. Identify the Top Ten Aspects of the Health Care Experience that Require Your Immediate Attention. Using the priority listing generated in Task 3, note the top ten aspects of your health care operation requiring immediate improvement as rated by your customers. Convene your Customer Satisfaction Leadership Council to share this information and analyze what it means to your organization.

Table 3.10. *Sample Priority Listing.*

Measured Activity	r rank	m rank	Priority Index
1. Informed about delays	8	1	9
2. Likelihood to recommend	2	8	10
3. Staff cared about you as a person	1	11	12
4. Adequacy of info to family/friends	4	10	14
5. Nurses informative re treatments	7	9	16
6. Nurses attentive to you	6	12	18
7. Waiting time to see doctor	17	3	20
8. Comfort of waiting room	21	4	25
9. Waiting time to treatment area	22	5	27
10. Doctors informative re treatment	14	13	27
11. Courtesy shown family/friends	5	22	27
12. Nurses' concern for privacy	10	18	28
13. Doctor's concern for comfort	12	17	29
14. Nurses took problems seriously	9	23	32
15. Privacy during registration	26	7	33
16. Doctors informative re home care	19	14	33
17. Convenience of parking	29	6	35
18. Doctor took problem seriously	15	20	35
19. Technical skill of nurses	11	26	37
20. Waiting time in X-ray	24	15	39
21. Skill in taking blood	23	16	39
22. Nurse courtesy	13	27	40
23. Let family/friends be with patient	16	25	41
24. Doctor's courtesy	18	24	42
25. Helpfulness of registration	25	21	46
26. Insurance-billing process	28	19	47
27. Courtesy of blood technician	20	28	48
28. Courtesy of X-ray technician	27	29	56

Look for trends in the types of measured activities in this top ten list. Are there numerous measured activities with the same themes, such as "waiting times" or "concern by staff?" Identify themes where improvement is needed and create active solutions that address the specifics of each theme represented.

Task 5. Research Each of the Top Ten Customer Satisfaction Priorities for Your Organization. The purpose of the research is to quantify, where possible, how extensive the problems are. For example, for item 1 in Table 3.10, "informed about delays," the goal is to find out exactly how long patients presently wait before they are advised of delays in the system. Do thirty minutes pass before patients are informed about a delay, or are they never informed about the delay, or something in between?

Then establish departmental or interdepartmental teams to create new, improved standards of performance for keeping patients informed about delays and, in addition, make changes to improve upon the service delivery to reduce the number of delays or amount of time spent waiting. In this case, the obvious solution is to increase the frequency with which patients are informed about delays in treatment. But go beyond the obvious, perhaps by explaining why the delays are occurring (if there is a reasonable excuse that the patient might understand). For example, a staff person might say to a patient who is waiting:

> *We apologize for the delay in getting your X-ray taken, Mr. Jones. An unexpected crisis has occurred and a young child arrived in the ER with massive injuries from an automobile accident. We should be able to do your X-ray in about fifteen minutes. Thank you for understanding. By the way, can I get you a drink of water or something to read while you're waiting?*

Patients should wait no more than fifteen minutes before receiving an update on the status of their delay. When delays become excessive, *excessive* defined as more than one hour, the option to reschedule the appointment for outpatients should be given, with the courtesy of paid transportation if public transportation is needed.

Task 6. Evaluate How Your Organization Compares to Other Comparable Health Care Organizations in Customer Satisfaction Ratings. Share with your department managers and Associates what your organization's satisfaction scores are compared to other health care providers, and share what each department's satisfaction scores are compared to the competition. Don't be surprised to find that a raw Customer Satisfaction score of 87 percent, which sounds like a good rating at first glance, actually translates into a ranking of 178 out of 456 competing hospitals in one database. Raw scores can be deceiving. Translating the raw score into a percentile score or comparative statistic is enlightening. What seemed to be a B report card with an 87 percent raw score suddenly becomes a C, or "average," score when viewed in comparison to other health care providers.

Use comparative and percentile translations to motivate people to a higher level of Customer service. Organizations that compare Customer Satisfaction ratings only to themselves or to others within their "system" of hospitals are operating in an artificial world. A comparison of this nature is like comparing speed records in a family of turtles. What does it mean if you are the fastest in a family of turtles? What does it mean if you are the best-rated organization in Customer Satisfaction among a lot of poor performers compared to industry standards?

As the battle for the top Customer Satisfaction scores continues to heat up, the ability to edge out competitors in top positions becomes more and more difficult to achieve. The difference between being rated number one nationally and being rated number forty-eight nationally in Customer Satisfaction can be as little as five raw points.

When delivering raw scores and comparative Customer Satisfaction information to managers and Associates, it is helpful and appropriate for the Customer satisfaction champion and other leaders to *show feelings* of disappointment if results are less than goals, *make statements* of encouragement and confidence in future performance, *set goals* for specific improvements in performance for each department specifically and for the organization in total, and *draw attention* to the importance of Customer Satisfaction measurement as a competitive advantage or disadvantage.

Task 7. Post Customer Satisfaction Ratings. Keep the message and motivation for continued and better Customer service constantly in front of staff and management. Post department-specific satisfaction results in each department and review them at the weekly staff meeting. Refer to Table 3.11 and Table 3.12 of this chapter for sample formats for satisfaction reporting.

Notice that the report contains not only the organization's current Customer Satisfaction ratings, but also the current week's ranking compared to all other organizations in the national database. Comparative data on this one-page report serves as a staff motivator for better performance. For example, the Patient Care rating of 90.54 percent may seem to be an excellent rating. But in comparison to 454 other hospitals in the national database, it rates as number fifty-two! It is a good performance level, but far from the goal of 98.4 percent, which is what is needed to be number one in the national database.

The sample report also indicates a quarterly cumulative ranking for the organization, which is a second comparison serving to inform and motivate staff to provide better Customer service. Again using the sample for Patient Care, we see that the Current Week Score of 90.54 percent, representing a ranking of fifty-two in the national database, is a lower, less desirable position than the organization had in the past quarter, as represented by the Current Quarter Cumulative Rank of forty-one and the Last Quarter Rank of twenty-seven. Obviously, something has changed and there is a downward trend in Customer Satisfaction ratings. Active management would focus immediate attention on what has changed in this area of performance.

Table 3.11. *Holy Cross Sample Customer Satisfaction Report.*

Why Strive for #1 Service?

"Excellent service is our primary consideration.
We must strive to be the best in that designation."

— Judy Henson —

Customer Satisfaction Scores
Week of January 10–16, 1997

	Current Week Score	Current Week Rank	Current Qtr. Cum. Rank	Last Qtr. Rank	Goal
Inpatient	87.14%	#51	#16	#6	96.6%
Neighborhd. afl.	89.90%	#7	#4	#5	94.5%
Outpatient	95.37%	#1	#4	#21	93.7%
1-day-surgery	92.10%	#27	#7	#15	96.7%
Emergency	89.34%	#10	#28	#11	90.7%
Home health	94.40%	#2	#4	#1	98.4%
Patient care	90.54%	#52	#41	#27	98.4%

Customer Service Tip of the Week

#1 SERVICE means having the kind of enthusiastic attitude
that makes our visitors feel warm and welcome
— no matter how cold it is outside!

Source: Holy Cross Hospital Customer Satisfaction ratings. Used with permission of Holy Cross Hospital.

Performance statistics of this nature are used by leadership and department managers to drive home the message of the degree of improved Customer Satisfaction that is needed for each department and section of the organization. It is not enough to say, "Our Customer Satisfaction levels are excellent." How "excellent" is "excellent," and compared to what? If you can't measure it, you can't manage it.

Notice that in Table 3.11, the core statistical information in the report is augmented at the top with words of wisdom from a Holy Cross Associate about Customer Satisfaction. Including an Associate's words of advice in this manner personalizes the report while providing an opportunity to highlight, recognize, and share Associates' good thinking before the entire organization.

At the bottom of the page is a Customer Service Tip of the Week, or reminder of what is needed to make a difference in Customer Satisfaction ratings. Again, the tip is provided by a hospital Associate, thus adding Associate ownership to the message.

Task 8. Participate in a National Database of Health Care Satisfaction Measurements. If your organization is not participating in a Customer Satisfaction measurement database that includes hundreds of competing hospitals, make the move to become part of a leading national database. (Recommendations for databases are found earlier in this chapter.) *Excellence* is a relative rating determined by the Customer, and you need to know how your organization is performing relative to others in order to compete in the new dimensions of health care management.

The second Holy Cross sample Customer Satisfaction report (Table 3.12) shows the primary components of a health care experience in the sequence in which the experience generally occurs, starting with admission to the hospital and progressing through nursing care, tests, and treatments, and concluding with discharge, final ratings, and the "likelihood to recommend."

Table 3.12. *Holy Cross Hospital Inpatient Survey Points.*

		Raw Score	Rank	To Be #1 Nationally
	Week of January 10–16, 1997			
A	Admissions	83.10	306	97.30
B	Your room	84.85	29	94.50
C	Diet and meals	82.25	33	91.80
D	Nursing care	90.54	52	98.40
E	Tests and treatment	86.82	83	95.80
F	Other services	87.69	196	98.30
G	Visitors and family	86.87	164	96.90
H	Your physician	86.91	132	95.10
I	Discharge	87.04	60	96.20
J	Some final ratings	86.77	176	98.50
	Mean	**87.14**	**51**	**96.60**
K	Likelihood of recommend.	86.89	249	99.40

The above points listed under this period are based upon the return of 65 patient surveys.

The rank will fluctuate due to other hospitals in Press, Ganey, raising or lowering their scores.

Our rank for this week is #51 out of 456 competing hospitals.

Source: Holy Cross Hospital Customer Satisfaction ratings. Used with permission of Holy Cross Hospital.

Notice that the Raw Score, Rank, and what is needed To Be #1 Nationally are again reported for each segment of the health care experience, as well as the Likelihood of Recommendation. In this particular example, a raw score of 86.69 percent for likelihood to recommend places this organization in the 249th position, or slightly over the fiftieth percentile marker in the national database of 456 hospitals. At first blush, management might think that a score of 86.69 percent was reasonably good, but in the context of how other hospitals are performing nationally, it is little more than average.

A final comment on this sample report focuses on the notation: "The rank will fluctuate due to other hospitals in Press, Ganey, raising or lowering their scores." Without comparative information determining how your organization's performance stacks up against that of competing organizations, there is no benchmark for how much improvement is needed to be considered *excellent.* As Customer Satisfaction ratings take on increasing influence in the health care business arena, the standard for what is *average* or mediocre performance will continue to rise. It is and will become increasingly difficult to motivate staff to improve Customer Satisfaction when their perception of their performance level is distorted, as it can easily be if only raw scores are used to gauge performance levels.

Task 9. Break Out Patient Satisfaction Measurements by Specific Departments. Refer to the following sample report of patient care satisfaction ratings by unit, Table 3.13, as a guideline for the types of information to be shared. Use this information to make immediate changes in management behaviors. Department leaders who consistently have the lowest satisfaction ratings should be assigned a Customer Satisfaction SWAT team or mentor for assistance in making quick improvements. Should a trend of poor satisfaction performance persist after various forms of assistance have been provided, it is possible that such a manager should be reassigned to a nonmanagerial role.

Use this information as a basis for executive discussions and decisions regarding the framework of unacceptable managerial performance levels. At what point should that manager no longer be a manager? A number of suggestions are provided in this Task and earlier in this chapter. Your executive team must make their own determination of performance break-off points. However, beware of performance standards that are too lenient or too wishy-washy. Performance that is measurable is manageable. Set the perimeters and manage within them. Specific structure and standardized approaches for how people will be managed benefit the organization and are easier for people to deal with.

Table 3.13. *Patient Care by Units.*

Week of January 10–16, 1997						
		Raw Score				
		Last Week		This Week		
Unit	Room #	%	Rank	%	Rank	# Returned
CICI & SICU		94.2		88.76		21
EFC	(300–325)	87.5	202	94.79	3	2
REHAB	(326–349)	82.81	345	85.37	293	6
4-ASU	(400–412)	88.52	157	97.35	2	8
4-A	(415–527)	78.33	371	93.64	5	5
4-B	(430–457)	80.35	368	72.3	456	7
5-A	(500–518)	98.1	2	90.44	57	6
5-B RESP	(530-542)	100	1	82.83	345	5
5-B TELE	(545–555)	98.48	1	90.83	46	5
6A NORTH	(601–612)	100	1	89.58	93	4
6-B	(632–657)	79.16	370	91.95	15	17
Total Surveys			62			65

OUT OF 456
COMPETING HOSPITALS
these are our weekly
NURSING CARE RANKS
for this week

Source: Holy Cross Hospital. Used with permission of Holy Cross Hospital.

Task 10. Break Out Customer Satisfaction Measures by Specific Key Performance Areas. Some Customer expectations should become indisputable and be made standards of performance for the organization. For example, patient call lights should be answered quickly. How quickly? You decide. We recommend a timeframe of no more than three minutes. That means the patient will be responded to within three minutes of pushing the call light button. That is a specific, uniform standard of performance that can be measured.

Other Customer expectations include the timeframe in which the telephone is answered and how long elapses from the moment a Customer is put on hold to the moment someone gets back to them. We recommend a standard of no more than thirty seconds. That means that when a person is put on hold, someone will get back to them at least every thirty seconds to let them know the status of their call.

Your Task is to identify what specific standards of performance your organization will adopt and how you will measure the performance of each department. Remember, if you cannot measure it, you cannot manage it. Table 3.14 shows how Holy Cross Hospital compiles this type of performance information and then uses it to determine the top performers—those to whom others within the organization go for quick assistance in one special area of performance, responding to call lights.

Earlier we emphasized the need to know performance levels for patient satisfaction for each segment of the health care experience; that is, admissions, food service, nursing, etc. Equally important is information collected from each subset of performing departments.

There are three primary values found in reporting individual departmental satisfaction statistics. First, leading performers can be recognized and rewarded for their success and results. Recognition, reward, and reinforcement, the 3Rs, are valuable motivators for continued high performance levels. Second, internal comparisons with reasonably like types of services—for example, nursing units to nursing units—provide sources for internal benchmarking and immediate team support. Departments with lower satisfaction scores can look to those with higher scores and benchmark best practices. Often, specific management practices found in one top-performing unit are copied and transplanted to other units, thus resulting in some immediate improvement in performance. Sometimes it is a matter of how work systems are laid out on one unit versus another unit that enables staff to respond more quickly and easily to patient needs. Internal comparisons point to the best performers from which others should study, steal, and implement their best ideas.

Table 3.14. *Call Lights.*

		Week of January 10–16, 1997			
		Promptness		**Attitude**	
	Room #	**Raw Score**	**Rank**	**Raw Score**	**Rank**
ECF	(300–325)	87.5	112	87.5	201
REHAB	(326–349)	80.00	338	80	338
4-ASU	(400–412)	96.42	2	96.42	3
4-A	(415–527)	85.00	212	95	3
4-B	(430–457)	75.00	372	85	291
5-A	(500–518)	91.66	9	83.33	168
5-B RESP	(530–542)	75.00	372	87.5	201
5-B TEL	(545–555)	90.00	31	85.00	291
6A NORTH	(601–614)	100	1	100	1
6-B	(632–657)	87.5	112	91.17	46
Mean Score		**86.80**	**141**	**89.09**	**131**

Our rank is out of 424 competing hospitals

Promptness in responding to the call button.
#1 National Rank = 98.1 Raw Score

Nurses' attitude toward your calling them.
#1 National Rank = 98.7 Raw Score

Source: Holy Cross Hospital Customer Satisfaction ratings. Used with permission of Holy Cross Hospital.

Third, reporting individual department statistics creates an internal competitive situation among departments within a division. When four of the ten nursing departments are performing at top satisfaction levels, as shown in Table 3.13, there is inherent pressure for the remaining six lesser performers to improve. In this particular example you can see the result of the internal pressure to improve. Four of the five lowest performing departments in "Last week's ranking" moved to top performing status in "This week's rank." One of the five worst ranking departments last week, 4-B in this case, slipped to a ranking of 456, or last place nationally. The comparative data sounds a wake-up call for the management of this department and the leadership of the organization. Attention should focus intensely on this unit and the circumstances surrounding a performance rating that is consistently sinking, and sinking deeply.

Internal competition is a subset of organizational competition. Each department leader and staff want their performance levels to be greater than those of their colleagues. Because improvement of departmental performance is part of improving organizational performance, there is also a sense of camaraderie in healthy competition. In this case, it would not be unusual for department leaders from top-performing departments, such as 5-B TEL and 5A, to immediately offer support and assistance to consistently lower-performing units such as REHAB and 4-B.

Task 11. Review Customer Satisfaction Measurement Data to Assure that It Breaks Out Certain Business Operations in Separate and Distinct Databases. The basic business operations and distinct areas of Customer Satisfaction that require measurement include the following:

- Ambulatory surgery: registration, lab, X-ray, EKG, nursing, physician, other services
- Inpatient services: admissions process, patient's room, diet and meals, nursing care, tests and treatments, visitors and family, physician, discharge, likelihood to recommend
- Emergency Room: registration, nurses, physicians, tests, family and friends
- Outpatient departments (free-standing or hospital-based): arthritis, eye laser, foot clinic, audiology, gastroscopy, cardiac testing, lab, X-ray, EKG, MRI, mammography, nuclear medicine, cast room, obstetrics, chemotherapy, occupational therapy, colonoscopy, physical therapy, CT scan, registration, cystoscopy, ultrasound, ENT (ears, nose, and throat), other

- Home health: arranging for home health care, dealing with the home health care nurses, non-nursing staff, therapists
- Neighborhood affiliates: phone, reception, care, tests and treatments

You may wish to include other measured activities within one or more of the service lines. What is provided here is the starting point.

If your Customer Satisfaction data are not broken out into specific departments, identifying weak performers and the extent of problems they represent will be difficult. Facts are friendly, and in a highly competitive field such as health care, those with the facts are those with an advantage. These are data that you can't afford not to have.

Task 12. Review the Frequency and Volume of Customer Satisfaction Feedback. The more frequently you request Customer Satisfaction measurement from your vendor, the more costly it is to the organization. More work equals more cost. Consequently, cost-conscious administrators order Customer Satisfaction measurement reports on a quarterly basis. They rationalize that Customer Satisfaction ratings do not change dramatically in a short time, or that things have not changed at their hospital or clinic or medical practice, therefore Customer Satisfaction ratings should not be changing. Wrong. If things are not changing in your organization, it is predictable that your Customer Satisfaction ratings will be changing—for the worse.

Customer demands and expectations are on the rise at somewhat alarming rates. The rate of increase in Customer expectations is so great that one wonders when Customer expectations will become so extreme as to be impossible to fulfill. Fortunately, we are still nowhere near that point.

Change and improvement are the lifeblood of an organization's survival. Customers, including patients and physicians, are fickle. What was exceptional today may not even be acceptable tomorrow. With so many variables to manage—including patients with changing, unique needs, staff turnover, changing job descriptions, and physician turnover—keeping the formula for successful Customer Satisfaction in balance is difficult without frequent feedback as to where to make adjustments in performance. Quarterly feedback is useless. By the time the information is available, the environment and all its variables have changed several times over. Staff become less accountable as time elapses between the point of service and the receipt of negative feedback. Excuses like, "I don't remember it that way. . ."; or "Things have changed since then . . ." make dealing with the data difficult.

Monthly feedback is better, but still leaves much to be desired. By the time monthly data arrive, they are still almost too old to do anything with. What is more important, dissatisfied Customers have completed their stay without the organization having an opportunity to make adjustments and improvements to their overall experience. Patients and physicians on the brink of defection are more difficult to recover after time elapses.

Organizations that are serious about Customer Satisfaction management track key measurements weekly, making adjustments as performance levels fluctuate. With the help of weekly satisfaction feedback, underperforming areas can be rapidly corrected, and most patients and physicians on the edge of dissatisfaction can be salvaged or recovered before the end of their stay. What would otherwise have been an unhappy experience can be transformed into a satisfactory experience. Weekly data make it possible to fine-tune organization performance constantly by never allowing deteriorating performance to fall much before it is quickly recovered. However, weekly information gathered through a Customer Satisfaction measurement vendor is exceptionally expensive and not necessarily recommended.

Your organization can collect Customer Satisfaction information weekly, tabulate results in-house to identify "dog" and star performers, make appropriate organizational changes, and forward this information on to your measurement vendor for inclusion in the monthly report. This allows you to use information in a timely manner without increasing your cost.

Warning: Most Customer Satisfaction measurement firms will give discouraging words to this practice, claiming it is a distorted methodology. Remember, as vendors they are concerned with the scientific validity of the total methodology, and any deviation from their highly controlled model is frowned upon. The fact is, you need the information, and whatever potential distortion a modified methodology presents, it is minimal and worth it. Customer Satisfaction ratings are *an indicator* of performance, not an exact science. It is more important that you have information that you need when you need it than it is to have "more scientifically valid" information at a time when it does you little good.

Task 13. Measure Customer Satisfaction Data for Free-Standing Clinics. Specific performance data for each free-standing clinic will help direct your organization's energy and resources to improve specific performance areas to make a difference for your organization. Composite information as provided in this chapter is helpful in a general way but may not necessarily reflect the specific needs of your organization to perpetuate growth. Free-standing clinics represent additional market share and revenue as a stand-alone facility and as a feeder system or referral source to the hospital, ER, and other hospital-related physicians. It is a reflective situation in which the reputation of one segment of the business, the free-standing clinic, reflects upon and influences Customer perceptions of other parts of the organization, such as the ER and inpatient facility. Therefore, it is essential to the well-being of the entire organization that Customer Satisfaction in free-standing clinics is very high.

Task 14. Measure Customer Satisfaction for Physician Practices. Increase the number of physician practices engaged in measuring Customer Satisfaction feedback. Health care organizations can motivate physician practices to engage in Customer Satisfaction measurement by

- Subsidizing the cost of measurement as a benefit of being associated with your organization and in exchange for feedback results on the practice
- Including participation in feedback as a condition of affiliation with your organization

- Using physician leadership to communicate the value of measurement data and the process

When patients experience a satisfying continuum of care from physician office staff through hospital admission, discharge, and follow-up, the overall experience will be memorably more pleasant. All too often hospitals embrace extraordinary Customer Satisfaction initiatives but do not connect physician office staffs to the need for an integrated experience. A small irritation that starts at any point in an experience is typically carried emotionally through to the end of that experience. This means that if patients become irritated with the duplication of information given initially to the physician's office and requested again by the hospital at admission, this small irritation can color the entire experience, thus making other situations less tolerable than they might otherwise have been.

Think of individual patients as having something like a virtual irritation tank, where personal irritations are stored away without episode. Some people's tanks are bigger than others', meaning that some people can tolerate more irritations than others before they become totally disenchanted with the experience. Each time a patient rubs up against an annoying situation either with the physician staff or the hospital staff, their little irritation tank gets a little fuller until they finally can't and won't tolerate further irritations—they've reached their maximum level of annoyance. Now they're just plain upset and unhappy.

When physician office staff are not equally committed to providing outstanding service as the hospital, not only within the walls of the physician practice but as a partner with your organization in providing a continuum of care from physician to hospital and back to physician, you are fighting an uphill battle. Physician office staffs must partner with the hospital to problem-solve in the name of service excellence. Discuss how to deal with physicians or physician office staffs with less than desirable service skills, and how to enhance the average standards of Customer Satisfaction performance among all physician practices.

Task 15. Analyze Patient Satisfaction Statistics. Dig deep into the statistics for Customer Satisfaction measurement and search for relationships among various types of patients and their satisfaction levels. Consider gender, age group, and insurance types to determine whether there is a distinctive difference in ratings based on components of these variables. Trends that you see will have to be investigated further. Identify what is contributing to the trends, and how you can use this information to improve Customer Satisfaction ratings. Answers to these questions are found in one-on-one research with patients.

Translate the differences you find by gender, age, and insurance types into specific performance-based training for Associates. If Associates know what makes one profile of patient happy, they can adapt to that type of patient. Such mini-customization based on patient profile types will significantly affect overall satisfaction ratings.

NOTES

1. Resources: Press, Ganey Associates, 1657 Commerce Drive, South Bend, Indiana 46628, (219) 232–3387; Parkside Associates, 205 W. Touhy Avenue, Suite 204, Park Ridge, IL 60068, (847) 698–4825; The Picker Institute, 1295 Boylston Street, Boston, MA 02215, (617) 667–2388.
2. Jerry Seibert, Jan Strohmeyer, and Raymond Carey. "Evaluating the Physician Office Visit: In Pursuit of a Valid and Reliable Measure of Quality Improvement Efforts." *Journal of Ambulatory Care,* 1996, pp. 17–37.

Measurement Tools That Work

Chapter FOUR

Your Customer wants to tell you something. Are you listening?

Winning organizations believe they can continue to achieve higher and higher levels of Customer Satisfaction until they have reached national top-ranked status, and then perhaps advance even further by keeping one step ahead of aggressive competitors. Unless your organization is the top-rated organization in the country (or, for some industries, in the global market), there is room to advance.

MEANINGFUL MEASUREMENT

The problem with Customer Satisfaction measurement is that it is intangible and, as such, difficult to measure. A snapshot of Customer Satisfaction taken at any one point in time is a loose measure of past Customer opinions and, perhaps, intent to reuse your services in the future, which is an opinion subject to change.

Customer Satisfaction measurement tools are used for two primary purposes: as an internal report card on performance, and as an external report card on performance. Keeping these purposes in perspective is important. The most popular use of Customer Satisfaction data is as an internal report card on organizational performance. This use provides a source of specific opportunities to improve Customer Satisfaction.

The second, and growing, use of Customer Satisfaction data is as an external report card for employer coalitions and managed care providers to assess the probability that any one health care organization will provide an excellent health care experience for those enrolled in their health care plan. Stability of enrollment for managed care organizations, and satisfaction with health care providers, are essential factors in the formula for success for managed care organizations and employer coalitions. High Customer Satisfaction ratings are desirable. They translate to a stable enrollment in managed care health care plans. Lower Customer Satisfaction ratings are undesirable, as they cause instability in health plan enrollment, a dangerous situation for managed care providers, which depend on stability as one of the cornerstones of building a sustainable managed care business.

The bottom line for managed care organizations seems to be that high Customer Satisfaction must coexist with cost-effective delivery in order for a health care provider to be considered a desirable participant in a managed care delivery system. The good news about Customer Satisfaction opinions is that they can easily be changed by changing the way staff deal with patients. Patients do not typically hold grudges. If they have had a mediocre experience at your organization in the past, and this visit is exceptional, they will tell you it was exceptional. The bad news about Customer Satisfaction opinions is that they can easily be changed by changing the way staff deal with patients. This means that patients and physicians arriving at your organization with an initial positive impression can leave with a negative opinion if the experience leaves something to be desired. Consequently, it is essential to know how Customers perceive the health care experience at critical points in time *during* the experience, rather than after the experience.

Alternative Approaches to Measuring Customer Satisfaction. To direct and effect improvements in real-time behaviors and work systems, we must largely rely on Customers to tell us where they see our performance to be deficient. The following ten methods for mining information, used in concert, will uncover where additional changes in personal behaviors and work systems need to be made to better serve the Customer.

Postdischarge Mailed Surveys. Postdischarge surveys are the most popular source for gathering data on patient satisfaction but the least effective for making change. The lack of timeliness of information is the greatest downfall of this approach. Even monthly data collection yields information reported some six weeks after the experience has taken place—too long for people to remember the situation clearly, and enough time for staff to cloud the issues with lame excuses such as, "We already changed that."

The lag time between time of incidence and time of report can cause your organization to fall from grace or make it impossible to scramble up from the bleak pits of Customer opinion. If your organization relies heavily on postdischarge paper surveys, at least order them monthly and compile internal results weekly. Internal weekly compilations identify weak spots sooner relative to the point of service, thus allowing corrections to be made rapidly, before further damage to Customer Satisfaction occurs.

Those who elect to use this approach to measuring satisfaction should augment it with two or three additional approaches in order to gain further insight into what is truly meant by the limited and stiff data provided by postdischarge survey results. No one source of feedback is entirely representative of Customer perceptions. An assembly of data from various sources creates a more credible and complete picture.

Be selective in the choice of vendors for administering postdischarge surveys. The quality of vendor and measurement instruments are imperative to the validity of the results. Home-grown survey instruments that are not statistically validated will probably provide a skewed result that should not be trusted.

Statistically validated survey instruments offer substantially more credible results; results that you can be comfortable knowing are a reasonably true picture of organizational performance. See the checklist under Selecting Measurement Tools and Services further on in this chapter for an assessment of how your Customer Satisfaction measurement tools and vendor measure up.

To sum up, the single greatest mistake that most organizations make in Customer Satisfaction management is relying solely on postdischarge paper satisfaction surveys to gauge Customer Satisfaction. Although these surveys are a good way of gaining an overall macro-feeling for levels and trends in Customer Satisfaction, they are a long way from providing timely information essential for moving an *above average* experience to an *exceptional* experience, or a *good* experience to an *above average* one. Effective Customer Satisfaction requires real-time involvement by all staff, volunteers, and physicians.

Surveys Administered at Discharge. Surveys administered at the time of discharge are more likely to reflect the true nature of the recent experience without the influence of outside sources. Some such surveys are administered verbally and provide an opportunity for a skilled interviewer to pinpoint highlights of the experience as well as note any less-than-optimal experiences. One-to-one interaction further enhances the sense of relationship, which is essential to long-term business with each Customer.

The difficulty with this approach is that it takes time and requires skilled interviewers. If Customer Satisfaction information is valued, however, the investment in time should not be seen as a barrier, and interview skills can be taught.

The one-to-one exchange provides one last opportunity for the organization to engage in recovery specific to a Customer's unsatisfactory experience before that Customer leaves the premises. It provides one last opportunity to create a positive experience—and to win Customer loyalty.

Postdischarge Telephone Surveys. Telephone surveys are good feedback mechanisms for the same reasons that interviews administered at the time of discharge are good sources of feedback. They allow the interviewer to gauge the intensity of comments made, probe into problematic situations, and possibly recover service in situations where the incidence was particularly annoying, and undiscovered.

However, like interviews at the point of discharge, telephone surveys are costly to engage, and being conducted after the fact allows for a number of negative influences to take effect without the benefit of immediate opportunities to recover the service. Nonetheless, such an opportunity, even if it is delayed, is possible with postdischarge telephone follow-up work.

Focus Groups. Focus groups are effective for seeking detailed aspects of a particular experience. The synergy of the group helps provide ideas in areas that otherwise may never have been explored via a standardized survey document. Further, focus groups allow you to gauge the intensity of Customer feelings regarding various issues, hear points and counterpoints of view presented by members of the same group, and explore the group's problem-solving potential.

Survey Return Rates. Survey return rates provide some indication of the amount of variation in Customer thinking. When survey return rates are considerably less than expected, the question "why" has to be answered. If all patients/Customers were thinking alike, then why are they not participating in your survey as the others are?

The reasons for small survey return rates can be "all over the map," from administrative problems such as an unappealing survey or cover letter that does not engage the patient by providing sufficient reason to participate, to the extreme interpretation that patient opinions are highly negative and rather than share negative feelings, patients choose to say nothing at all. The point is, when postdischarge survey response rates are low, the internal value that administration places on the content of the responses received may also decline, thus begging the questions, "Why the poor response rate? How quickly can we improve it?"

Customer satisfaction survey organizations conduct regression analysis and other calculations to determine the minimum number of surveys that must be returned in order to statistically ensure that the content of the returned surveys truly represents the opinions of the majority of customers.

Regardless of statistical correlations, low response rates represent an indication of something unfavorable either in the survey administrative process or in Customer opinions.

Rates of Business Growth. Business indicators are often indicators of Customer Satisfaction. Although they cannot and should not be used in isolation as Customer Satisfaction indicators, business indicators frequently parallel Customer Satisfaction ratings. For example, when data indicate a downward slide in Customer Satisfaction, it would not be unusual to see a corresponding slip in the volume or quality of business being conducted by the organization.

The reality is that rates of business growth or decline are an outcome of Customer satisfaction. Not until Customers become dissatisfied do they go elsewhere; this represents a decline in business volume or market share, which is a key business indicator. If satisfaction rates are booming, referral rates and repeat business will be on the rise and an increase in business volume will be seen. The longer the delay in receiving Customer Satisfaction feedback data, the more vulnerable the organization is to Customer defection. By the time long-awaited Customer Satisfaction feedback reaches you, Customers will have already voted with their feet, and efforts to recover service at this point are most difficult to implement and least likely to succeed.

The best advice for use of business growth statistics is to take them seriously at the point that they initially begin to change. If business volume is declining, do not accept excuses and borrow time. Look for corrective action plans to implement immediately. Too many executives are eager to offer explanations if business volume is not what it should be. Meanwhile, time marches on regardless of these explanations, and soon it is too late to recover defecting Customers.

Customer Complaint and Compliment Letters. As Customer Satisfaction improves, the number of complimentary letters addressed to the CEO should increase and the number of complaint letters should decrease.

One CEO reported that the number of complaint letters dropped by 50 percent following installation of their Total Customer Satisfaction strategy.

Track your ratios. The trend should be upward numbers of complimentary letters and declining numbers of complaints. Even though the 3C Card makes it easy for patients and visitors to issue complaints, it is equally easy for them to submit a compliment.

Physician Behaviors. As the Total Customer Satisfaction strategy unfurls within the organization, administration should hear far fewer complaints from physicians. Happier, more satisfied patients will be making more positive statements to their physicians relative to the total health care experience. This translates into more satisfied physicians who have fewer gripes to make to hospital staff. When the patient is happy, the doctor is happy. Overall physician satisfaction should rise noticeably.

Listening. Staff and management with keen listening skills will hear both positive and negative casual comments from patients, physicians, and visitors. As a result of staffs' keen listening, problem situations can be converted into opportunities for improvement in work systems and behaviors.

One Customer complaint should be enough for staff to initiate change. Two complaints of the same nature are enough to put a priority on the need to change. Three or more complaints of the same nature demand management attention.

Listening is the single most rapid source of feedback; therefore, it is the most valuable source of feedback in terms of identifying opportunities for service recovery. Keep the listening posts open and responsive. Optimal listening posts include patient comments to staff and family members, physician criticisms and compliments to staff, and complaints of staff among themselves.

Comparative Databases. Comparative databases put your service ratings into perspective and provide some direction for where to look for benchmarking opportunities within the health care industry. For example, if the Customer rating for call light response time is at the fiftieth percentile for your organization, then you know that a significant amount of improvement in call light response time is needed. And you can use the top-rated organizations in the database as benchmarking organizations.

SELECTING MEASUREMENT TOOLS AND SERVICES

Not all tools and vendors for Customer Satisfaction measurement are equal. Substantial variances exist among even the most prominent suppliers. It is not our objective in this book to promote one vendor over another, but rather to outline qualities against which to evaluate various vendors.

The following qualities are a *must have* from any vendor measuring Customer Satisfaction. Do not allow sales and marketing staff to persuade you differently. These are core, nonnegotiable requirements.

- Large, comparable client database
- Alternative reporting formats
- Statistical correlations for each survey question
- "Can do" attitude and research ability
- On-site support as needed
- Forward thinking organization
- Cooperative and flexible staff
- Timeliness of data
- Client training and development and user groups
- Good cost-value relationship

Large, Comparable Client Database. A large database of health care organizations specializing in your line of business is necessary to assure that extreme and unusual ratings from a smaller population of patients do not distort the overall picture of performance. "Specializing in your line of business" means organizations that have a profile like yours, that is, the same type of business and same size of organization.

Ask to see your vendor's list of current participants, and check references from this list. Thousands of responses to identical survey questions are needed for the vendor to create statistically valid results—far more responses than even a large health care provider can accumulate in a reasonable period.

Hundreds of like health care businesses should be actively participating in the vendor's database in order to meet this standard. Past clients who have not been active in twenty-four months or more are not to be included in the count of active participants. The delivery of health care is changing at lightning speed, so the only good data are current data. This requirement alone will limit the number of measurement vendors available for selection. Do not discount the value of this quality. Local, small boutique organizations, local marketing research organizations, and home-grown surveys rarely can provide this valuable information.

Alternative Reporting Formats. Providers that are inflexible in their reporting format and availability of data will not necessarily help you solve problems or provide valuable information. Business problems can be solved only when credible information is available to dig into the problem.

Seek vendors with the capability of producing ad hoc specialty reports when you need them. Inquire as to what specific kinds of information they can report on demand and how much lead time is required before the reports are available. Remember, timing and data hold answers to achieving your goals.

Statistical Correlations for Each Survey Question. Not all measured qualities contribute equally to rating the overall health care experience or the potential growth of business. To an untrained measurement person it would seem rational that one could draw certain inferences from accumulated raw data. For example, if the consistently lowest-rated item on your internally designed survey was the "quality of food service," an untrained eye might think that "quality of food service," or any of the five lowest-rated items in the raw data, is where to invest your efforts. In fact, quality factors rated lowest in the raw data summary may very well be the last place to focus resources if your intention is to make changes that will positively influence the likelihood of recommending your hospital. But you would never know this unless each survey question is statistically correlated to a key desired behavior, such as likelihood to recommend.

This is one of the reasons we see health care organizations erroneously focusing on typically low-correlation items such as quality of food. Great sums of money and personal effort are funneled into better cuisine and menu options at the expense of attention to relationship-building skills—the highly valued item according to the Customer population. Then administration wonders why Customer Satisfaction ratings for likelihood to recommend their organization aren't moving up.

You should want to know what the top ten qualities are that most highly correlate with the likelihood to recommend your organization because priority and attention given to these factors will have a payoff. Avoid measurement organizations that cannot explain how correlations were conducted or will not provide statistical supporting information on their explanations. Many organizations have slick marketing presentations and promise effective information that a noninformed individual might easily buy into.

"Can Do" Attitude and Research Ability. Only vendors with positive, problem-solving attitudes—people interested in conducting further research for your organization and providing greater insights to data relationships, causes, and effects—should be considered. Not all measurement vendors have the capability to conduct research on special issues of their own interest or research projects you may wish to commission. Find out which research projects potential vendors have conducted in the past twelve to fifteen months, and what their ability is to conduct research requested by your organization. Assess whether the vendor organization is free-thinking, looking for better ways of collecting, managing, and utilizing the data, or simply processing information in and out of a database.

On-Site Support as Needed. Statistical reports are not always easy to read and interpret. Vendor support for reading, interpreting, and problem-solving results from data is essential to the data's usefulness. Expert support staff provided by the vendor should be made available for you on-site at your facility at no additional cost.

The quality of vendor support is also an item for evaluation. Too often, trainees are slotted into Customer service roles, where experts should be. Although they are ambitious and filled with potential, trainees too frequently lack the essential life experiences that are necessary to solve your organization's problems quickly and effectively. Consequently, their value is limited.

Explore the profile of the person assigned to serve your account, including details of their background in the field of satisfaction measurement. Seek only senior, experienced people with a range of problem-solving experiences to draw upon. Do not hesitate to require more talented staff to serve your account if you feel that those assigned to you are not serving all your needs.

Forward Thinking. Measurement vendors should serve as a source of professional development in the categories of management and of utilization of data. If you or your staff tend to be the only sources of new thoughts or ideas for Customer Satisfaction research, your measurement service is not providing the full range of services that you need.

Possible interview questions to use in evaluating a Customer Satisfaction measurement representative include the following:

- Describe your greatest challenge in Customer Satisfaction management. How did you manage it? What were the final results?
- Describe the most creative research projects you have been involved in during the past year.
- What was the least worthwhile research project you have been associated with and why?

Watch for signs of new thinking in the vendor's staff and leadership. If you do not see creative thinking, look for another representative.

Cooperative and Flexible. Some approaches to the use of measurement data suggested here, as well as those created by your staff, may not be in keeping with the pure methodology that a measurement vendor will want to impose on you.

Question: Is your vendor willing to work with new thinking and hybrid approaches to using the data that you want to implement, or will they be condemning and critical? Remember to consider all opinions, but also remember that scientifically correct data collection that is not timely is of limited value to you.

Timeliness of Data. What the vendor considers timely, and what actually is timely in terms of making an impact on Customers and implementing change in the organization, are frequently worlds apart. When you speak of monthly data, you should mean how quickly after the close of the end of the month will you get your data? If it takes more than seven business days to return a summary of data, then it takes too long. If it is standard practice to provide data to other clients on a slower calendar, so be it. But for you, data for the month end must be in your hands no later than seven business days, inclusive of mailing delivery time, following the end of the month. Sooner is better.

It is time to better manage vendor relationships. Remember, satisfaction measurement data quickly deteriorate in value with the passing of time.

Aged data are meaningless. To most measurement vendors, your timing requests will be novel. Generally, they will resist by offering many excuses.

As a New American Health Care Organization you know more about how Customer Satisfaction management should take place. Make processing demands, then problem solve without compromising your deadlines.

Client Training and Development and User Groups. Sharing ideas for improving Customer Satisfaction is one of the most valuable sources of rapid, effective improvement in performance. Use measurement vendors that provide active user groups and opportunities for annual or more frequent developmental workshops. Exhibit 4.1 is a quick and easy assessment tool to see how your Customer Satisfaction measurement vendor measures up. If you answer "sometimes" to two or more items or "never" to one or more items in Exhibit 4.1, it is time to investigate alternative providers.

Good Cost-Value Relationship. Pricing for Customer Satisfaction measurement data covers a wide range. There is a spread in pricing for services offered by the top three market share leaders in the industry. When evaluating potential vendors for this service, do not make your decision based on the low-cost provider. Instead, evaluate each vendor on all the qualities provided in this chapter and then look at their pricing. Do not let a few dollars of additional cost prevent your organization from getting the valuable, credible, and timely information it needs to build business.

Several of the top vendors in this field have made arrangements with state hospital associations for preferred pricing packages for their member organizations. Check your state, regional, and national associations for preferred pricing packages. If that does not help get the cost into a range that is reasonably affordable for your organization, there is always the option of group-purchasing through your affiliated organizations, such as the Veterans Hospital Administration and other purchasing arrangements, and by negotiating directly with the vendor. Someone once said, "You don't get what you deserve, you get what you negotiate." So negotiate!

Exhibit 4.1. *Vendor Checklist.*

How Does Your Customer Satisfaction Measurement Vendor Measure Up?

Assess your current Customer Satisfaction vendor performance on each of the following items.

	Always	Sometimes	Never
1. Are experienced resource staff available to help you on-site at your facility, if requested and at no cost?			
2. Are additional research projects or results of such projects available to you from your measurement vendor?			
3. Is the measurement vendor a "forward thinker," and do they have a can-do attitude?			
4. Is pricing cost effective?			
5. Are results available and provided to you within seven days of the end of the measurement period, including delivery time?			
6. Are alternative reporting formats and additional detailed data available to you upon demand?			
7. Is the survey instrument statistically sound and tested?			
8. Is there a large database of comparable, active clients?			

ACTION PLAN FOR TOTAL CUSTOMER SATISFACTION

Task 1. Evaluate Customer Satisfaction Measurement Vendors. Does your current vendor measure up to the qualities listed in Exhibit 4.1? If not, can they provide what is missing? Few vendors will be able to meet all the demands we suggest, but some larger, national services will more closely fit the profile of what your organization needs.

Do not let cost or a historical relationship with a vendor be a deterrent to obtaining highly credible Customer Satisfaction data. Some organizations make the mistake of staying with a measurement vendor even though they do not provide all the qualities of service that are desirable because the particular vendor has a great deal of historical data on your organization. This behavior assumes that historical data is more important than the creation of a valuable, new, high-quality database. Wrong.

If a new provider is needed, start over with one that can meet the qualities listed in Exhibit 4.1. The value of the information provided, even with a short history, will be of greater value to the organization than unusable historic data.

Task 2: Check Timeliness of Customer Satisfaction Report Results. Insist on a maximum of seven calendar days after the end of the reporting period as your standard of performance for the vendor. If this is not their usual standard but they are willing to try to meet it, your relationship is on the right track. Hold the vendor to your agreed-upon standard of performance.

Another point of concern is the timeliness of the data included in each report. If the report is issued within the timeframe you want but a third of that month's data is not included in the vendor's report but rolled over to the following month, there is a quality problem to be resolved with the vendor. Timeliness and accuracy of data is the name of the game, and a delay to the following month ages that data, substantially reduces the value of it, and distorts the performance behavior for the period listed in the report.

Task 3: Build Added Value into Your Vendor Relationship. What additional pieces of research do you need so you can better understand what your various Customers want in order to be fully satisfied and consider their health care experience to be exceptional? Work with your satisfaction measurement vendor to identify how and where you can collect this information. It is possible that they may already have some of this data on record and can easily share it with you, or they may consider conducting the research on your behalf and that of other clients they serve.

Work together to collect the data, then use it to make changes in the way you serve various types of Customers.

Task 4. Assess Various Methods of Collecting Customer Satisfaction Data in Your Organization. Satisfaction measurement via post-discharge surveys is but one means of collecting data on Customer Satisfaction. Alone, this method will not provide enough information to move your organization into a top position. Multiple methods and channels of data collection, both formal and informal, are needed along with a variety of rates and types of feedback.

Conduct an informal audit within your organization to determine which channels and means of collecting Customer Satisfaction data are routinely used in various departments. Use the brief survey in Exhibit 4.2 to collect the data. Departments that are using only one method or channel of data collection require additional support in terms of adding and activating at least one, possibly two, more channels of communication, depending on the number of Customers served by that department.

Exhibit 4.2. *Department Survey.*

Sample Survey

The purpose of this brief survey is to identify what methods and channels of Customer Satisfaction feedback are used by each department in order to determine where additional Customer Satisfaction measurement support may be needed. Please complete the following survey and return it to Administration.

We use the following methods or channels of communication to collect information on Customer Satisfaction levels and to make changes as needed.

____ 1. Postdischarge paper survey form (Press, Ganey or other provider).

____ 2. One-on-one customer interactions where we ask the Customer how well we are doing, and if there is anything else we can do for them to improve their experience.

____ 3. 3C Card: Comments, concerns, and compliments.

____ 4. Routine conversations with Customers that turn into problem-solving ideas.

____ 5. Telephone interviews postdischarge.

____ 6. Focus groups.

____ 7. Other ____

____

Chapter FIVE

Calculating the Cost of Dissatisfied Customers

The number one reason people leave an organization is that their problem was not resolved.

Have you ever heard someone, in some other hospital (because it never happens at your hospital) respond to a patient complaint with, "Well, she's the only one—we've never had anybody say that before," or "This person is a special case, nobody else has ever complained about this"? Here is the statistic: One out of twenty-five people who are unhappy with your organization will tell you. Twenty-four will not.

Why won't they tell you? What is wrong with the other twenty-four? What is going on in their heads? They are unhappy over something, but they are not going to say. They do not like the bill. They do not like the service. They do not like the attitude. They do not like the food. Whatever it is they are unhappy about, they do not tell you.

WHY PATIENTS DO NOT SHARE THEIR COMPLAINTS

The most frequently cited reasons for many patients' reluctance to complain include the following:

- They have given up. They do not tell you what is wrong because they have already given up on you. Their image of you to start with is that you are not going to respond. Their thinking goes something like this: "Your staff do not seem to respond to a reasonable request much less an unreasonable one. So why bother to set yourself up for rejection?"

- Fear. Patients are often afraid to speak up because they do not want to be seen as complainers. If a patient is viewed as a complainer, the caregiver might passively-aggressively ignore him when the patient calls for a need, pass them off to someone else, then to someone else, thus letting the patient suffer needlessly.
- Protection. People might not tell management that they are unhappy because they are trying to protect someone, keeping the staff out of trouble. As a patient, you are not sure that management will handle the situation right, and you do not want to make things worse. Patients have enough to handle without adding conflict among staff and supervisors to their list of concerns.
- Revenge. Revenge is an interesting motivation for withholding information. It is a passive-aggressive way of letting the negative consequence of a problem situation occur when it could otherwise have been avoided.

An example of withholding information occurred at my community hospital in the suburbs of Chicago. I sat in the visitors' lounge fuming over several incidents that had occurred within the past few hours at the hospital. I had not said anything yet, and the person sitting across from me said, "It looks like you are somewhat agitated."

I said, "That is a real understatement."

He said, "Me too. I'm an attorney."

I thought, "Oh my. You just never know who the agitated person is, what their connections are, or who is watching the situation." I said, "What are you going to do? Are you going sue them over your unhappiness?"

He said, "No. But I have spotted four or five things that they are doing that could get them into serious legal difficulty. I am so angry with them right now that I have decided that by way of vengeance, I am not going to tell them."

"Oh my," I thought again.

Reservation of comments may not reveal a lack of strength but rather a perception that your operation is out of control. The client keeps quiet just to let the situation go right through the roof. Kind of a nasty attitude.

For whatever set of reasons, most people will not tell you when they are unhappy or dissatisfied. They are afraid that they will not get good care, so they put up with bad situations.

Short-Sighted Management

Here is a story I think you will enjoy. It makes the point succinctly. It is about a man, one of the 4 percent of patients who are willing to speak out. His story made the national press. Everybody read it. I thought you would enjoy hearing about it, too.

The story is about his experience with his bank, that hallmark of excellent service in our society. This bank did not have its own parking lot. It had a city parking lot that sat adjacent to the bank. The deal was that you would bring your parking receipt into the bank, and the bank clerk would pick up her little rubber stamp and—Voomp!—stamp your ticket for you so you did not have to pay for your parking. That was it. Voomp! She stamps the little parking ticket, and it is over.

The Customer in this story had banked at this financial institution for twenty years. After twenty years of "Voomp!" stamping parking tickets, the bank figured, "Let's change what our Customer expects. Let's not ask them what they want, let's just change what the Customer expects."

So, our Customer comes into the bank and presents his ticket for validation. The clerk says, "I am sorry sir, I cannot validate your parking ticket."

He replies, "What do you mean, you cannot validate my parking ticket? I have been coming here for twenty years, and you have been validating my parking ticket. There's the rubber stamp, just pick it up and stamp the ticket."

Get the picture? He is not asking for a lot. There's the stamp. Just pick it up and use it. It is not like he is asking for a special change in policy. This is a little thing. It is no big deal.

"I am sorry," the bank clerk repeats. "It has to do with the kind of transaction that you have given to the bank this morning."

"Pardon me?" he responds.

She says, "You wrote a check this morning and took funds out of the bank."

Now, we have all been there. You kind of sense that you have just left the real world and now you are in some fantasy world. Like smart Customers do, this smart gentleman said to himself, "I will try to right this situation by applying some logic." He said to the bank clerk, "Try this one on for size. The reason I could write a check today is because earlier I put money into the bank!"

Then the clerk again replies, "I am sorry sir, it is our policy."

Policy! What is a policy? Somebody wrote something down. If it is written down, then it must be true, it must be a policy. And of course, the word *policy* has as its root word, *police,* so you see policy has in it the concept of enforcement of written standards. And this man has asked the bank to violate enforcement of written standards.

What do you imagine the response by the Customer was? Did the Customer say, "Oh my gosh! Policy! If only I had realized! Forgive me. Boy, am I out of line!"

The word *policy* has this effect on many, many Customers. It is like taking a big red cap and putting it in front of a bull, because the person who says, "It is our policy," has basically said, "I am not going to think, and I am not interested in you. This is my little moment of power in which I dismiss your concerns."

Do not ever use the word *policy* with a Customer. It is like using a swear word. If there is, in fact, a policy (and there are some policies that are legitimate), just do not use the word. What you might say instead is, "I am real sorry, but there are some reasons we have been told that we cannot do this. I am wondering if there is something else that I can do to help work through the need that you have." In this way, you maintain a picture of being open, not simply being stupid and unwilling to think.

The basic rule is that you never use the word *policy* with a Customer. Why? Because people have been "behavior-modified" over dozens of experiences in which lamebrains have used this word. Now they are accustomed to responding in a negative way to statements about *policy*.

Think about this. Do you know what the most important policy in health care is? The most important policy in health care is *to serve Customers.* That is our policy. If it is not your policy, you need to change and make it your policy. The policy is to figure out a way to make Customers' requests happen for them, if there is any way at all that you can.

Now back to the story. Our Customer, having tried logic only to see that the clerk was not interested in logic and was retreating into policy, could have berated the clerk. But he was a little more classy than that, and he probably figured that she did not make the policy, so again thinking logically and rationally and trying to be courteous in this awkward situation, he asks, "May I speak to the manager?"

At this point, the Customer is assuming that he must have in front of him a board-certified cretin, and that the only thing that is necessary to solve this problem is to get a person of true intelligence involved. Some people think that people of true intelligence are the people in management. So he begins to think that when he gets a management person out there he or she will wave the magic wand, pixie dust will appear, and the parking problem will go away. "I will get them to do the unbelievably hard work of stamping my parking receipt!"

The manager is now summoned forth. (At about this point you can see why a lot of people do not bother to tell you what is wrong.) The manager arrives. He listens to both sides of the situation, and then he turns to the Customer and says, "I am sorry sir, the young lady has explained the situation correctly. It is our policy."

End of game. Or is it? The Customer thinks, "What more can you do? Well, nothing, because I'm just a Customer. I cannot do anything." By the way, the name of this bank was the Old National Bank. The *Old National Bank*—somehow it all fits. It all goes together, the bank name and the performance.

The story does not end here. A news story appeared in the newspaper later about the competing bank, a bank called Seafirst Bank. The manager of Seafirst Bank instructed tellers to be *kind* to their new Customers. "Be a kinder, gentler bank."

An article that appeared in the Seafirst Bank company newsletter told the story. You see, the frustrated Old National Bank Customer decided to move his account to the Seafirst Bank. It was no small account. The first check he deposited to Seafirst Bank was for one million dollars as an opening deposit to the account. What does the phrase the "first check" imply? Of course, it implies there is more coming. Thirty-six million additional dollars worth of deposits migrated from Old National Bank to Seafirst Bank, whose employees are going to be kinder and gentler to their new Customer.

Don't worry. It was not all bad news for Old National Bank. You see, they saved the $1.00 cost of the parking validation. The interest they would have earned on the thirty-seven million dollars that was moved from the Old National Bank to the Seafirst Bank would have paid to *buy* the parking lot for all their Customers. That is short-sighted management.

Why short-sighted management? Managements typically fail because they do not have a philosophy. They do not see their work as a mission to serve. Or because their philosophy does not hold the Customer as a number-one priority, they do not see the Customer as a person of power. They are focusing on the finance report—a myopic management.

WHY CUSTOMERS DEFECT

Unhappy Customers quit, and they quit for particular reasons. The number-one reason that people leave an organization is because their problem was not resolved.

In the preceding story about the bank Customer, the Customer did not leave the organization because one bank had a nicer lobby than the other, or because the interest rate was greater at one bank than the other. He left the bank because when he had a problem, he could not get anyone to see that his problem was important.

BROADCASTING BAD NEWS

A lot of hospitals are worried in this competitive era about what their competition is doing. Should you be worried about your competitor? About 10 percent of your worry should be about what your competitor is doing, and the other 90 percent of your worry should be focused on your business, and what you need to be doing for the Customers that you've got. What do you think your Customers want? *Answer:* they want an active, interested, "concerned about my problems" attitude from your organization. They do not care much about another big billboard marketing campaign from your organization.

Notice something. An unhappy Customer will tell somebody about their unhappiness. Rebecca L. Morgan, author of *Calming Upset Customers,* cites the following statistics: Unhappy Customers tell, on average, twelve other people about the unfortunate experience. Each of those twelve people tell, on average, five other people. That means that for every one unhappy Customer, seventy-two people hear a negative story about your organization.

On the flip side, people who had a good experience do not talk about their experience to many other people.

Hypothetical Case

Let's take a hypothetical case. There are a hundred patients visiting your organization on any given day. Ninety-two of the hundred patients had a positive experience.

Let's make the most generous assumption, let's say that each of the ninety-two patients that had a good experience told one other person. This means that there were ninety-two positive messages broadcast about your organization.

At the same time, eight patients had a less than satisfactory experience. Each of the eight told twelve others, which means that there are ninety-six negative messages about your organization being broadcast in the first tier of communication. As each of those ninety-six tell five others, a total of 576 people are hearing a negative message about your organization.

So, for every one unhappy Customer, you will need at least twelve happy Customers just to break even on the number of negative and positive messages being broadcast in the community. To say it another way, when your Customer Satisfaction scores indicate that less than 92 percent of patients are rating you as less than *above average*, there is more negative buzz, broadcasting, or press about your organization occurring than there is positive broadcasting. This means that when the new neighbor comes to town and inquires about your organization to friends and neighbors, that neighbor is more likely to hear a negative message about your organization than a positive one.

Why is it that we like to tell unhappy stories? We just do. People listen to these tales of woe. There is a little bit of Clint Eastwood in all of us, "Go ahead, make my day." So, we tell the unfortunate story at coffee break in the afternoon, and everyone laughs. The next time we tell it to somebody, we add a few more details, and the story just got worse. Then pretty soon, by the time it gets to the Christmas party, people are saying, "Hey, come tell us that story!" You have gained a reputation on this story, and it is being broadcast to anyone who will listen.

People love to hear about bad things that happen to other people. We just love dishing the dirt! It is the only reason tabloid papers and soap opera stories exist. For some reason, we're all like little radio stations. And we have learned that our audience likes listening to bad stories and gossip.

True Story

It just happens that in my town, there was a guy that did a real good job with story telling. His name was Mike Roykol, a past columnist for the *Chicago Tribune.* This guy did not have a tongue, he had a sword. It turns out that forty-five years ago General Motors sold Mr. Roykol his first new car, the cheapest Chevy model they made at the time. The transmission was bad, and Mike got a lemon of a car.

General Motors and the dealership would not fix it. Mike told the story in grueling detail in a newspaper article, with millions of readers tuning in.

Now, how long is Mike's memory? How long is Mike going to remember that he bought a lemon of a car that the manufacturer would not stand behind? How long was Mike's radio station going to be broadcasting this story? Maybe twenty years. Maybe longer. In 1997, a decade or more after the original incident, Mike Roykol wrote a newspaper column blasting a General Motors product. In the column he vowed that someday he might buy another GM product. "Sure I will," he said, "The day they find that old Chevy and replace the transmission." You see, unhappy memories do not fade, they just age—sharply.

Now think about that little old lady patient, the one you think has no power. When she leaves your organization and goes back to the retirement home, she will tell sixty of her good friends why your organization is such a pit to go to. And she will tell her kids, and she will tell her doctor, and she will tell—you get the picture. People are like radio stations broadcasting their daily life experiences. And as with the networks, bad news gets more coverage than good news.

Doctors tell management, "Do not worry about what you going to do for us until you have fixed all the problems irritating our patients." Although patients may not be telling you all of the things that irritate them about your organization, assuredly they are telling their doctor about them!

You probably are not going to be able to satisfy every single person completely. Some people can't be pleased, no matter how hard you try. But you better be hitting high numbers of people who are happy.

When organizations rank in the eightieth percentile range in Customer Satisfaction, they think they are doing OK but, in fact, they are losing it. The number of negative stories told about that organization in the community will be greater than the number of positive stories being told about that organization.

Don't feel burdened by this message—feel challenged by it. It is not a negative message. The fact is, if you're going to do a good job with Customer Satisfaction, you have to understand how people really are, how they feel, and how they respond to you.

SERVICE RECOVERY

Service recovery is the idea that an unhappy Customer can be salvaged or *recovered* and returned to being a happy Customer. In most cases, this can happen if the problems causing Customer dissatisfaction are resolved, the Customer is satisfied, and you have recovered what otherwise would have been a lost Customer. But there is only so much time. Today you have an opportunity to build a better organization. If you do make a mistake, the majority of patients (70 percent) will probably do business with you again if you eventually resolve the problem. However, a whopping 95 percent of Customers will do business with you again if you resolve the issue on the spot. The difference between 95 and 70 percent translates to tens of millions of dollars in revenue for a single health care provider. The difference is simply in the timing of the solution. Fix it now and salvage the Customer relationship or fix it later and lose some of your Customers.

Time and resourcefulness are your best friends in neutralizing a bad situation and winning back an unhappy Customer. See Figure 5.1 for a graphic illustration of the service recovery–time relationship.

If Old National Bank, in the story cited earlier in this chapter, had called the Customer, John Barrier, at home on the evening of the incident and said, "Mr. Barrier, I do not know what happened today, but I am the person that the branch manager reports to, and I want you to know that you have our apology. You will not be faced with this situation again," there would have been a 70 percent chance that Mr. Barrier might not have taken his money out of the bank. But they did not do that. They did not resolve the Customer's problem.

Customer-perceived problems cannot be ignored. They have to be resolved quickly. Listen and respond. The next time a patient lifts the lid on the meal tray and says "Ugh!"—what will you do? Maybe the food *is* no good. Or maybe the patient's biological chemistry is off because he is sick,

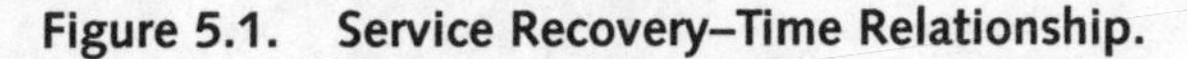

Figure 5.1. Service Recovery–Time Relationship.

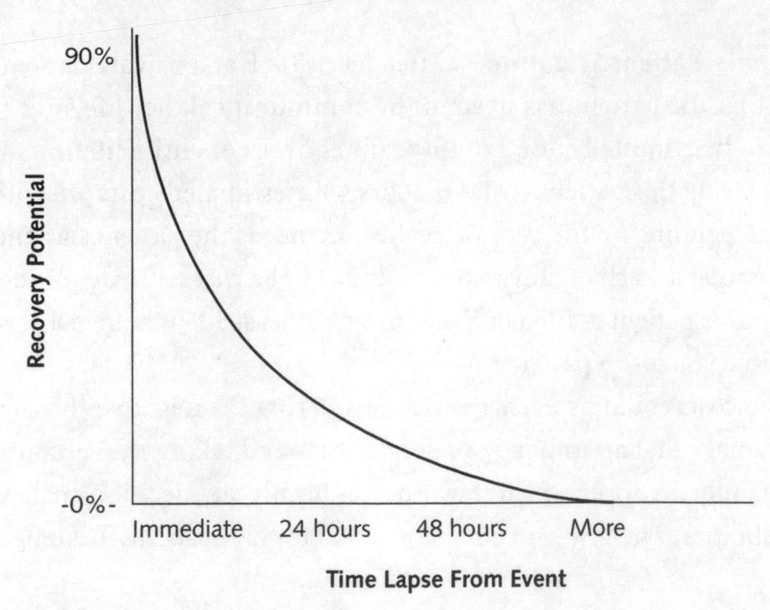

and it just does not taste good to him that day. What should be done, right then?

Realizing the situation, you say, "I am going to get you something else. There will not be any charge for this meal." Resolve the problem on the spot. We are not interested in giving out free meals, but we *are* interested in protecting our relationship with the Customer.

ECONOMIC COST OF ONE LOST CUSTOMER

We have seen how much good work is required just to catch up and break even with one unhappy Customer. But what is the big deal about losing *one* unhappy patient, *one* unhappy, grumpy physician, or *one* troubling, bureaucratic payer? After all it is only *one.*

We asked one chief financial officer (CFO) to estimate what it would cost if they were to lose a Customer. He worked out the following ballpark estimates based on a number of assumptions. Let's look at three cases: a single patient situation, a single physician situation, and a single payer situation.

Single Patient Situation. First, let us look at a private patient. Assume that the patient has lived in the community all her life, and she is going to be admitted a total of three times over her entire lifetime. What would losing this patient cost? Of course, the estimated costs are within a range depending on the type of health care needs the patient has and the costs unique to each organization. In this case the cost estimate for the lifetime of one patient is $38,000. That means at least $38,000 in lost revenue each time you lose a patient.

The costs could be even greater considering the negative "broadcasting" damage that an unhappy patient creates and taking into account the other family lives over which she or he has health care decision-making responsibilities. The low-end cost of $38,000 for an individual can become four times that amount, or about $152,000, if all members of the average four-member family are considered.

A Single Payer. Supposing it is the payer who becomes unhappy. In this case the CFO used the profile of a small community employer with 200 Associates to produce the following estimates. Most Associates have a spouse and dependents, therefore a total of 500 covered lives was used in the calculation. Assuming there is one admission over the life of that contract for each of the 500 covered lives, what would losing that contract mean to the hospital? According to this CFO's calculation, it would cost about $51 million in lost revenues.

A Single Physician. A final scenario is the loss of one physician. Let's assume this physician provides the hospital with three admissions per week about forty-five weeks out of the year, and is going to be in the area and admitting patients over her entire practice lifetime. What would losing that physician mean to the organization? According to the CFO, it would mean an estimated loss of $6 million in revenue.

Your figures and calculations may be different, but the economic point remains the same: The loss of one physician, payer, or patient has a dramatically negative impact on revenues and profitability. Lose too many and it can literally bankrupt an organization.

NEW CUSTOMERS CAN'T BE BOUGHT

The notion that you can just go out and find new patients, new payers, or new physicians, assumes that there is an endless supply. To the contrary, the supply is not endless and competition is more intense than it has ever been.

If you can create and nurture patient, physician, and payer relationships, then today's appendectomy will positively influence expectations for next year's gall bladder operation, and the patient's whole family and all their friends will be positively influenced to select your organization for their health care needs.

If, on the other hand, you screw up with one of those encounters, you cut off that entire chain of future business. The cost can be drastic. You can make more money on Customers who are with you over time than you can on one-time Customers. Whatever profit is made in the first year or first encounter with a Customer is typically added to, or grows over time, thus increasing the profitability that your organization receives from that particular Customer (see Figure 5.2).

True Story

Let me use my husband as an example. Once upon a time he was a loyal American Express card carrier. Now his card is cut up into small pieces. That means he's not using it anymore. For twenty-five years he didn't leave home without it.

When ordering merchandise over the phone the little numbers that he would have to read to use the card ended with three digits "007."

You have to know where he is in life. The hair is gone. The chest has slid somewhere, and the 007 gives him that brief macho thing for an instant. Now, it's a stupid kind of thing, a nothing thing, an irrational thing, an idiosyncratic thing, but he did not like it when they changed his credit card number.

The fact is, American Express got a new computer system, so everybody got a new number. However, it took my husband twenty-

Figure 5.2. Profitability Components of One Customer.

Base service	Repeat business	Referrals	Money management	Price increases

five years to memorize his number, so first of all his nose was out of joint about that. Second, he does not get that macho 007 feeling.

Is this a silly thing? Of course! But Customers are full of silly things—and they have the money. They make the choices.

Of course we are not going to let this situation go easily. The first thing he does is write a letter: "Dear Customer Service, sure would appreciate it if you would give me a new number ending with 007."

Now, according to my math teachers back in high school, there are an infinite number of numeric combinations that can be made up, and still end in 007. You *can* find a 007 ending.

American Express does not have to pay for those numbers. They are all available for free. It is not like he was asking for something that would cost them anything. He is asking for something that would cost them zero money.

The letter goes off to American Express requesting a 007 ending for his credit card. No response. He calls on the phone and talks to the grand mucky-muck of Customer service at American Express. He writes to the grand pooh-bah of Customer service, "I know you can turn loose one of those 007 numbers you have," he says.

Their response, "Cannot do it. Our system automatically assigns the numbers." In other words, our system has no thought behind it.

He went at American Express three times for what is basically a nonsense request. By the time he made the third effort, it was too much. The first request was enough—the Moment of Truth. (A *Moment of Truth* is when a Customer rubs up against the organization.) The second time, "Oh geez, I have got to write a letter," he thinks. The third time? Well, three strikes and you're out in our society.

Now, my husband was not the only one charging on this American Express credit card. The cash stream on this little card was coming from all the people in his consulting company, and they charged about $250,000 a year on this card. That was ten years ago. What has it cost American Express in lost charges over the past ten years from this one little card alone? *Answer:* Ten times $250,000, or

$2,500,000 of revenue that has now been given to VISA! Why? Because American Express would not give him another 007 ending number.

Do you realize what market share is? It is one Customer that has been lost after another one that has been lost, after another . . . because of violation of things that matter to the Customer. American Express did not understand that the loyal Customer just keeps bringing you back more and more business. Loyal Customers mean that you do not have to go out and market as heavily, because you do not have to find a lot of new Customers. A few new ones is good, but keeping all the old ones builds business.

CUSTOMER DEFECTIONS

In the language of Quality control we talk about zero defects. In Customer service we talk about *zero defections.* Zero defects in the quality of our work, and *zero defections* in Customers are the goals.

Think of it this way: It is a matter of personal pride. If Customers come to you today and the next time they need health care they go somewhere else, what have they just said about you? "Not good enough," is what they have said. If they come to you and say it is great, and you hear, "This is the fourth time a member of my family has been here." Wow, you have done it. You have done the job, and you have done it right over and over. What a great success that is. It is those Customers that you are losing that you now have to focus your effort upon.

True Story

I will not tell you which hospital I go to, but I would like to tell you of an experience that I had with my local hospital. Would I recommend them to others? Well, maybe. So, why do I consider going back? I go back, temporarily, because my doctors are great and that is where they practice at this point. My loyalty is to my physician, and as a patient I'm working on changing my physician's loyalty to that hospital.

I do not have a loyalty to the hospital. They have not done anything extraordinary for me, yet. I am not against the organization. They are probably struggling real hard to get better, but they are your average, run-of-the-mill hospital. Not a lot to write home about.

During my last encounter with this hospital, I noticed that I was having several Moment-of-Truth experiences. The first Moment of Truth occurred when I arrived at the hospital. Did the hospital staff expect my arrival? If they did expect me and were prepared for my arrival, then they successfully passed that first Moment of Truth.

The patient does not see or know everything that is going on at your organization. They do not know what the data processing department is doing, or what food service or central processing is doing. They do know that when they rub up against something in the organization it is either going to be handled well, or it is not. The patient only knows about the events they directly experience at the hospital. These events are the Moments of Truth.

My doctor told me to go to the outpatient area of the hospital for this procedure. When I arrived, there were no signs showing outpatients where to go. There was a big sign for emergency, but nothing for outpatient. No big deal. I could handle it.

When I walked in, the greeting I received was not, "Hello. We are so glad you are here. We want to do whatever we can to make your stay here a pleasant one." I received no greeting at all. So I looked for the desk.

There were two signs over the only apparent desk. One sign said "outpatient cashier," and the other one said "X-ray registration." Well, I was not there for X-ray, and I was not there to pay cash. I thought I was supposed to get service before I paid the bill. So, I went to "X-ray registration." The person there did not say, "Hello, how are you?" He said, "Not here, over there!" pointing a finger down the hall. It was not a big thing, but it was a Moment of Truth. So, I went "over there," as he directed.

Low and behold, they did know I was coming! My name was on a piece of paper, and the piece of paper literally looked like it had been crumpled up and taken out of the waste can and smoothed out. My name and other names had been written on it in pencil. It was not a computer report. It was more like the lined sheet of paper my kid uses for middle school homework assignments. My name looked like an afterthought on the paper. It was not a big thing, but I wondered.

Of course, they wanted my insurance card. When they asked for the insurance card, I said, "But I have been here for other services. You should keep a record of my insurance information." They replied with the standard, "It is our policy to always ask for the information."

Then they took my insurance card and walked across the room, turned on the Xerox machine, and did this piece of work called copying. They do this hundreds of times every day. Every time a patient comes in, they do the same piece of work over and over again, walking to and from the Xerox machine, wasting time and energy.

Everywhere else I go, they don't have to do that. The grocery store has my banking information on a plastic card I keep on my key ring. They scan the key ring, scan the food, and "zap!" it is charged to my Visa account. No questions, no hassles, no waiting. Hotel chains have my credit card and personal preference information in their system so when I arrive, my preferences for type of room, bed size, refreshment, smoking versus nonsmoking are already taken care of. No hassles, no questions, no waiting. Likewise, the auto dealer has a history of my car and its repairs and services.

Here, at the hospital, where it really counts, they do not seem to know much about me at all, even though I have been a patient here several times before. These hospital people, with their crumpled piece of paper, trudging about doing the same piece of work over and over, present a different image. It is not a big thing. But images are made up of a lot of little snapshots. Pictures.

More to the Story

You see, it was first thing in the morning. The light on the answering machine behind the hospital desk was blinking, and a staff person pushed the button to listen to the messages. The first message was from some very frustrated person saying, "Why don't you people answer the phone?" In unison, the hospital staff, all four of them listening to the message, laughed. The ten of us patients on the other side of the counter weren't laughing. It wasn't that we thought this was horrible, or that we had even made a judgment about it, but we had one set of feelings, and some of us identified with the frustrated telephone caller.

Do you know what we did? We just stood there, looking at each other in wonderment. We did not look at the staff, we just looked at each other in disbelief. Could this behavior be for real? There was a little gritting of the teeth going on with some of the patients as they observed the hospital staff's behavior. It was not a big thing, just another Moment of Truth. But as I encountered the organization in these tiny ways, I was beginning to get a sense of something that I was not totally comfortable with.

Finally I got to the patient care unit. There was a kid behind the desk, and he said to me, "I have never done this before." Now, I did not know what it was that he was going do that he had "never done before," but I was not sure I wanted to have anybody doing something to me that he had not done before. Do you want to be the first case that the brain surgeon operates on? I did not want to know this.

Well, it turned out that it was the first time he had filled out this form. But you see, this was the third time I had filled out this form. It was no big thing, but these little Moments of Truth were like snowflakes beginning to add up. If you put a lot of snowflakes together, you can get a pretty big snowball.

One of the good things about this particular experience was that there was not much waiting. I came in, went through the admission process, gave a quick patient history, and "boom!" I was down on the patient unit and ushered into the patient dressing room.

In the patient dressing room all of the lockers were being used by the staff. There were locks on the lockers, so the fact is, there was no patient dressing room. What was labeled "patient dressing room" was a staff dressing room with a patient dressing room label on it. It was no big thing, just another Moment of Truth.

The hospital had thoughtfully provided for me by giving me a grocery bag to put my clothes in. It was not a brand new grocery bag, but an old grocery bag with grease spots on the side. Somebody trucked this bag in from home, and said, "Here, this is for your clothes."

I was thinking, "Will an old grocery bag provide adequate security for my watch and wedding ring?" About now I was becoming a touch irritated. No anger or big-time irritation, just a little annoyed. In my head I was thinking, "At these rates, don't you think I could get a new bag?"

As I undressed and put the patient gown on I noticed that they didn't have a patient gown to cover all of me, so they gave me two gowns. "Hmmm. Twice the laundry cost, no wonder health care is out of control in its costs," I said to myself.

Then they gave me a wonderful set of slippers. These slippers were so good, I still have them. They were cheap on the bag, but they gave me great slippers! The slippers came in a plastic bag. I took the slippers out of the plastic bag, but then there was a piece of refuse to dispose of. What was I supposed to do with the plastic paper? There was no trash can. I was not angry that there was no trash can, it was no big thing, but having worked for nurses as a young orderly, I knew that I was not supposed to just throw trash around. So, I was thinking, if you cannot manage trash, can you manage health care?

Why is it that no one has seen this operation from the point of view that I have? *Answer:* They do not go into the changing room and do what patients have to do. They are out of touch with the world patients are experiencing.

Have you ever walked into a restaurant or a store, and you see something immediately that is wrong? A bad attitude, bad lighting? You see it just like that! And the people who have been there for twenty years do not see it. It is amazing. Then, when you point it out, they pretend that it does not exist. That is how it was at this hospital, and at many hospitals that I visit.

Back to the Story

I dressed in two gowns, and I had everything in the bag. I opened the dressing room door and—whoops!—I went right out into the waiting room where all the dressed people were. Not only were the gowns not big enough around, but they were also a little short! There I was, the cold winds blowing through my legs.

I whisked around into the service area, where I thought things would immediately get better. I supposed that they could have installed a door from the changing room to the clinical service area so gowned patients would not have to walk through the dressed waiting area, but that would have been cost. And if it was a choice between cost for a one-time expense and embarrassment every time for every single Customer, well, they picked the second option. It is no big thing, but it was starting to get bigger.

I arrived in the treatment area, and there was some good news. A wonderful nurse came over and asked me to sit down. Instead of standing above me and giving me an orientation, she sat down on a chair next to me. I must tell you that I was absolutely amazed at my own reaction. I felt that she was on my team. She was sitting with me, side by side, looking at the treatment areas.

She said, "We are going to put you on one of those beds, and we are going to . . ." It was kind of like being in a football huddle, all getting the play-by-play information together. I thought, "Ooh, that was positive—a positive Moment of Truth." Bad news, though, the same person who did so well with her bedside manner could not hit my vein to insert the IV. She tried once, and said, "I am sorry." She tried again, and she was very apologetic. Her hands were trembling a little bit, and she missed again. "No problem," she said, "some days it is hard to find." Then, a third time and a miss. It was not a little thing anymore.

In came another nurse, who inserted the IV just as the first nurse apologized to me, saying, "I am new here."

I started thinking, "There is high turnover here. Probably because of poor supervision or lousy management." What was I doing?—reaching for assumptions. I was coming to a conclusion about lousy management based on this one morning's experience.

Justified? Totally unjustified. But therein lies the power of Moments of Truth. Each Moment of Truth, positive or negative, helps create an overall image of the organization for the Customers. When you manage the Moments of Truth positively, you create a positive impression in the Customer's mind.

ACTION PLAN FOR TOTAL CUSTOMER SATISFACTION

Task 1. Get a Stream-of-Consciousness Log Going. In an organized fashion, conduct mini-focus-type groups with each of the various departments in the organization or health system. Pick a few patients, staff, or physicians from each department. Choose departments that routinely work closely together. Give participants a pad and pencil and ask them to write down the events and feelings that patients are reporting and wondering about. Participants should feel free to add their own observations. The lists that are generated should be reasonably lengthy, at least twenty to thirty items.

For example, as I sat in the preoperative preparation room at a hospital, I noted and listed the following items in the first ten minutes:

- Patients say, "Oh! That's cold," when they have to lie down on the gurney. (Maybe a warming blanket would be a good idea to relieve this reaction.)
- There is no place to put patients' clothes. Patients are required to undress and put their clothes in a very nice plastic bag, but there is nowhere to store the plastic bag. Should you take it with you to surgery, ask a stranger to hold it, or just leave it there on the floor in the middle of the preoperative area and hope it is there when you return?
- Nurses are so frustrated with the length of time it takes material management staff to deliver a small supply of patient identification bracelets that they are clocking the amount of time they are put on hold on the telephone, waiting for someone to get back to them. Staff have a running bet for how long they will be on hold, depending on what day of the week it is! "The current waiting time for a Tuesday is twelve minutes," reports one nurse, frustrated at the wait just to get patient identification bracelets so they can continue preparation for outpatient surgery. That is a good chunk of unproductive, frustration-raising time.
- A physician makes a lengthy personal telephone call, maybe ten to fifteen minutes long, and using a loud, booming voice that is impossible for patients to ignore! How annoying to others trying to carry on a private, personal conversation.

You get the idea. Look around and be constructively critical. What improvements can be made? This is a subjective assignment. Make no apologies. Review the log and start making changes.

The fact is, if someone had asked me what I noticed as I sat for hours in the preoperative room, I could have pointed out a number of possible improvements during my visit.

Task 2. Test Your Department's Responsiveness to Customers' Needs and Moments of Truth. Create a counterfeit patient or Customer name and personally experience the services provided by your organization or department. Experience the major aspects of the services provided as well as the little things. Track the responsiveness of the organization to you as a hypothetical patient/Customer from admission, through discharge, to follow-up.

Note where improvements in people processes, work processes, and the physical plant can be made. What improvements in image need to be made? Assume that all reasonable requests for improvements can be made. Look for reasonable improvements that only a patient or Customer would see. Question every aspect of the experience. Do not accept rationalizations for situations that contribute to a less than excellent experience.

Points of disorganization, unprofessional approaches to work systems, and innocent comments by staff that lead patients to form unfavorable impressions are all fair game. If you owned this department or this organization, what changes would you make?

Repeat this process every six months.

Task 3. Calculate the Economic Cost of a Lost Customer. With the assistance of the finance staff, calculate the economic cost that the loss of one patient would mean to your organization. Do the same to determine the cost of losing one physician and one contract. Share these statistical facts with staff and educate them as to the impact of losing a patient. They will be amazed at the financial impact.

Then calculate the economic cost of the same losses for your department. If you manage the physical therapy department, for instance, what kind of economic loss would be encountered if one patient were lost? If one referring physician were lost? If one contract were lost? Bringing the calculation closer to home—specifically what it would mean to your department staff— it is likely to have a greater impact on your effort to communicate.

Task 4. Implement Customer-for-a-Day Program. Associates who have had a personal health care experience in a hospital or clinic tend to be more understanding and also more critical of the experience and each of its components. This being the case, it is beneficial to Associates' understanding as well as to improving Customer Satisfaction if a patient-like experience can be provided for each Associate. First-hand, personal experiences are more enlightening than reading or hearing about a situation.

The Customer-for-a-day experience is valuable for personal development, but to gain its full value it must become a basis for action to improve the organization. To transform the experience into action, each Customer-for-a-day should be required to identify at least four or more problems that need to be addressed. It is not necessary to have the solution to the problems, but simply to identify them, then turn each problem into a Do-It-Group (DIG) or Just-Do-It-Group (JDI) to make rapid improvements in the work systems that will then benefit Customers.

To administer this program, one Associate each week is assigned to act as a Customer. Obviously, coordinating this program will take some planning. During the time that an Associate is assigned to be in the Customer-for-a-day role, colleagues are to pitch in to cover the workload. Overtime is not an option for this program. With everyone participating, the revolving workload works out to be the same for all Associates covering for one another. A sense of camaraderie should develop among staff. Everyone in the department wins because the problems that are identified and resolved actually benefit all departmental staff and patients.

If Customer experiences are more lengthy and complex, and it is necessary to invest more than one day in the Customer-for-a-day role in order to gain full exposure to all the potential improvements that might be made, select one of your more innovative and detail-oriented staff for that assignment. Your investment in time and effort will be greater, and therefore you want to assure that the return on that investment is as great as possible.

The specific core items that those in the Customer-for-a-day role should be looking for are listed below. Before sending anyone into the Customer-for-a-day role, review the following list and add more items that are specific to the type of Customer(s) that you have. Present this list to the Associate before he begins the assignment. If the Associate knows what he is looking for, it is more likely that you will get the kinds of results that you want.

Tools, services, people or systems that are not in place when needed. This list is usually very long. Watch staff as they search for supplies and pace back and forth from one end of the department or desk to the other doing small tasks that should be centered into one work area. What is missing? What should be there for smooth administration of the procedure? What would make the entire process much smoother?

Waiting periods. Where did the Customer experience waiting periods of five minutes or more in the process? Waiting for any reason is still waiting and therefore eligible for this list. Did they wait for staff, equipment, test results, or some other reason? For each waiting period, note the amount of time the patient waited and what they were waiting for.

Customer annoyances. In what situations did the Customer appear to become somewhat annoyed? You can tell by their body language, tone of voice, and messages sent.

The annoyance could be rooted in any number of reasons. Your job is to note if and when the Customer became annoyed, what it was that seemed to create the annoyance, and what could be done to avoid this situation in the future. Think solutions. There is always a solution.

Customer comments. What comments did the Customer make along the way that represent anything other than a compliment? For example, off-the-cuff comments about the environment, staff, process, equipment, or just plain wishes are helpful insights. Take note of these comments and what the Customer was referring to when she made the comment. Include your observations of what can be done to improve upon the situations that elicited unfavorable comments from Customers.

When the Associate has completed the Customer-for-a-day assignment, she should share the highlights (good things she learned about Customer Satisfaction) and spotlights (things that need to be corrected or that need additional attention) with other staff at the departmental meeting. DIGS and problem-solving groups should be established to address each spotlight area. Implement solutions to the problems as soon as possible.

Chapter
SIX

How to Win and Retain Customer Loyalty

In an age of expanding Customer expectations, a satisfied Customer is not enough.

Americans are accustomed to "Satisfaction guarantees" for everything from consumable foods to durable products and personal services. When a service provider or product manufacturer creates a service or product, it should meet a standard of excellence that the company is willing to stand behind—no exceptions.

AN ISSUE OF GUARANTEES

One of the industries to understand this dynamic more recently is higher education. In the September 17, 1997 issue of *USA Today,* the University of Miami College of Engineering was quoted as touting "Satisfaction guaranteed or 50 percent off your next purchase."

Lewis Temares, dean of engineering, pledges a year's free tuition for graduate school to any student who graduates and does not have a job within six months. The package is worth $17,000. Temares has obtained $500,000 in donations to support the guarantee. The goal is to not have to spend any of the $500,000. Responses from incoming freshmen are generally along the lines of, "It is comforting to know that our future is one of the university's main interests."

What's behind Temares's thinking?

If we are good, we are not going to have takers. And if there are takers, it is going to mean something's the matter. It is a way to drive change.

If there can be guarantees in higher education, why can't there be guarantees in health care?

GUARANTEES COME TO HEALTH CARE

The average business spends six times more money on marketing, trying to find and recruit new Customers, than it does on working to keep the Customers that it has.

Notice hospitals that have big marketing programs directed at recruiting new Customers. I am not against big marketing programs. I just find it interesting to observe where the emphasis of financial investment is being placed. Health care organizations are running major marketing campaigns, yet they have no quality or Satisfaction guarantees that they are willing to offer to their current or prospective Customers. New American Health Care Organizations, however, continuously challenge and upgrade their present level of Customer Satisfaction.

One Texas hospital challenged their admissions office to process a patient admission in three minutes or less. If the admission process was not completed in three minutes or less, the hospital took $100 off the bill. Boom! Customers looked at their watches! They were timing the process. They were not feeling inconvenienced any more. The staff were willing to put their money where their mouth was. When you occasionally have to pay money out on some guarantees, motivation is created to change the system and make improvements, not to change the guarantee.

It is time that health care organizations start offering some guarantees, as other businesses do. Hospitals cannot guarantee clinical recoveries, but they can guarantee that the food will be up to standard, that the cleanliness of the room will be to standard, that the admissions process will be rapid, and that staff will be friendly, for starters.

The goal is to not pay out money. So for every guarantee that must be redeemed in cash, there is a moment of learning and a motivation to change the system.

WHERE WE'RE DOING GOOD WORK

What is it that Customers desire—what do they value most? Look again at Table 3.3. As we discussed in Chapter Three, certain themes seem to come out of this list, particularly in the top ten issues most closely correlated with the likelihood of patients' recommending a hospital. Big issues as identified by Customers include courtesy, attitude, sensitivity, and information; the primary dynamic that is being described in this measurement is *relationship*.

Notice that none of the items said, "You made me better. You made me healthier." It is almost as if there is a great wisdom in patients, who seem to be thinking, "I hope that you will do your best for me technically. I hope that you will make my problem go away, or ameliorate it in some fashion. But if you cannot do that, could you at least do this?" There is a kind of nobility that comes out of this profile of Customers.

The relationships of patient and staff, and patient and physician, matter. Relationship is *really* a big deal for the patient. It is not a little "extra." It is a real, core need.

WHY RELATIONSHIPS ARE IMPORTANT

How does a person feel going through medical treatment? Why is this relationship stuff so important? What is happening to patients' inner life when they are undergoing medical treatment? What is going on that causes these things to be so important? What are they thinking?

They are thinking, "I am losing control." Anxiety, fear, insecurity, and anger set in. They are uninformed, not knowledgeable about what is happening to them. They are stripped of nearly all personal control and come under the authority of doctors, nurses, and others with whom they have little or no initial relationship. Their life and their future are now in the hands of strangers.

Health care involves a more complex emotional situation than any other type of business. Concern, sensitivity, information, and all the items on the list of satisfiers help alleviate these scary feelings of anxiety, fear, and insecurity and help people feel that someone is there with them. *It's a human thing.*

In some organizations the pendulum has swung too far in the direction of high tech and low touch. We are losing the *human thing,* and thus losing the Customer. Health care must be *both* high tech and high touch.

Believe all the data you can find on Customer Satisfaction, but that won't be enough to get excellent ratings. One of the actions that Holy Cross Hospital took was to meet with patients within the first hour of their visit. They said, "We want this to be an excellent experience for you, and we want to get an excellent rating from you on our Customer Satisfaction rating scale. Can you tell me what it is you are looking for, or what it is that you want to have happen?"

From the Customer, who has the power, they get a list of some of the things that the patient really needs. These notes go into the patient chart. At the end of the patient stay, before the patient leaves, staff revisit the patient in the patient's room and say, "We said early on that we wanted to earn an 'excellent' rating from you on this experience. How well did we do? What one or two things could we have done better in your eyes?"

So remember, in addition to a post health care experience survey, live communication with real people might just be a good thing.

Here is another example of benchmarking against the Marriott. I stayed recently at a Radisson Hotel. Next to the bed they had a Customer response card. Most hotels have that, as do most hospitals. But do people want that? The Marriott has a little card there too, but they also use another system. They have a piece of plastic that sticks to the front of your TV. I will guarantee you that everybody is going to see that sign if it is on the front of the

TV. Do you have TVs in your patient rooms? What message might you put there that you would want everybody to see?

At the Marriott, because you are an "Honored Guest," they want you to be able to reach them at any time, so they list all the ways you can reach someone. They have a guest relations Associate on duty twenty-four hours a day, and "here's the number to call!" Or, you can respond on the TV interactive system. The message goes on to say, "Exceeding your expectations is our priority." That is how you get to be the number-one-rated hotel among frequent business travelers.

The Marriott message is not exactly the message you would want to have on your TV, but it is an excellent example of having more than one way to get feedback from patients.

FEEDBACK LOOPS

Feedback is constantly being provided to your department or organization from various Customers, visitors, family members, vendors, and others who experience your operation in some form at some point in time. The feedback is either good or it is bad. There is really no middle-of-the-road rating.

It is good if the patient is saying, "This is the best hospital that I have ever been treated in." You know that you are doing well. You are delivering the kind of service that you want to deliver. If the physician is saying, "This is the best hospital that I've ever practiced medicine in," you know that your operation is satisfying the physician constituency. If Associates are saying, "This is the best hospital that I've ever worked in," you know that you're delivering excellent internal service to your colleagues and Customer departments. When the feedback from Customers is less than excellent, it is a message to change the work process (see Figure 6.1).

Figure 6.1 shows a standard, quality-improvement kind of thinking. The process represents you in your department or area of responsibility. The 7 Ms, or manpower, money, minutes, mission, methods, materials, and

Figure 6.1. Customer Feedback Loops.

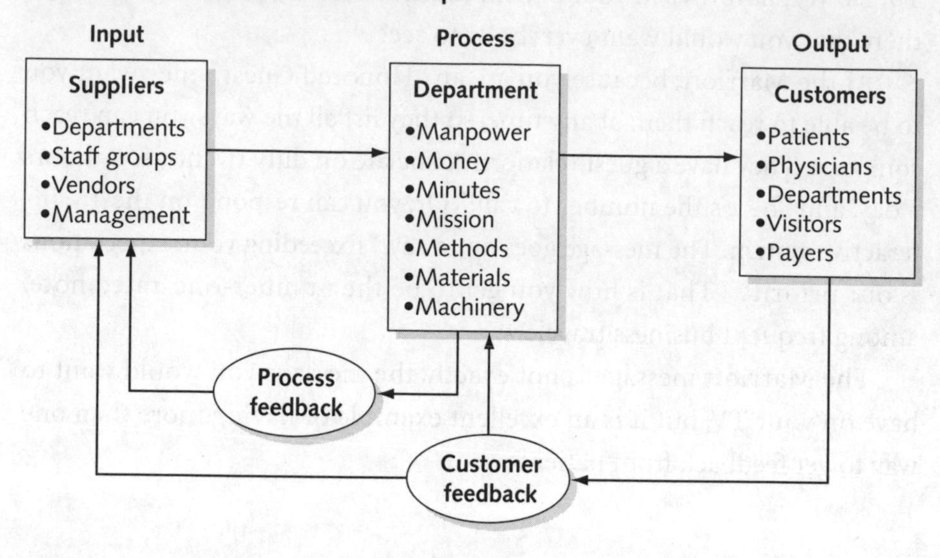

machinery, are the resources you use to get the work done or the service delivered. But to a large degree you rely on input from other people within or outside the organization, who are your suppliers. Suppliers either help you perform your service well, or they make it impossible for you to perform your service well.

A supplier can be a commercial provider from outside or it can be another department internally supplying you with what you need. Some people in the input process may do work and hand it to you in your department for further work. If they did not give you what you needed in terms of a product to work with, it is a lot harder for your to do your job. For example, if a patient goes through Admitting and is annoyed by the process and thinks your organization is discourteous, when he arrives on the nursing floor, you will hear the nursing staff say, "You can't believe how upset he is. I have to take ten minutes to calm him down before we can get started on care."

We really need our suppliers to do their jobs well. But our suppliers may not even know how they are doing. Suppliers need feedback from the departments they serve as well as the Customer constituency.

Let's look downstream from your department. The work you do gets moved to the next department or person. The output from your department is equal to the input to another department. Processes that you carry out in your department feed into the system. To know how well it worked, you have to get feedback from real people. The problem is that most managers understand this logic but have difficulty putting the knowledge into practice. In other words, they don't collect satisfaction feedback from their Customers. Some departments receive some level of Customer satisfaction feedback, but only because patient satisfaction surveying is a function that administration manages and mandates. It is rarely something that department leaders have undertaken to help themselves improve their performance levels.

In all fairness, Customer feedback is a time-consuming process for department managers to undertake, and there have been few role models in the health care industry to show them the way. However, that excuse belongs to yesterday. The Tasks in this book provide department managers, executives, and CEOs with a step-by-step process to focus the limited resources of time, money, and attention efficiently to improve Customer Satisfaction.

THE SHOCKING TRUTH ABOUT CUSTOMER LOYALTY

Many people are misled by the results of their Customer Satisfaction measurements and feedback. They tend to think that if they are performing at *above average* levels or greater, their Customers will probably be loyal to them.

What I am about to show you cost the Xerox company about a million dollars worth of research to find out. They spent a great deal of time, effort, and resources to understand exactly where their Customers stood on the issue of loyalty. What the research showed jarred them into a new level of performance. As you read about Xerox, visualize how these behaviors appear in your organization. Consider what changes you will need to make in order to properly manage and retain Customer loyalty. You may be shocked by reality.

Xerox and Customer Loyalty

Xerox is a company that at one time "owned" the copier market. They really didn't have any competitors. But they fell into a period of decline, and all kinds of competitors came into the market to take market share. Xerox was an organization that had been preeminent and lost it.

Now, of course, Xerox has come back. They are much stronger and much more aware. They will tell you that much of their success stems from having restructured their organization along the lines that Customers requested. Here's what they found out that startled them into a new level of performance.

Xerox had a five-point Customer Satisfaction rating scale. Like a lot of people in hospitals, they thought that a performance level rated from *above average* to *excellent* was a good one to have. It was not, as the facts will bear out.

Their old Customer Satisfaction performance goal was to have 90 percent of their Customers give them a rating of either 4 or 5, *above average* or *excellent.* Here is what they learned about what those ratings actually mean.

Zone of Defection. Customers who rate at the extreme low end of the scale are the ones who will tell twelve or more people how terrible their experience was. They may tell twenty to forty people. These kinds of unhappy

Customers are termed *terrorists.* They have a vendetta. When they are unhappy, they are really going to do a job on your reputation.

A ratings range from 1 to 3.6 is the zone of defection. Customers giving these ratings would just as soon buy Canon equipment or another competitor's brand the next time they buy as they would Xerox's. They have no loyalty whatsoever. (See Figure 6.2.)

Zone of Indifference. Notice that people rating the performance as average, or even some aspects of performance as *above average,* were also very likely to defect. There is no brand loyalty even this high on the rating scale. People who gave Xerox ratings of between 3 and 4 and who even said they were satisfied were nevertheless in a *zone of indifference.* These people would not necessarily seek out a competitor's product, but whether they

Figure 6.2. Customer Loyalty.

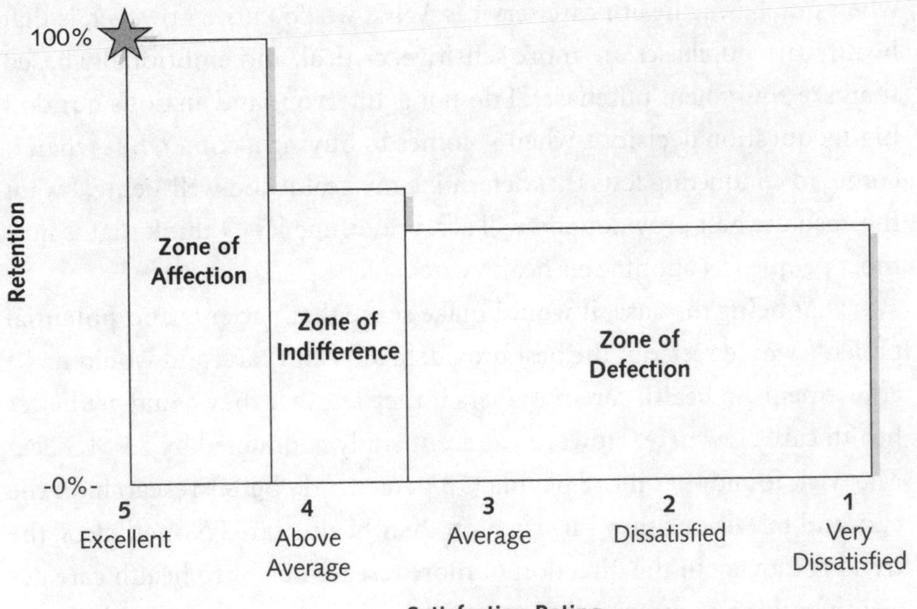

bought from Xerox or the competition depended on what deals were being offered. These people, even some of those who rated Xerox as high as 5, or *excellent*, were on the fence.

Zone of Affection. There was also a group of people who rated Xerox's performance as high as possible. We call these *the fans* of the organization. They are in a zone of affection. Their feelings toward the organization are very positive. Xerox researchers referred to these people as *apostles*, because just as the apostles of old, these Customers went forth praising the organization, trying to convert friends and colleagues. They are an unpaid sales force: "Oh, you have to get a Xerox!" they say.

Correlation to Health Care

We do not know whether Xerox's research results are directly applicable to the health care industry because we don't know whether people behave the same when it comes to buying capital equipment like a copier as they do when purchasing health care services. What we do know, however, is that health care purchases are more sensitive, critical, and emotionally based than are equipment purchases. I do not get nervous and anxious nor do I highly question decisions when it comes to buying a copier, but when it comes to conducting tests that determine my health and well-being, I want the absolute best provider and will accept nothing less. I think that is how most people feel about their health care.

That being the case, it would make sense that patients and potential patients would seek out the best providers of health care, and would make adjustments in health care providers if they felt that they could get better health care elsewhere. However, a recent study conducted by KPMG Peat Marwick found that more people (75 percent) do better research on the cars and televisions they buy than on their health care.[1] Nonetheless, the trend is moving in the direction of more research prior to health care decision making as more and more information becomes available to the public on results and satisfaction levels among health care providers.

Likelihood of Purchase

Now, what was the likelihood of purchase? People who rated Xerox a 4, or *above average,* were one-sixth as likely to buy another piece of Xerox equipment as the people who rated them 5, or *excellent.* To put it another way, people who rated them as 5 were six times more likely to buy their product again than people who rated them as 4.

Knowing this, what type of rating do you want for your health care organization? Look at your Customer Satisfaction feedback data and consider the volume of *good* or *above average* versus *excellent* ratings. You do not want to be a *good* hospital, because being *good* or *above average* puts Customers in a zone of indifference. They are saying it nicely, but you have not won them. It is kind of like when you were dating. You had a nice date, but let's face it, there was no commitment. Do you understand? "And by the way, I will be busy the next time you call for a date." That is what we are talking about. Or maybe you went on a date, and your date said, "Hey, this date has been a 4 on the rating scale. That is not where you want to be." Can I translate this any other way to get it across?

CUSTOMER EXPECTATIONS VERSUS REALITY

The art of designing, developing, and delivering distinctive Customer Satisfaction is a special practice with unique problems and opportunities. It requires that all staff be skilled in watching a process unfold and evaluating its unfolding against the perceived judgment of Customers.

Services such as health care cannot be demonstrated or sampled prior to purchase the way one can test drive an automobile, sample cuisine, or observe another's haircut. Patients cannot sample a tonsillectomy or heart catheterization before undertaking it. They must use other means of determining what kind of experience they might have with the provider.

One way that Customers select a provider is by listening to the recommendations of trusted people—family, friends, and physicians. If close, trusted family members recommend a physician or facility, the patient will probably select it, at least for the first encounter.

The second way that many Customers use to select a provider is through dynamic communication with their physician and other caregivers. This communication stems from the patients' desire to understand and learn more about what is happening to them, as well as to provide feedback for caregivers to respond to clinically.

Think of the last back massage your significant other gave to you. After a long exhausting day, a short back massage feels so good. You direct the other's ministrations by providing constant feedback, "Oh, that feels really good there," or "Up a little higher and to the left." With active feedback, the result of your massage is more positive than if you had not directed the other's efforts. Similar dynamics are operating, though more seriously, in the health care environment.

Making the patient knowledgeable enough to specify the services they need, and making them comfortable enough to provide feedback during and after health care delivery, is a form of Customer education. The more complex the health care service is, the more important patient education becomes. Ironically, patient education is one of the areas that health care providers are weakest in, and it is one of the first areas to be cut in efforts to manage costs—a serious tactical error.

THE CORRELATION OF PATIENT EDUCATION TO PATIENT SATISFACTION

A Customer's expectations and perception of a service are integral to his or her satisfaction levels. The closer the experience resembles expectations, the more satisfied the Customer will be. Therefore, early education on what to expect in each step or stage of the process shapes the Customer's expectations to be closer to reality. The more closely the experience resembles expectations, the more satisfied the Customer will be.

To the extent that most clinical outcomes rely on how well patients follow physician's post-treatment instructions, patient education again plays a dominant role in overall satisfaction. When patients understand why certain behaviors are prescribed and required and the ramifications if protocols are not followed, they are more likely to follow through on instructions and therefore to have better outcomes. Yet even with this knowledge, health care organizations still are not making patient education and follow-up a high enough priority.

True Story

Recently, a close friend of mine went to the doctor for her annual physical exam. Several days after the exam a lab technician called and reported that her cholesterol level was high and she would have to take medication. That was pretty much the end of the communication from the lab tech.

Only through persistent questioning by the patient was she able to find out how high the "high cholesterol" level was. Was it dangerously high, or borderline high? Just a little high, or drop-dead high? How long would she have to take the medication? What would the medication do for her? Did it have any side effects?

SERVICE RECOVERY AND HOW TO MAKE IT WORK FOR YOU

Service recovery refers to the effort and actions associated with correcting a less than *excellent* Customer experience or situation. When things do not go as planned, and Customer Satisfaction is at risk, service recovery includes all actions that would be taken to recover a positive impression of your organization in the eyes of that Customer.

Life doesn't always go exactly as planned. Unexpected variables can make what should be a positive situation become questionable just as quick as the blink of an eye. The good news is that when service events go wrong, they are generally correctable. The problem is that people usually do not see that the situation has gone sour, or they do not know what to do to correct the situation, or they do not feel that they have the power to save it.

Service recovery must be undertaken as quickly and as soon after the unfortunate event as possible. The more quickly you fix a problem, the more likely you are to recover from it. The longer it takes for the organization to recognize a problem and act upon it, the less likely it is that you can fully recover from it.

Let's say that a patient's dinner is delivered and the food is unacceptable for some reason. If the Associate to whom the patient complains takes immediate action to replace disagreeable food with something more appealing, it is likely that the patient will forget about the unfortunate experience altogether, or may even have a *more positive* impression of the organization because of staff's rapid responsiveness to her needs.

Many situations are not as easily addressed as unacceptable food, yet the principle of recovery remains the same. For example, a patient's dentures are misplaced. We don't know whether it is the patient's fault or staff's neglect, they are simply gone. Rather than drag out the process of lengthy paperwork, insurance filings, and other administrative deeds done before the dentures are replaced, why not quickly conduct a thorough search assuring the patient that if they are not found, the organization will quickly have them replaced?

The fact is the organization will probably replace the dentures anyhow, so why not tell the patient that you will take care of the problem right then, and follow up with behind-the-scenes administration and paperwork for insurance purposes. By acting on the patient's behalf quickly, the situation is corrected, and the organization recovers from what otherwise might be an unnecessarily damaging situation.

In order to effect rapid service recovery, Associates must be empowered to make decisions on the spot. Certainly, the extent of Associates' empowerment has to be limited and directed in line with organizational values and expectations. This requires training and a simple set of rules for behavior.

- Rule number one. If the Customer is unhappy it's because of an unmet need. If you can meet that need, and the cost is less than about $200, do it quickly.
- Rule number two. If the cost of service recovery is more than about $200, tell the Customer that you are working on getting a solution as quickly as possible. Then contact the supervisor in charge, who should have authority to execute solutions costing up to $1000 on the spot.

Service recovery processes must be delivered from bureaucracy. Timeliness is the key. It is cheaper to spend $100 to correct a situation quickly than pay the cost of correcting the negative publicity attached to an unhappy Customer over a longer term. The kicker is that the organization usually ends up paying for the missing or damaged goods anyhow—just later, when service recovery has less impact on Customer loyalty.

If you think that Customers are going to go back to their home touting the story of free new dentures, well they might—under the banner of how wonderful your organization was to handle this important denture problem so quickly. If you think there will be a run on denture claims from people scamming the hospital for new dentures, think again.

John Sharpe, vice president of Four Seasons Hotels, states that the Customer may not always be right, but staff are encouraged to err on the side of the Customer.

No one will ever criticize a staffer for making a guest happy.

How well does your organization manage service recovery? How much can be gained by installing better service recovery practices, policies, and training?

Service Recovery—A True Story

The doorman at Toronto Four Seasons Hotel, neglected to load a darting guest's briefcase into the taxi. Upon discovering the forgotten briefcase, the doorman called the guest as he arrived in Washington D.C. and found that he desperately needed the briefcase for a morning meeting. The doorman hopped on a plane and returned the briefcase to the guest in Washington D.C. without first securing approval from his boss.

Traveling across country is beyond what would be needed in most health care situations. But if we took that thinking and applied it to Associates working in daily health care, it might sound something like the following true story at Trinity Hospital in Chicago.

Service Recovery—Another True Story

A department manager at Trinity Hospital received feedback about an unhappy patient following the patient's discharge. Upon receipt of this disappointing information, the department manager immediately contacted the patient at his home stating that she understood that he was unhappy. Rather than becoming involved in a problematic situation over the telephone, she invited him to join her as her guest for lunch at a restaurant of his choosing to discuss the situation.

The patient was favorably impressed that he garnered such attention, and he agreed to meet with the department manager. At the conclusion of lunch, the problems in the work system were clear to the hospital manager, and the patient had received an apology, a complimentary lunch, the undivided attention of the manager, and a promise that the situation would be corrected. In short, an otherwise defecting Customer was recovered.

On the surface it seems that just one patient or Customer was saved in this situation. In fact, many potential defecting Customers were salvaged by correcting problems in the system that were identified by the patient. The best protection against Customer defection is immediate correction of problems.

If I were to ask the question, true or false, "Customer satisfaction is everyone's responsibility," 99 percent of managers and executives would get the answer right: "True." However, the greatest pitfall to effective service delivery is untrained and ineffective staff. They simply do not know how to act in a way that garners Customer Satisfaction. Executives and managers have not managed the daily delivery of Customer satisfaction closely enough.

To adjust service delivery constantly in order to highly satisfy Customers in their infinite variety requires a fully trained, flexible staff that understands Customer Satisfaction objectives and the boundaries within which they can operate. To develop such a staff, the organization must undertake the following five, specific actions:

Devote as much time to service training as to technical training. Include scripted responses and behaviors to the top twelve most frequently experienced situations on their jobs, including

- What to do and say when a patient is angry
- What to do and say when a physician is angry
- What to do and say when a family member is angry
- What to do and say when patient education questions are asked
- What to do and say when family makes requests contrary to your policy and practice

Make service recovery easy. Make it easy for Associates to correct Customers' irritations and annoyances and to submit and implement new ideas for improving work systems and other activities that support improved Customer satisfaction.

Bureaucratic, cumbersome systems defeat the effort and won't be used anyway. It is really not difficult to handle most service recovery situations, and there is not much risk in allowing Associates some level of latitude in guiding service recovery. Keys to success in service recovery are found in a well-defined program with financial limitations, scripted responses, thorough training, specific time frames for behavior, and a tracking record of incidents from which trends can be assessed and improvements made.

Drive out fear of mistakes. Clinical mistakes are intolerable, but individual errors in judgment resulting in over-serving the Customer should be tolerated. Extraordinary service requires risk-taking. Without it you will never be able to separate effective service practices from poor ones. Associates should not fear making decisions in support of Customer Satisfaction, within prescribed limits. Organizations filled with fear are frozen and ineffective in providing extraordinary Customer Satisfaction. Drive fear out of your organization.

Praise and encourage Associates who challenge traditional ways of doing things. Rather than eroding your organizational values, new approaches are likely to strengthen them. Provide reward, recognition, and reinforcement for new thinking and behaviors that move the organization toward higher levels of Customer Satisfaction.

Train, train, train. Training is the basis of success. Do not let anyone make Customer contact until she or he is thoroughly schooled in your service values, the Customer's situation, and the proper "keep them happy" attitude.

William Martin, author of *Managing Quality Service,* lists the following seven essential traits of good service staff:

- Personal appearance
- "Keep them happy" attitude

- Attentiveness
- Tactfulness
- Guidance
- Persuasiveness
- Gracious problem solving

Training alone is not the answer to extraordinary Customer Satisfaction. Stellar performers possess equally superb technical and people skills. They have the "can do" and "keep them happy" attitudes, and demonstrate a full range of controlled emotions appropriate for each situation, including compassion, empathy, happiness, and understanding. In addition, they work in organizations where there is a structured, easy process for Associates to deliver Customer Satisfaction—a rewarding experience for the Associate and a winning experience for the Customer and the organization.

Are your staff skilled at sharing appropriate emotions with patients? Do they have the ability to share in the joy of good news to a patient or Customer? Do they have the ability to feel the pain of bad news delivered to a patient or Customer, or are they robotic and unfeeling?

THE VALUE OF PROBLEM-SOLVING SKILLS

Effective problem-solving skills can turn Customer satisfaction into a competitive advantage. At the Center for Studies in Creativity at Buffalo State University in New York, twenty students who had problem-solving skills were matched with an equal number without such skills. They were given a real-life marketing problem: Devise ways to bring more off-season guests to a sea-level hotel.

By conducting the experiment at a local TV station, the students could be observed during the process. Observers could decipher which skills and talents were consistently used by each group of students to achieve the level of results performed.

The results of the experiment indicated that the students with problem-solving skills and training smiled more, supported others' ideas more, criticized less, and generated more useful ideas during the exercise. When studied for quality, the study found that groups of students trained in problem-solving skills outperformed those who were not trained in these skills by about three to one. In other words, those trained in problem-solving skills were three times more effective than those who were not trained in problem-solving skills.

Then observers asked, "What happens if we train people to turn a complaint into a problem statement," where problem-solving skills can be used? The results were identical. Teams that were trained on how to convert a complaint into a problem statement and then use the problem-solving skills that they were taught came up with twenty to thirty usable marketing ideas whereas untrained groups could think of only five or six.

MEASURING AN ASSOCIATE'S SERVICE POTENTIAL

The essence of Customer Satisfaction lies half in work systems that support and deliver products and services, and half in people who interface with Customers and work systems. The importance of selecting the right kind of people for Customer interface is crucial to superior Customer Satisfaction ratings. The following tips are offered for measuring Associates' service potential.

- Ask open-ended interview questions with nonobvious answers. For example: What responsibilities did you like best in your last job? Which did you like least? What types of Customers do you prefer to work with routinely? What are the characteristics of Customers who provide the greatest challenge to your skills, and how do you manage the situation? What types of results have you been able to achieve? What would you do differently?

- Listen to each response. Stimulate conversation that will give you insight to the candidates' value judgments by asking how they might handle a difficult, but typical Customer situation found in your organization. Provide numerous and varied examples. Test their thinking to see whether it is their personal core values that you are hearing in their responses or coached interview responses.
- Dig for reasons. Search out why candidates selected one course of action over another. Ask them to describe a number of challenging or difficult situations in their previous employment as well as in their personal life. Probe for what they felt the difficult part of the situation was, and why they felt it was difficult. Correlate their responses to your health care situation. How likely is it that they will experience a similar situation in your organization? Are their responses acceptable to you? Look for a match between their values and decision-making judgments to those desired by your organization.
- Conduct a thorough personal evaluation of Customer Satisfaction competencies. See Exhibit 6.1 for guidelines, and add the additional qualities you find necessary for success in your organization.

For a more detailed and explicit service excellence assessment tool, contact Management House, Inc., for a supply of the *Inventory on Customer Satisfaction Skills for Health Care Providers.*

RETAINING AND GROWING PATIENT REVENUES

For years health care organizations have discussed plans to expand their community involvement as a way of extending their organizational influence in the community. They talk about expanding wellness services provided by the hospital as a means of creating a more diverse and larger Customer base, but few organizations have done a good job with this. And few health care organizations have developed mature tactical plans for

Exhibit 6.1. *Customer Satisfaction Competencies Checklist.*

- ☐ Does s/he like people?
- ☐ Does s/he have problem-solving skills?
- ☐ Is there a genuine desire to be sociable?
- ☐ Are they comfortable among strangers?
- ☐ Are they emotionally in control?
- ☐ Is there a sense of trust?
- ☐ Can they communicate simply and effectively?
- ☐ Do they have high self-esteem?
- ☐ Do they exhibit sensitivity toward others?
- ☐ Is there a track record of competitiveness?
- ☐ Do they have a sense of belonging to a group or place?

significant community involvement. One reason they have yet to do a bang-up job in this area is that the Associate population does not have a clear understanding of the future financial value of Customer retention.

It costs less to sell new products and services to existing Customers than it does to sell them to new Customers, and profit margins on follow-up products and services are usually greater. See Figure 6.3 for a picture of why Customers are more valuable over time.

Notice that the base profit in Figure 6.3 from delivery of services and products represents a sizable foundation upon which increased sales over the years are built, and it becomes more significant as time goes on. Added to these base sales are future services that you will provide to these same Customers, which now represent a zero acquisition cost. On top of these profits are the additional dollars realized when cost squeezing occurs, which should be a natural by-product of repeat customers. For example, if the admission and record-keeping processes are efficient, each time a repeat Cus-

Figure 6.3. **Why Loyal Customers Are Profitable.**

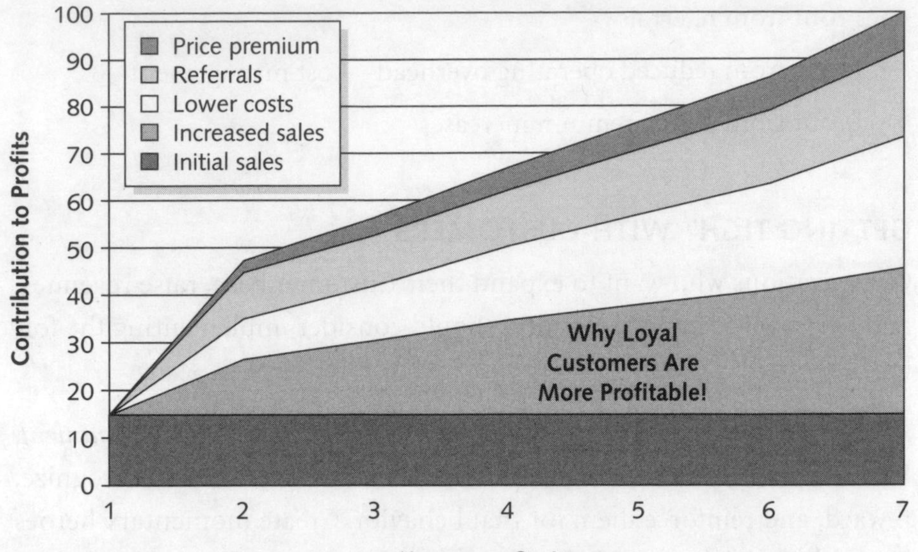

Profit price premium—top and small; profit from referrals— second from top and slightly larger; profit from reduced operating costs—third from top and larger; base profit from increased sales over time—largest.

Source: Adapted from Frederick F. Reichheld and W. Earl Sasser, Jr., "Zero Defections: Quality Comes to Service," *Harvard Business Review,* September–October, 1990.

tomer comes to your facility the amount of staff time and resources needed to process the admission, insurance, and payment records should be considerably less because you would already have this information on file.

Doing it once means that there is more profitability from reduced administrative overhead costs. Topping it off is additional profit that may come from price premium adjustments while cost management is simultaneously in place.

By maximizing Customer Satisfaction you positively influence four of the five sources of profit:

- Profit from increased services over time
- Profit from referrals
- Profit from reduced operating overhead—cost management
- Profit from price premium increases

GETTING TIGHT WITH CUSTOMERS

Organizations who want to expand their Customer base, raise revenues, and improve Customer retention should consider implementing the following ideas.

Reward staff for Customer retention as well as for Customer recruitment. When Associates deliver an exceptional job in service recovery, recognize, reward, and reinforce them for that behavior. Create momentary heroes out of them. With so much focus on recruiting new Customers, who's paying attention to retaining the current Customers?

Be visible and active in the community. I often hear that one of the strategic initiatives announced by executives for the coming year will be greater involvement with the community. Executives attend seminars on how to do this, make announcements that they are going to do it, but then the snap, crackle, and pop of the initiative sizzles to a little of this or a little of that at the local health fair—and that's it.

The objective is to create a true relationship between the community and your facility. To do this requires the *active and routine* involvement of all Associates in some aspect of the community. From management's point of view, the task is to direct enough resources into the high-priority areas first and then further develop the balance of areas of interest.

The type of involvement referenced here is definitely more than the annual Christmas party for the nursing home residents or the blood-pressure reading at the local health fair. What we are talking about is a comprehensive, integrated designed effort to make a difference and to build strong relationships with all components of the local community.

Become involved with retirement homes, including providing preventative, educational, social and clinical programs routinely on site for residents. These seniors will come to think of your organization as a part of their family, not just their medical supplier.

Become actively involved with the larger employers or employer coalitions, not only in terms of negotiating health insurance coverage but also as a provider of wellness programs on site for their employees.

Get to the kids, as they are the future of your business. Use the rehabilitation department and sport medicine areas to combine and provide on-site support for school systems, summer camps, and athletic activities throughout the community. The referral pattern will grow from these community involvements. And don't forget the little kids. Link up with child care centers to provide for wellness and health management needs for young children. Market safety items such as car seats, bike helmets, and vitamins through day care centers as well as provide learning opportunities for young children. The list can go on and on. You get the idea—comprehensive, routine, active involvement with all aspects of the community. The objective is to become a part of every aspect of living in the community and to build relationships.

Aggressively pursue preventative medicine. Many health care organizations gave away the lucrative business of health clubs and other business opportunities in preventative personal health management. If you do not have your own fitness facility, then partner with a local one in an active role. Promote preventative analysis services such as heart disease prevention, flu shots, weight management, smoking cessation classes, stress management classes, and other education and testing services. Actively schedule and remind patients of follow-up services needed. Aggressively help Customers manage their health.

Become a life learning center. In addition to providing support groups for medical diagnoses such as diabetes, cancer, and others, expand the educational component to include pre-retirement planning, teaching a second language in multicultural areas, computer skills, parenting skills, teen-management skills, and other such topics. Connect with the community on every level of learning.

Develop Customer incentives for retention. Everybody understands the concept of frequent flier miles, why not adapt it to a wide range of health care preventative services in exchange for discounted pricing? For example, a given number of hours of volunteer service with the health care organization translates into reduced pricing for home health care, if and when needed. Shorter lengths of stay mean patients need more assistance when they get home, thus home health care becomes increasingly valuable. The idea is to tie present and future Customers into loyal Customers—people who are committed to using your organization for a wide range of services.

Organize senior clubs and teen clubs. Pull senior patients together for social as well as functional purposes. Organize trips and social events. Provide discounted services on travel, insurance, and other basic living and recreational commodities. Act as the local chapter of the American Association of Retired Persons. Create a reason for coming together.

For teens, the future adults and decision makers for health care, the approach is somewhat different. Through local schools and churches construct programs that offer teens insight into health care professions through career "shadow days" when teens "shadow" various professionals in the organization. Offer schools and churches the opportunity to assign teens to your facility for community contributions. Become actively engaged with local schools and churches. These are gathering places of people who, by their very nature, want to do good for the community and others.

Gather feedback from defectors. They left for a reason. Talent lies in listening to what defectors have to say about your organization without becoming defensive, and taking immediate action based on what they tell you, without exception. Invest the time and resources needed to investigate what events or situations, large or small, led to the Customer's decision to seek health care services somewhere else. To understand this information is to realize what must change for the future viability of your organization.

Manage customer data. Do you know who your current patients are and how often you are seeing them? If you are not seeing them as often as you should be, then ask the Customer what the barriers are to more frequent, appropriate use of your services.

When Customers disappear, they have defected, and there is at least one reason behind each defection. Usually there is more than one reason. If the Customer responds to the question of why they defected with a somewhat superficial explanation such as, "I thought I would try XYZ hospital this time," then probe a little further by asking, "What is it about XYZ hospital that you find more appealing?" Get to the root of the defection, then recover that Customer by correcting the misperceptions, or correcting the situation that lead to the defection. Fix the mistake.

Listen carefully to what Customers are saying verbally as well as what they may be saying "between the lines," and make necessary changes in your operations to avoid further defection. Approach every defected Customer with the attitude that you will do whatever is needed to recover that Customer. Barrier-bust your way to growth and progress.

Build a constellation of patients in the community. For many patients, the only relationships they have are with caregivers from your organization, and other support organizations they depend upon. Their family members are nonevents or nonexistent, and other supportive relationships have died or moved on.

Creating a relationship with Customers is a strong retention tool. It may be as simple as sending birthday and holiday cards to patients past and present. Your holiday card may be one of the only cards they receive. Loneliness affects more people than you might imagine. A simple relationship through special holidays may prove to be a powerful and inexpensive Customer retention tool.

The synergy created among a constellation of patients in the community will become self-perpetuating—a community within a community that grows stronger and stronger, a community that will lead your organization to more extensive services, greater profits, and stronger Customer loyalty.

Allow your imagination to race unbridled for ten minutes. We did, and came up with the following list of services and products that are natural extensions of the traditional health care community.

- Child care center and supporting services. Within your own high-quality child care center, or within other child care centers in the community, offer the following items for sale: vitamins, cold and allergy medications, safe toys, developmental software, safe infant clothing, classes on parenting. The idea is to connect natural extensions of your health care services to other related community services in an intermingling of relationships and benefits to the community. These extensions will strengthen your organization and its people in all aspects of community living.
- Special food service. You can sell prepackaged, frozen meals for special-diet patients to purchase and heat at home; for example, low-sodium, fat-free, low-cholesterol meals in a dish. Campbell Soup company and other commercial enterprises are cashing in on the need to provide specially prepared foods for special diets. This market is a natural extension of the food service operation already in place in hospitals. You have the knowledge, the kitchen, and the clients. What else does it take but a little initiative?
- Durable medical equipment. Sell it, rent it, lend it, repair it. Become the central source for any durable medical equipment need, short-term or long-term. Provide durable medical equipment on site at your facility; become a mini-medical mall of sorts. So often health care facilities offer a rather weak source for durable medical equipment via an arrangement with a local vendor that is operating at less than excellent standards of Customer service.

    Make equipment available on site, before the patient leaves the facility. Satellite facilities located in the community are convenient for Customers seeking replacement parts and service. The point is, capture the patient and the business on site, where and when they need the services and equipment the most. Once Customers have left your premises, you have lost control of the purchases or services. They may or may not visit your community medical equipment center. They may go home and find a second source for these services, thus becoming a lost Customer to your organization.

- Home alterations. Frequently alterations to Customer's residences are needed either permanently or temporarily in order to adapt their living space to their new temporary or permanent physical limitations. For example, ramps for wheelchairs, holding bars for baths, adjusted electrical outlets for people with disabilities, and other special construction projects are frequently needed. A true continuum of care would provide a source for these services, which constitute a natural extension of hospital services. Most larger health care facilities employ maintenance staff skilled in providing these basic services. Why not hire them out to patients who need their services? What? Create a revenue center out of a facility plant and maintenance? Yes! Make a revenue and service center.
- Delivery systems. Home health people are driving around the community regularly to conduct home health services. Why not add other delivery services to the distribution channel? For example, your hospital could deliver prescriptions, flowers, and specially prepared food.

Patients are buying these goods and services elsewhere. They could easily buy them from you. *Example:* Marriott Hotels are widely known for quality services; even room service food at the Marriott facility is better than average. When Marriott learned that a large number of guests were ordering carry-out pizza into their hotels, they recognized the need to partner with a quality pizza provider. Now, nearly all Marriott facilities offer Pizza Hut pizza on site. The Marriott and Pizza Hut partnership is the same concept as health care partnering with prescriptions, special diet foods, flowers, and twenty other ideas that you can identify. Think bigger, more grand. This is called *leveraging your Customer relationships.*

STAY CLOSE TO THE CUSTOMER

Staying close to the Customer is the number one secret to Customer retention. Tom Monaghan of Domino's Pizza gets close to his Customers by keeping senior managers and himself on the road visiting pizza stores every week. The average is two store visits per week per executive. Compensation for pizza makers is pegged to Customer Satisfaction ratings.

Privately held Domino's, the world's largest pizza delivery chain, pays 10,000 mystery shoppers $60 each to buy twelve pizzas throughout the year at its 5000+ stores and evaluate quality and service for each encounter. Domino's managers' compensation is based partly on these ratings. Customer service at Domino's Pizza does not end with an evaluation of external service. They also evaluate internal Customer service.

Companies are discovering that Associates who view one another as Customers usually treat actual patients or Customers better than those who do not value or understand the importance of internal Customer Satisfaction.

Good external Customer satisfaction requires good internal Customer satisfaction. To this end, Domino's 16 regional offices rate the services of corporate staff on the quality of service they get from headquarters. For example, did the sponsorship department of Pizza Ponies, popular miniature horse teams, appear on time for a store grand opening? Were pizza supplies delivered on time and in the quantity ordered? Were questions to corporate staff answered correctly and in a timely manner?

Every four weeks, Domino's hands out bonuses to every full-time corporate office Associate based partly on their internal Customer Satisfaction ratings. Pizza stores rate distribution, supplies, ingredients, and numerous support activities provided by corporate staff.

If we were to ask hospital department managers to evaluate the quality and value of services provided by health care corporate departments such as finance, communications, marketing, and others, how do you think they would fare? Based on the casual comments that I hear in hundreds of health care organizations that I visit each year, my guess is that most service delivery departments have no idea what corporate departments even do, never mind how well they do it. What does that tell us about the value and contributions of corporate health care departments?

The following six approaches will help you to stay close to your Customer.

- *Think of yourself as a Customer.* What are the fundamental elements you would want if you were the Customer? Mirror those elements and standards of performance to all those you serve.
- *Generate awareness.* Make every Associate aware of your vision and exactly how they should perform to make that vision a reality. Leave no behaviors to chance. Program the behavior of each job in great detail. Avoid any variance in behaviors and performance levels.
- *Monitor service.* Watch internally to make sure that Associates treat one another as Customers. Internal service mirrors external service. Accept nothing less than the desired internal and external service-oriented behavior from all Associates.
- *Listen to everyone in the distribution chain.* Associates in the distribution chain have heard the various Customers in the chain speak. Respond positively to any problem presented by anyone in your distribution chain. Horst Schulze, president of Ritz Carlton Hotels, says,

  Keep listening to your Customer because they change. And if you have 100 percent Satisfaction then you have to make sure that you keep listening and are ready to change just in case they [Customers] change their expectations. Then you can change with them.

- *Prune bureaucracy so Customers can talk directly to you.* Create multiple listening posts so you can hear directly from Customers about what they are thinking. The farther you are from the Customer's lips, the less you will hear.
- *Stay in touch after the service is delivered.* Build on the relationship that is already born if you want to extend your business and services. If tangential services are unavailable, include Customers in social, recognition,

problem-solving, and education activities sponsored by your organization to keep Customers linked to your organization.

Getting Close to the Customer—A True Story

In 1988, Motorola had revenues of $8.25 billion. It was clear that they had to prune bureaucracy in order to get closer to the Customer and create a competitive advantage. At that time, chairman Robert Galvin visited Customers and heard that Motorola was hard to do business with. Galvin realized that he had work to do and agreed that Total Customer Satisfaction should be the topic of executive action plans for 1988. Realizing that they had been "driven by cost savings instead of taking care of the Customer," Galvin made immediate and drastic changes.

All executives were given pagers so any corporate Customer could reach them day or night, any day of the week. Field service crews were now authorized to repair Customers' defective pagers and mobile phones on the spot without office approval if the expense was less than $1000. Previously all repairs had to be authorized through the corporate office before repair work could be done. The company was revamped so that buyer satisfaction figured into every manager's bonus. The time between a Customer's need and delivery of service was squeezed to zero. As Motorola's response time improved, so did their Customer Satisfaction ratings.

ACTION PLAN FOR TOTAL CUSTOMER SATISFACTION STRATEGY

Task 1. Chart Trends in Customer Satisfaction Statistics. Month by month or quarter by quarter, by department, and for the entire organization, chart the trends in Customer satisfaction statistics. How many units or departments show 92 percent or more of Customers reporting that the department delivered *excellent* service? How many have Customer ratings indicating that they would recommend your services to friends and family? If less than 92 percent of your Customers are reporting your performance as *excellent,* you are losing ground and eventually will lose market share. Take a good, long look at the detailed statistics. High Customer Satisfaction with one part or department in the health care delivery system can be totally negated by poor satisfaction with another part or department.

Task 2. Identify Customers and Their Needs. With the participation of staff, each department is to identify who their Customers are and what they have to deliver to each Customer in order to be viewed as providing *excellent* service. The list of Customers should include internal and external Customers.

This list might include physicians, referral organizations, patients, or internal departments. Post that list in your departmental communication center. Below the name of each Customer group, list what these particular Customers expect from you.

We have found that Customers want open communication, fear-reducing relationships, and timely service. Be specific in your definitions of what *your* Customers want from you. *Timely service* as a definition of what is wanted is too abstract. Define exactly what *timely* means to each Customer. Does it mean within ten minutes, within thirty minutes, or as soon as it is requested? Be specific. What does a *fear-reducing relationship* mean? What do Customers fear? How can these fearful situations be transformed into fearless situations?

Keep this information posted as a continuous reminder and reference for Associates. Review this information on Customer identification and service needs in your orientation of new Associates. Players must know what the goal is if they are to make a touchdown.

You might use the following headings to organize your thinking: Customer/Department Name, Service Needs, Contact Person.

Task 3. Identify Your Departmental Suppliers, and What You Need from Them. Include not only the product or service needed, but when you need them to be delivered. Evaluate whether you are getting what you need to maximize service to your Customers or whether there is some improvement in performance required.

If you are not getting the type of service needed from your suppliers, call individual meetings with your vendors to discuss exactly what it is that you do need. Be prepared to problem solve, or in extreme situations, change vendors if they are unable to meet your needs. No longer should you accept what the vendor has to offer if it is not good enough for you or your Customer. Take positive control of vendor relationships and performances.

Task 4. Collect Customer Feedback. We deal with patient satisfaction feedback in several chapters, but patients are not the only Customers from whom feedback is needed. Departments serving internal Customers other than patients also need feedback on their performance. A simple internal Customer Satisfaction survey used uniformly by internal departments serving internal Customers works best. For example, materials management and human resources departments support internal Customers and need feedback on their performance. Notice that feedback from the Customer teaches the provider what their business is. Exhibit 6.2 provides a sample form to evaluate internal Customer Satisfaction. Internal Customer Satisfaction surveys should be short and routinely administered, ideally every forty-five to sixty days.

Departments, such as material management, that serve a large number of internal Customers, need to survey only a sampling of Customers every period. They might sample two or three nursing units each survey period rather than every nursing unit every period. A rotating survey process provides enough feedback to make necessary improvements to performance, yet does not overwhelm heavy users such as nursing departments with endless surveys.

Exhibit 6.2. *Sample Internal Customer Satisfaction Survey.*

Thinking of your working relationship with the _______________ department, how would you rate their treatment of you as a Customer on the following items?

Please assign each of the following statements a rating from one (1) to four (4) which best describes your feelings about services provided by that department.

Almost Never	Occasionally	Frequently	Almost Always
1	2	3	4

Customer Satisfaction

1 2 3 4 1. They quickly respond to my Customer complaints.

1 2 3 4 2. They maintain good communications with me as a Customer.

1 2 3 4 3. Their attitude is of wanting to serve the Customer.

1 2 3 4 4. They actively improve services to meet Customer needs.

Quality

1 2 3 4 5. The work they do for us meets quality standards.

1 2 3 4 6. Attitude of their staff is aggressive for high quality.

1 2 3 4 7. Problems in quality are immediately responded to.

1 2 3 4 8. Quality standards are as good or better than other units.

Productivity

1 2 3 4 9. Timely results can be counted on from this group.

1 2 3 4 10. The department stays focused on Key Result Areas.

1 2 3 4 11. Problems in quality are immediately responded to.

1 2 3 4 12. They go out of their way to minimize bureaucracy and red tape.

Economic

1 2 3 4 13. Solutions they provide make economic sense.

1 2 3 4 14. They ask for ideas to reduce inefficiency and cost.

1 2 3 4 15. They control costs without being "penny-wise and pound-foolish."

1 2 3 4 16. They run things in a business-like fashion.

Innovation

1 2 3 4 17. Ideas are encouraged and implemented.

1 2 3 4 18. They suggest ideas to us and work with us to solve problems.

1 2 3 4 19. They are reasonably accessible and open to change.

1 2 3 4 20. When needed, they make clear decisions to reduce confusion.

Exhibit 6.2. *Sample Internal Customer Satisfaction Survey, cont'd.*

People Growth

1 2 3 4 21. The staff is competent and knowledgeable.

1 2 3 4 22. The staff show good morale and spirit, and are actively engaged.

1 2 3 4 23. They treat me with respect and appreciate my efforts.

1 2 3 4 24. They seem to work well as a team.

Organization Climate

1 2 3 4 25. These folks live our corporate values.

1 2 3 4 26. They encourage interdepartmental teamwork.

1 2 3 4 27. The manager upholds our general management philosophy.

1 2 3 4 28. They deal with problems quickly and decisively.

Comments

29. From my perspective, Customer service could be better if:

____

30. As a Customer/peer, I need your help to:

____

31. It would be a big help if your staff interacted with me in the following way:

____

32. To add to your department excellence, may I suggest:

____

____

But administration of internal Customer Satisfaction surveys is not enough. Action must follow and changes be made—now. To assure that efforts to improve internal Customer Satisfaction are just as active as for external Customer Satisfaction, structure and accountability measures need to be added to the assignment of conducting the research. We recommend that each internal service department use the feedback from internal satisfaction surveys to identify the top three or four problem service areas each month, and undertake an action plan to implement needed changes. This is the concept of continuous improvement put into action. There will always be the poorer performance areas, as no department is totally perfect day in and day out.

Problem areas and corresponding corrective action should be tracked by the department manager and reported to the supervisor every quarter. If we cannot measure an action, we cannot manage it. This is one way to measure how much change and improvement is occurring in the arena of internal Customer Satisfaction management.

The internal Customer Satisfaction survey shown in Exhibit 6.2 is a good place to start. Add additional criteria specific to your department to make it an optimally meaningful instrument for you.

Once the internal Customer Satisfaction survey has been in place for six months and refined to better fit your organization, Customer Satisfaction ratings should be built into the organization's structure for evaluating Associate performance.

It is not uncommon to find organizations building compensation practices around Customer Satisfaction ratings as provided by patients. A natural extension of that thinking is to include internal Customer Satisfaction measurement as a part of the overall Customer Satisfaction measurement process. *Remember:* Internal Customer satisfaction mirrors external Customer Satisfaction.

Task 5. Create a Customer Satisfaction Mentoring System. An effective Customer Satisfaction mentoring system pairs department managers who are more expert at delivering *excellent* Customer Satisfaction ratings to work with, or mentor, department managers with lower or mediocre satisfaction ratings. Mentoring should be viewed as a professional development opportunity not as a license for criticism, unless progress does not occur.

To assure utilization of the mentoring process, establish a Customer Satisfaction threshold below which a Customer Satisfaction mentor would be assigned should any departmental rating fall. For example, any department performing at a level of 10 percent or more below the satisfaction goal should have the assistance of a Customer Satisfaction mentor. Or the break point for determining whether a mentor is needed might be determined by a ranking system. The five departments with the lowest Customer Satisfaction performance levels in the organization, providing that the performance level is below the goal, will receive the assistance of a mentor. Another spin on this idea could be that any department that performs in the lower 25 percent of the organization for three or more consecutive months receives a new manager for that department.

A mentoring system provides uniformity in application of the performance standards as well as standardizing how unacceptable Customer Satisfaction ratings will be managed. It is a means of installing structure in the organization without becoming punitive.

Task 6. Evaluate and Rejuvenate Organizational Community Involvement. How often and to what extent is your organization actively involved, not just represented, in community events and organizations? Using information and ideas provided in this chapter, create a tactical plan that will bring your organization into the forefront of activities with seniors, working parents, employers, teens, and children in your community. These new and strengthened relationships will build loyalty to your organization.

Active involvement in the community, for our purposes, is defined as providing a service to another organization and coordinating services provided by others that will then benefit your Customers. Beware of substituting representation on a committee or task force for participation, leadership, and activity.

Task 7. Assess Ease of Customer Problem Solving. How easy is it for a patient, physician, or other Customer to reach someone in administration with immediate problem-solving authority? If it takes more than one phone call, it is not easy enough. Squeeze the bureaucracy and hierarchy out of problem solving. Give the supervisor in charge the authority, training, and guidelines to solve any problem at the time of occurrence.

Task 8. Use Customer Defection Information to Improve Performance. By tracking information on Customer defection you can uncover the keys to better management of the organization and Customer Satisfaction. Defecting Customers will tell you exactly what is wrong with the organization—if you are willing to listen.

Begin by installing a system to gather information on Customer defection that will tell you where defections are occurring and exactly who the defectors are. Then, boost efforts to salvage as many of the defectors as is possible. The economic gain of salvaging a lost Customer is well worth the cost of staff and resources.

When contact with the defector is made, be direct in asking why they left your organization. Be ready to take notes and ask specific questions. For example, what part of the experience was particularly unpleasing? Chances are, you will not have to ask. Defected Customers will tell you readily, as they are not planning on coming back.

This is the opportunity to recover from the situation. Provide whatever is needed to save this Customer. If the overall experience was legitimately a bad one, substantially reduce the cost of the experience and offer to redo whatever is needed to provide a satisfactory experience at what, in essence, will be a greatly reduced cost. Think of the positive publicity you will receive. More important, think of the future income that you have salvaged and the bad press that was avoided.

Finally, turn this costly experience into a problem-solving opportunity. Fix the system with the information provided by the Customer. After all, you are not interested in giving away revenue, and now you have the solution to the problem. All you have to do is implement it!

NOTE

1. Deanna Bellandi. "Consumer's First." *Modern Health Care,* January 26, 1998, p. 30.

Chapter
SEVEN

The Irrational Nature of Customer Satisfaction

Sweating the Small Stuff

Be prepared to respond to unreasonable requests.

This last holiday season we all went through a number of experiences as Customers—good ones and bad ones. Think back to some good experiences in stores or with services you received—when you walked into the store or called a service on the phone, and they did the right thing. You felt good about the experience, and you want to give them an ad right now. You want to tell your family and friends about the outstanding experience that you had.

Now, think back on another kind of shopping experience that you had in the last thirty days—one that was not so great. There are probably many more of these than there are of outstandingly positive experiences. A negative experience is value subtracted.

CUSTOMER SATISFACTION AS A CORE PHILOSOPHY

Older than the American Revolution is a store that is still in business in Philadelphia, a store call Wannamaker's. It is the first department store of its kind. John Wannamaker, founder, said something about the Customer that every one of us has memorized. In 1768 he said,

The Customer is always right.

Linguists, people who study language, tell us that if you look at statements that people have memorized, they reveal something about the core values of the people. The problem is that this commonly quoted statement, "The Customer is always right," may not be an entirely true statement. Have you ever seen a wrong Customer? Have you ever been a wrong Customer? What is it about the statement, since it is not literally true, that we have all nonetheless, bought? Even if the words are not literally true, why is it that we buy it as a philosophy? *Answer:* It is good business.

People in business like to equivocate on this. The Harvard Business School conducted a study in which they sent this statement, "The Customer is always right," to Fortune 1000 company presidents and asked what each CEO thought about it. A majority of CEOs gave responses like Ken Olsen's, then at Digital Equipment. They said something like, "Well, yea, uh, we agree. . . . We generally buy it, but. . . ." They added a qualifier.

Ken Olsen, like John Opel at IBM, thought that the computer Customer needed big computer boxes. Meanwhile the Customer was saying, "We don't want a big computer box. We want a little computer box with big computing power inside."

IBM and Digital Equipment Corporation lost huge market share because they did not understand that the Customer is right. What Customers say they want is what they want. And the Customer was right. Ken Olsen is no longer working with Digital Equipment Corporation.

The statement, "The Customer is always right," is not literally true, so these CEOs, being intellectually honest, responded to the Harvard Business School study question with a qualifying "but" and came up with a list of exceptions. There were a few fanatics, a minority of executives, who said, "Yep, that's the way it is." And we saw people like Stew Leonard and others who unequivocably instilled the practice that the Customer is always right into every aspect of their business operations, and watched their business—Stew Leonard's Dairy in Norwalk, Conn.—grow to be one of the most profitable grocery stores in sales per square foot anywhere in the United States.

Consider this example. Mobile Corporation's most recent rating lists thirty-five Five-Star hotels in the United States. Seventeen of the thirty-five hotels on that list, or nearly half of all Five-Star rated hotels, are owned by one chain, the Four Seasons.

Four Seasons Associates are taught to respond to unreasonable Customer requests. Some people would say, "I am willing to listen and respond." But are you willing to respond to an *unreasonable* request? Four Seasons Hotel management teach staff to respond to *unreasonable* Customer requests. Well, a lot of people would say that is foolish, because the Customer is not always right, and that to believe so is an extreme position. It is almost fanatical, isn't it? But everybody who wants to explain it away is not on the Five-Star list.

CUSTOMER SATISFACTION IN THE NEW AMERICAN HEALTH CARE ORGANIZATION

Our concept of an organization is contrarian in relation to other organizations in the industry. We are not interested in running a hospital the way our competitors run their organizations. New American Health Care Organizations have a Four Seasons mentality. It is different from everybody else in the pack. They want to be at the top of the heap in service and quality. Health care organizations can adopt a Four Seasons mentality without adopting a Four Seasons budget. What we are talking about adopting is a service attitude, not material luxuries. Let's learn how we are going to respond.

Admittedly, that "The Customer is always right" is not literally true. By adopting the philosophy as if it were literally true, you are going to take a risk. If you go with the literal interpretation, the risk is that you might overserve the Customer or patient. You might serve people who do not deserve it. You might serve people who probably ought to be shown the door. You might, in fact, spend some money and effort and time that other hospitals would not see the value in. So there is a risk. You could be wheel-spinning. But those who do not adopt this philosophy are taking a risk, too. They are taking the risk of underserving. The consequence of underserving is that you will not go far enough, and you will leave too many people with the short end of the stick.

Either way, there is a risk. If you overserve and respond to unreasonable Customer requests, you are one kind of extremist. If you are too conservative and do not go far enough, you are another kind of extremist. Look at your organization's value statement. What do the words tell you to do? Which way should you place the bet? I submit to you the notion that the very nature of health care directs you to take the risk to overserve. If you do what the excellent companies do, you will achieve what excellent companies achieve.

True Story

There was a story in the newspaper about an organization in my home town of Chicago. It was about one of our local institutions, First Chicago Bank. The story was widely spread. Perhaps you will recall what the bank tried to do. Since the beginning of banking, there has never been a fee for conducting banking business with a teller. This newspaper article reported that First Chicago Bank was introducing a $3 charge to deal with one of their live tellers! Come in and talk to Linda, teller at First Chicago. That will be $3! What was the Customers' reaction? No way! This article about the notion of a fee-for-bank-teller service kicked off a wicked teller-fee backlash.

Competitors were quick to respond. For Example, Bell Federal Savings, which has an office across the street from First Chicago Bank, said they were going to put a sign, "Free tellers." Harris Bank said they were going to pay Customers $1.50 if they asked whether the bank charged teller fees. The point is that competitors were quick to respond to Customers' anger about First Chicago's nickel-and-dime approach.

Think of it, First Chicago Bank was imposing a charge to do what? Deposit Customers' money upon which they made more money! Here they had a $3 item that then turned them into the joke of the month. It was a national publicity disaster. Jay Leno, host of the "Tonight Show," made jokes asking whether Customers could talk dirty to a teller for an extra $.95. Then the absurdity of the idea made the cartoon strip, *Sylvia*.

Nobody was going to go with it. What were they thinking? Who approved that? Somebody in management thought this was a good idea! Banks have a reputation that is either real good, or not so good. Once these Scrooge banking characters decided to charge $3 to talk to a teller, the "not so good" reputation just ballooned. Of course, this all wound up with a follow-up article, "First Chicago Tries to Save Face."

Hard Choices

We can take the core lesson of this banking incident, apply it to a health care organization, and ask, "What are some of the simple things that Customers are encountering at your organization that they don't like?" We mean little things, not a big deal. For example, charging for TV viewing.

No hotel in the United States charges for TV, nor does any organization in the United States charge to watch TV. Yet like the bank, some health care organizations are nickel and diming patients and creating irritating situations year after year, Customer after Customer. They are on a glide path to a crash with that kind of thinking.

To create exceptional Customer Satisfaction, your organization needs to think differently. Your point of view should be that if the Customer is always right—if we are really willing to risk the possibility of overserving and really willing to put our organization behind those words—then everyone must be tuned in to the philosophy and how to turn philosophy into action and results. You might even say, "Geez, sometimes we might lose some revenue if we overserve." You sure might—and at the same time you will stop irritating people. Which do you want more? A little more revenue, or happy Customers? "Oh, you mean, there are going to be hard choices?" Yes.

In the book *Creating the New American Hospital: A Time for Greatness,* we said that the New American Health Care Organization is basically an amalgam of ideas. We borrowed all the good ideas we could from management books, and all the experiences of great management teams trying to run great organizations. We said we would borrow only from the best: only from a Four Seasons Hotel, a General Electric, a Disney, or a Southwest Airlines. And we would bring those ideas in-house and adapt them to health care.

As you select and adapt winning organizations' behaviors, there will be hard choices to make. Would your organization cash out the TV rental contract and stop irritating Customers now, or wait until another five years pass, the contract expires, and another 5,000 patients leave the organization with an overwhelming irritation at the nickel and diming?

Controlling Communication

One way of improving the overall cheerfulness of an organization is to eliminate the unhappy, bad talk and bad attitudes that have a way of being contagious if they are not managed.

Peter Ubel of the Center for Bio Ethics, University of Pennsylvania, was interested in quantifying or measuring the amount of negativity actually occurring in the hospital. He wondered how many negative comments could be heard if you got on an elevator in a typical hospital. Turning curiosity into action and research, he went for 259 elevator rides in five Pennsylvania hospitals and just waited for people to talk. Every time a staff person said something negative he noted it.

The results were surprising. In 14 percent of those elevator rides, which were generally less than 60 seconds long, he overheard some negative comments. Although his approach was not thoroughly scientific, as a sampling he was getting real quick pictures of each of the five organizations.

Think about this when you are on an elevator. You only have a few minutes to be with the person you are with, and what you decide to do is vent your feelings. But would you have trust in a doctor if you overhead him say, "I have to learn how to use the stupid piece of new equipment sometime, so it might as well be tonight"? This was a comment Peter Ubel heard on an elevator. Or how about this comment from a staff worker, "I worked sixteen hours yesterday, went home, had a beer, and before I knew it, I was back here. I don't think I can make it all night." Or this comment, heard from a nurse, "He must have been on drugs last night, he couldn't even read a chart."

If a patient comes into your health care organization, is full of fear and all the other strong feelings discussed previously, and they hear comments like this, now what?

Hospital Associates must learn that their negative comments not only violate patient confidentiality, but also reflect poorly on their profession and on their organization, which, in turn, adversely affects Customer Satisfaction ratings, and may cause others to worry about their organization's clinical competency.[1]

If we were walking through a hall of your organization, or if we were in the cafeteria, what kinds of comments would we hear? Would we hear any of this kind of thing? Would we hear negativity? Again, that's just the human thing. People in your organization are probably not any worse than those anywhere else, but the jobs in your organization call for them to be *better than other people.*

Happy, Healthy, Positive Communication

Think about what they do at Disney. At Disney, staff are not referred to as Associates but as cast members. They are told to consider themselves as being onstage, or playing a role, whenever they are in the eye of the public. The very words that a cast member speaks are dictated. The playwright wants you to say certain things and wants you not to say other things. So at Disney, cast members may not say negative things about other departments, other people, or Customers if they have done something wrong. They do not say anything negative when they are onstage, meaning in a publicly visible area.

Offstage is any area where members of the public are not found—say, a cast member lunch room or a manager's office. It is not a free-speech environment where cast members can run their mouths any way they want and any time they want.

Adopting the practice of being onstage or in character, which for health care Associates might translate to being in the professional role, is not only a good business idea, it also contributes to the holistic healing environment, because Customers hear and see only happy, positive, healthy communication.

Now, we are not saying to Associates that they have to shut up. We are saying that if they see anything wrong in the system, they can attack it, but the way to attack it is through the Do-It-Group (DIG) process. (See *Creating the New American Hospital: A Time for Greatness* for details on DIGs).

DIGs represent a system open to Associate complaints and recommendations for improvement. By using the DIG process, we are encouraging Associates to talk to management about issues that are important to them. Associates are not being asked to stifle themselves; they are simply being asked to control communication for the benefit of people who are in extreme situations.

What do you think? If Customers say they are more satisfied when they hear positive communication among staff and see a good attitude, should this become a standard of behavior for all staff in your organization? This would literally mean having to talk with all staff members, probably in training sessions, where you explain the idea to them, ask them what they think about it, point out that they have the opportunity to and are invited to air their feelings about things that are wrong, but that they cannot do that in certain places.

Competing on Patient Climate

Not every organization can be the Mayo Clinic or the University of Chicago Hospital in terms of technology and financial resources. St. Joseph's Hospital, Houston, Texas, found themselves in this situation.

St. Joseph's Hospital was located two miles down the road from the Texas Medical Center. Huge. How does a small community hospital in the middle of downtown Houston compete against the mighty Texas Medical Center? One answer is that they out-friendly them. And that is how the St. Joseph Hospital marketing campaign ran for some period of time.

Patient satisfaction ratings at St. Joseph got to be higher than those at competing organizations. So, do you need the technology? Yes, but apparently that is not all you need.

What Customers want is technical medical care, but they also want to be taken care of in their inner life. They want to be respected, communicated with, informed, and cared about. Patients are not just a piece of flesh on a gurney that staff have the liberty of talking over as if their words had no impact on the patient.

SATISFACTION-SUCCESS CYCLE

In Chapter One we explained the concept of the Satisfaction-Success Cycle, an adaptation from the service-profit-value chain concept introduced by Leon Schlesinger. If we look at that concept again (see Figure 1.1) and start at the end of the chain, which is the business results we want to produce, and work our way toward the start of the chain, you can see that the product that health care organizations produce—a courteous, caring, compassionate healing experience—is produced only from one source: Associates.

An environment with excessive Associate turnover is not particularly productive. Associate retention and productivity are directly linked. The chief learning officer for Sears reports,

It's not guesswork or theory anymore. We have built an empirical model that says unless you have a trained literate work force, and give them decision-making authority, you don't get satisfied customers, no matter how good the merchandise is. The right work force creates customer satisfaction, and that produces superior financial performance.

For years I have been trying to get the message across that Associate turnover in hospitals must stop. Turnover costs the organization more than recruitment and overtime. There are additional costs of lost productivity, lower quality, lost training investment, and lower Customer Satisfaction. Do you know why people turn over? People leave an organization because the workplace is not good enough to stay in.

Associate Retention Equals Productivity

Tenured people are far more productive than the new kid that is wandering around the organization looking for the bathroom. New Associates are simply not as productive as experienced ones. It takes time to become productive. What tenured people are able to produce feeds directly into profitably. They know the work systems, with all the inefficiencies, and how to work around them. They have developed relationships instrumental to efficient operations. They know best how to make the system work. So what can be done to reduce turnover and retain knowledgeable, motivated staff?

In the airline industry, the people at Southwest Airlines (SWA) absolutely blow the profitability picture sky high—they are way off the map compared with competitors. SWA staff are so efficient, so productive, that they need fewer staff per plane and fewer staff per passenger to provide transportation safely and satisfactorily. Where does that productivity come from? It comes from low Associate turnover—the lowest turnover rate in the airlines industry.

Health care organizations have to hang on to their good people. These good people learned their tasks in order to be productive. Their productivity creates the service or product with which the Customer is then satisfied—for this service or product they'll want to stick around.

Why would Associates want to stay at your organization? They have to be satisfied with the job life if they are going to stay employed with your organization. When Associates are satisfied, there is a chance you will be able to create high Customer Satisfaction. Customer Satisfaction cannot be achieved until Associate Satisfaction is achieved. And Customer retention cannot be achieved until Associate retention is achieved. Can you see the relationship in Figure 1.1?

Associate Satisfaction = Associate Retention =
Customer Satisfaction = Customer Retention

The dynamics of Associate and Customer Satisfaction are undoubtably interrelated and dependent upon one another. In the past you might have seen them as disconnected or unrelated. We see them as a direct, linear connection; one is directly dependent upon the other. This means that first you have to manage Associate Satisfaction, then you can manage Customer Satisfaction.

In the book *Nuts: Southwest Airlines Crazy Recipe for Success,* Herb Kelleher, CEO of Southwest Airlines, shares his philosophy on the priority of Customers and Associates. He says that the Customer comes second, and the Associate comes first. For the purpose of the organization, the Customer is first because to serve the Customer is the organization's sole purpose. But in order to fulfill the Customers' needs, the organization must first manage the Associates' situation. Southwest Airlines understands that.

Southwest Airlines is not putting Customers down. They are saying that the organization cannot do its number-one job— satisfy Customers—unless Associates are first satisfied. Customers who are disrespectful of SWA Associates are escorted off SWA planes, because Associate Satisfaction is a priority and disrespect creates an unsatisfactory working environment.

Does the leadership of your organization tolerate disrespectful behaviors toward physicians or Associates? Leadership must first deal with the needs of the work force if they expect the work force to deal with the needs of the Customer.

What the health care work force needs is more recognition and more training so they can do more and be more productive. They need the right kind of leadership, and they need to select the right kind of people to work in a health care organization. You do not need Associates or physicians with a bad attitude. Move the bad attitudes out so others do not have to listen to them anymore and their unhappy attitude does not influence the productivity and attitude of people who want to work hard for patients.

What we are trying to do in the Total Customer Satisfaction strategy is create an organizational culture supported by selection of the right types of people, then nourish these good people with the 3Rs—recognition, reward, and reinforcement—for work well done.

Customers Provide Clues

If the Customer was King, and the king said, "Jump," you would respond, "How high?"

The saying, "Customer is King," comes from Marshall Field, a major Chicago area retailer. Field originally had a women's haberdashery store during the era when no merchant in the United States put price tags on merchandise. People would haggle for everything. You might go into a store and see some lovely gloves. You would pick them up and fondle them, but you had no idea what they cost. So, you would have to ask someone, "How much are these gloves?"

One day a Customer told Fields that it was a little uncomfortable having to ask how much items cost. For Mrs. Got Rocks, merchandise without prices is not a problem. But for most of us, it is a little awkward, and we wish we did not have to go through that experience.

Now, the Customer did not come up and say to Fields, "Why don't you put little stickies with a price on the products." The Customer did not give him the answer. Customers give you clues by stating what they are feeling or thinking. And if you are smart, you will listen and figure out how you can respond to that message.

So, Marshall Fields came up with the idea of putting little signs on sticks that stood by each rack. It was an instant sensation. Everybody told their friends, and masses of people rushed to Marshall Fields' store to see the marked merchandise. As he watched the crowds coming in, he thought to himself, "Little signs? Hmmmm."

Later, Fields coined another phrase, which they still teach to staff people at Marshall Fields Department Stores. It is called, "Give the lady what she wants." Do not tell her why you cannot do it. In order to "give the lady what she wants," Fields Associates learn to "stop thinking that you know it all."

Because health care staff are technically knowledgeable, and they do know a great deal, to "stop thinking that you know it all" will be a new, learned skill. Here is the problem. The more you know, the more you come to trust your gut judgment. When you were young and naive in a career, you asked others how to do this or that. After you learned and gained experience, you found that others were coming to you and asking how to do this or that. Now, you think that you are the expert.

Unfortunately, a room full of experts get to a point that they stop asking the Customer, "Is this the way you would like it?" or "Is this what you would like me to do?" and they start thinking that they already know the answers to the questions.

We are becoming insular in our communications and not tuned in the way we used to be tuned in. Act like your younger, naive self. Reserve judgment. Ask the questions, "How did it go for you today?" and "What could we change to make this even better?"

True Story—The Proof Rock Restaurant

Proof Rock Restaurant, Dixie Rock Restaurants, and Black-eyed Pea Restaurants are owned by the same corporate organization. They are all extraordinarily successful business entities. What makes these organizations different from the hundreds of other competing organizations? Let us start with a picture of the president of the firm with his board of directors—children ages seven to twelve. If you can figure out what seven- to twelve-year-olds want, then you will know where mom and dad will be going for dinner. Do you understand the purpose of this? In other words, the dining preferences of children drive family restaurant choices the way Customer Satisfaction drives present health care Customers to recommend your organization to friends and family.

The Proof Rock Restaurant board of directors meets every ninety days, all expenses paid. Just a couple of days of input are needed. What can a seven- to twelve-year-old tell you about a hospital? This is what they told the president of Proof Rock Restaurant about dining.

They said, McDonald's was losing it. What does that mean, McDonald's is losing it? The kids said, "The games are too simple. I've got a computer, all the kids have a computer, and they give us simple paper games and scratch and sniff stuff," reports one advisor.

What has happened? Sophistication of our children has happened. They want more than simplistic, elementary games. The board went on to say, "You have to have more interesting games."

Management asked the kids for ideas and after fifteen minutes of thinking, this is what the kids offered. "You need to bury a treasure chest somewhere in the community. A real live chest. Put really neat prizes in it. Then you will need to have a map, and give a new clue to the location of the treasure chest every week. That way the kids will keep coming back to get new clues. Forget the 101 Dalmatian toys at McDonald's. We are not coming back 101 times to get little toys, but we will go back five or six times to get new treasure chest clues." They went on to describe the incentive further, "The number one prize in the chest should be a trip to Disney for the whole family."

That is the plan that Proof Rock Restaurant put into effect, and traffic in the restaurant went up 30 percent. Wham! Just like that! Who would have guessed? Did that idea come from some consultant? No, it came from a group of seven- to twelve-year-old Customers.

Is Anybody Listening?

In an article entitled, "Listen Doctors,"[2] Physician Insurers Association reported on the results of their research on common factors contributing to medical malpractice claims. They started by taking just one diagnosis and looking at it in depth. The selected diagnosis was breast cancer, and this is what they found.

Nearly 70 percent of breast cancer cases stemmed from delayed diagnosis of the cancer. They were mostly cases in which the woman herself found a lump in her breast, went to the doctor, and the doctor did not consider the lump to be a problem.

Get this picture. Here is an educated woman. She conducts a self-examination and something is not quite right. Now what does she know? She is not a doctor. But she is an expert on her own body. She knows exactly how it feels. She knows exactly what the densities are.

Now, she goes to the physician, most likely a male physician, and she tries to communicate to the doctor that she does not think this is right, but the "expert" doctor does not tune in. The headline says, "If the physician would listen they could avoid 70 percent of the lawsuits." Wow! The power of listening pays off for the patient and the physician.

Still Not Listening—Another True Story

Here is an example from the *Hawaii Advertiser.* A Honolulu clinical psychologist has been awarded $1,485,000 from Kaiser Permanent for failure to administer a screening that could have detected her breast cancer at an early curable stage.

The woman found the tumor herself, and the doctor failed to listen to what the patient was saying, resulting in more serious damages to the patient. You get the idea. This is real stuff. What seems irrational to the physician and staff is very real and important to the patient.

Here is another story from *Modern Health Care,* "Hospitals Forgetting to Query Customers in Quality Process." Hospitals ploughed ahead and did a lot of quality improvement work, but only 3 percent of hospitals asked the Customer what they would like to see improved. So what were they improving?—only things that the experts thought should be improved; 97 percent of what was being improved was not listed by health care Customers as needing improvement. Meanwhile, expertly managed organizations like Southwest Airlines are asking Customers, "What do you want us to improve next?"

Service Quality Edge

Take a look at this through the patient's eyes. Is it just me or are people driving crazier on the expressways than they were five years ago? Is it just me or is there a degradation of manners and civility?

The results of a survey of 534 senior and middle management executives indicate that 52 percent of the executives thought that service in the booming service economy had gotten better, while 39 percent thought it had gotten worse.[3] Service quality now becomes the greatest competitive weapon you can bring into the organization. Our patients are telling us the same thing. If I walk into your organization and see civility, kindness, and love that transforms Associate work into something truly excellent, your organization will be day-and-night different from society and from all other health care organizations. The experience of other organizations is that if you provide that day-and-night difference, you have a winner. Your Customers will write about it and talk about it, and they are right. It is different.

Here is what they said about it at Southwest Airlines

> *You know the Customer is kind of irrational about some things. If they see coffee stains on the flip down tray, then it means to them that engine maintenance isn't being done right.*

Translation: If I see some dust under the bed in the patient's room, and I complain about cleanliness as some Customers have, what do you think is going on in the patient's head? One thought might be, "Infection control in the operating room is no good."

If that is the way Customers think, not only should we be looking at all the big infection control issues, but we should also be looking at the little stuff that Customers see and understand, because they are going to think poorly about us if they see things being done incorrectly.

If you cannot manage the small stuff, like dust balls under the bed, how can you manage the big stuff? So maybe it is goofy, but even if it is goofy, you still have to respond to it because you do not want patients thinking that way. And if it is not goofy, and there is, in fact, a connection, all the more reason you should be managing the little stuff.

In a way, one does not have to be a great genius to be successful. You just have to listen to those ideas, and then do what you are told. If you are good at being servants to the Customer, you will be successful.

Differentiating Your Organization—A True Story

In closing, here is a true story about Carl Cornelius. Carl lived in a little town about seventy miles south of Dallas. He had a truck stop. One day a guy came into the truck stop in a big rig. The driver asked, "You got any beer?"

Carl said, "No." So off went the driver.

If Carl had been able to say "yes," the cash for the beer would have flown into Carl's pocket. So, Carl figured, if my Customer asked for it and if I had it, it would be a win for my Customer and a win for me. So, Carl asked his county clerk for a liquor license.

The clerk said he couldn't give Carl a liquor license because it is a dry county. Carl started to walk out, when the county clerk said, "Well, there is one way you can get a liquor license. If you had a town, and you voted in a liquor license within the city limits, then you could have one."

Carl asked, "Well, how many people does it take to form a village or town?" The answer was 150. You had to have 150 registered voters to become a town.

Now, there was a total of Carl, his wife, and a couple of guys running the gas pump in the area. But, there were four million people in Dallas, seventy miles away. The one greatest asset that Carl owned was about 4,000 acres of land outside of Dallas that he bought for about 5 cents an acre.

So, Carl put an ad into the Dallas paper offering free acres of homestead land if anyone wanted to come down and live there. Boom! People were down there—150 registered voters signed up to homestead on part of Carl's land, and he incorporated as a town. The town people met, and Carl was elected mayor. The first item of business was the liquor license. This is America. There is nothing impossible here.

Carl said he wanted to create something everlasting, and he also wanted to sell beer and wine in an otherwise dry area. "I just asked the truckers what they wanted, and they told me."

Today, Carl has a bar, a forty-two-foot swimming pool, and a cat fish pond (number-one-rated means of stress relief for men). He has a drive-through window. He has a chapel. He has showers, he has towels, a foot masseuse, and truck-stop chiropractor. He has a golf course. He has a day care center. You know why he has a day care center? For the truckers taking their grandchildren cross-country on summer vacation.

He has a restaurant, and how do you think he decorated the restaurant? He asked the truckers. As a result, he has pine paneling and many heads of dead animals hanging on the walls of the restaurant.

He has a convenience food store, and what do you think he stocks in the convenience store? He stocks the food that truckers ask for. The number-one-selling item for truckers is Vienna Sausage, a miracle of modern chemistry. When they have finished the Vienna Sausage, they will need some dessert. Of course, it would be vanilla pudding.

Carl also has a truck wash. Truck washes at truck stops have added remarkable value. Carl's Corner has become so remarkable that people talk about it. When you are down in the Southwest, Carl's Corner is a famous place.

Suppose there was a hospital that asked people what they wanted, and then delivered. If they couldn't deliver the request immediately, what list would the request be put on so that one year from now, or sometime in the near future, it will get done?

Economics follow Customer service excellence no matter what business you are in. Ask your Customers what they want. They will tell you. Then, do a good job providing it. If you do this across the board in every department in the organization, little by little you will start to transform the organization. No longer will you be like every other hospital, as Carl's is unlike every other truck stop. You will, in marketing terms, differentiate yourself.

One of the first ways you want to differentiate yourself is in courtesy and respect. What a warm, friendly, great place this is going to be. Then you are going to go and ask patients, physicians, and internal Customers for a listing of all the other things that you have not even started to think of.

Japanese television crews have been videotaping Carl's corner so they can teach Japanese people how to deliver Customer service. I worry about that. I do not want the Japanese studying Carl.

Peanut Butter Makes the Point

On the tables in the restaurants at Carl's Corner are salt and pepper and the usual condiments, including Tabasco sauce, A-l, catsup—and a jar of peanut butter. Peanut butter makes the point.

Have you experienced this? You go to a restaurant and they bring you the little basket of crackers and the little basket of stale rolls that you could probably pound a hole through the wall with. Then they bring you this kind of greasy yellow butter, and they bring you a drink. You are still waiting for something better to show up. How many of you would like to have the option of a little peanut butter right there, as an option to put on your roll or cracker if you want? Why is it that the only place you can get peanut butter on the table is at Carl's Corner? Because Carl asked.

Ask your Customers and visitors. You know every visitor is an expert: a lawyer, a contractor, a state legislator. They are people with power. What power or influence could they bring to the equation? What ideas could they provide for you?

ACTION PLAN FOR TOTAL CUSTOMER SATISFACTION

Task 1. Create Happy, Positive, Healthy Communications. With the assistance of the Training and Education Department or the Human Resources Department, develop a sixty to ninety minute training program around the idea of positive, healthy communication, and make it mandatory training and annual refresher training for all Associates.

Identify the specifics of what Associates can say in the presence of patients and physicians and what they cannot say unless they are in a designated problem-solving location such as a manager's office, Human Resources office, and other specifically defined locations in your organization. Include training in body language, appearance, and body movement. Show people how subtle positive communication from staff members can be a blessing in a patient's life. It may be the only communication that patient receives during that day. Why shouldn't it be pleasant and as positive as possible?

One of the reasons you are doing this is for your Customers. But you are also doing this for the whole team. When the whole team stops talking negatively, and you do not hear that negative haranguing all day long, wouldn't it be less of a drag on you? If every day that you came to work was a positive thing—gosh, that would be hard to take! Train your staff to button their lips in certain situations, and vent emotions and problems in a positive, change-oriented way in other appropriate, designated situations. That is what patients want.

Carry this Task one step further and conduct an audit of the type of communications, if any, that are found throughout the organization, including what is hung and written on the walls, in the halls, cafeteria, reception and waiting rooms, restrooms, supply rooms, receiving docks. Everywhere. If there are no communication messages happening, then maybe there should be. And if the messages that are in place are anything less than respectful and motivational, change them.

The other day I visited with a hospital manager in his office. On the wall next to the chair where I was seated was the exploded version of a cartoon. In the cartoon an office worker was portrayed backed up against a wall with a large hardware-type screw protruding through his chest. What kind of message is this? Not the kind that should be found in a health care organization. You might have a few of these hanging around your place.

Task 2. Develop Interpersonal Skills and New Thinking. Provide Associate training for improved interpersonal communication skills with patients and a new attitude of "doing all that is possible" to satisfy patient and physician requests.

There are limits in health care as to what can be done to totally satisfy a Customer. If it is medically possible—it is your responsibility to find a way to achieve it. For example, if the patient needs tea with honey to swallow the medication, then arrange for tea with honey. If the patient needs to see the doctor soon, make it happen.

Improved Associate interpersonal skills are needed to more effectively and empathetically communicate with patients and other Customers, deal with difficult people, and problem solve on-site. It is the responsibility of the organization to provide Associates with communication training. Script standardized responses to frequent patient or physician requests that are unreasonable to accommodate. Train staff on how to deliver these responses and what to do when the responses fall short of what the Customer is willing to accept. Should Associates debate conflicted situations, or should such situations be handled in another manner? If so, how? Show Associates how to respond to frequently encountered situations. Train, train, and train more until they are comfortable and effective in their communication skills.

Yes, training will take time and some money, but not as much as you might initially think. The payoff will be in improved Customer and Associate Satisfaction as staff feel better equipped to handle a variety of challenging situations confidently and successfully.

In addition to effective communication skills, Associates must learn to comfortably probe for clues from Customers that provide insight into how to create a more satisfying and exceptional experience while visiting your facility. It is more than a sincere, "May I help you?" or, "How can I help you?" It is the use of thoughtful, leading questions that help patients express to you how to make their visit most enjoyable. The following questions represent a starting point for probing for small ways to offer additional, value-added services:

- What time of day do you usually take your medicine? *Consideration:* People who routinely take medication usually take it on a schedule. Disruption of this simple routine can create significant chaos in their lives, although such a small and temporary change may not seem to be an issue to us. Attempting to maintain a medication schedule as close as possible to the one to which the patient is accustomed sends a positive, caring, value-centered message. When health care staff make special accommodations for Customers, even little ones, be sure to let the Customer know it in a kindly manner. If patients and physicians do not know that you have put extra effort into the experience, then you will not get those extra "brownie points" that add up over time and help nourish business growth.

- Is there any approach that makes it easier for you to take your medicine? For example, a spoon full of sugar to make the medicine go down. *Consideration:* Accommodating helpful health care aids is a way of demonstrating care and making health care management easier for everyone involved.
- Are you in need of hyper-allergenic pillows, towels? *Consideration:* Additional comfort factors.
- Would you like us to hold telephone calls or visitors after a certain hour? *Consideration:* Interruptions can be disruptive and counter-effective to the healing process. Yet this is a personal decision that requires each patient's input. Do not assume you know how patients want visitation handled.
- How often would like us to update family members on your progress? *Consideration:* Frequent communication reduces anxiety for family members, but too frequent communication is nonproductive for staff and can be agitating to recipients. Let the Customer help direct an appropriate frequency of updates to their family and visitors.

Create a standardized list of personal need questions that the patient care team can use for exploration with each patient. The list will be different for each nursing unit or delivery team. Questions that are appropriate for ortho or rehab patients will not be appropriate for cardiac patients, and so on. Nonetheless, there are some questions appropriate for each unit or patient type, and standardization of these questions assures that you are doing as much as possible for each patient.

Training is also needed for effective communication in the following circumstances:

- How to advise a patient or physician politely that you cannot accommodate their exact request.
- How to address and deal with angry, disrespectful, or difficult patients, visitors, and physicians.
- How to negotiate an acceptable solution to a difficult Customer problem.
- How to praise patients and motivate them to continue desirable behaviors.
- How to recognize unacceptable staff language and behaviors, along with a set of guidelines against which Associates can test any question or issue that might arise.
- Where and how Associates should voice concerns or problems.
- Seventeen things never to say in the presence of a patient.

  You don't look so good today.

  Whoops!

  This is my first time.

  I can't believe this.

  It is just not possible.

  No one does it this way, but . . .

  Too bad. Better luck next time.

  The doctor is not available.

  Our policy is . . .

The legal department (or administration) won't let us do that.

I am going to lunch now, I will finish this when I get back.

Wow! That looks different!

Little Lady . . .

Dude . . .

Honey . . .

Oh, it does not really hurt that much, now does it?

Sweetheart . . .

Task 3. Develop a Patient Preference Card. Information that the patient care team collects upon arrival of the patient, otherwise known as the "More than May I Help You?" questions, are to be incorporated in the patient preference card, which becomes a part of the patient's chart and automated patient information records used for future needs.

Adapt the idea of a Customer/patient profile as used by Four Seasons Hotels and other leading Customer-oriented hospitality organizations. Admittedly, it will require an investment in technology, since most automated health care systems were not designed with an integrated flow of information in mind. For immediate implementation, the "notes" section of the patient chart can serve as the site for this information. When information systems are updated, a special section for patient preferences can be integrated into the system.

Task 4. Adopt an Overserving Customer Philosophy. Make a commitment to overserve. Create an action plan for communicating and training Associates on what it means to overserve Customers. Define where specific limits lie and what staff behaviors and financial limitations Associates must operate within. Provide a smooth and rapid process for Associates to use when the amount of attention or resources required to satisfy a

Customer is beyond their authorized level. Bust the barriers of bureaucracy and time processing. They are slowing down business growth potential.

Task 5. Eliminate Joking Matters. With the management team, identify areas of the organization or behaviors within the organization that have become unfortunate topics of jokes or conversation. For example, broken equipment, silly protocols, and policies that no one follows, and so on, are often the sources of jokes and cutting remarks by Associates.

Your Task is to create an action plan for immediate change of undesirable individual or departmental performances. Change the root cause of the problem. Set a timeframe of thirty days for clean up. The objective is to eliminate negative comments within the walls of the organization. Patients and visitors are to hear nothing but happy, healthy, positive comments wherever they travel within the organization.

Some staff members are known for making razor-like remarks and witty jokes at the expense of other people or functions within the organization. Neither cutting remarks nor underperforming personal or departmental behavior is acceptable. Evaluate the legitimacy of the cutting comments, correct unacceptable behavior, and put a definite stop to unfavorable comments. Human Resources support may be needed if disciplinary behavior is involved. Specific language in the Human Resource disciplinary policy should be developed to put muscle behind this.

Task 6. Create Departmental Service Excellence Improvement Plans. Service Excellence improvement plans are a listing and prioritization of things to be done to the department, the health care process, or supporting elements of the health care experience that will result in an improved or enriched Customer experience. To create such a plan, each department leader is to install a process for continuously collecting thoughts, comments, and ideas from patients and visitors regarding how to make the health care experience more satisfying. Data collection takes place via a combination of formally structured and organized communications with patients, and an array of informal approaches including naive listening to what patients say directly to staff, family, and visitors.

Formal data collection is conducted by a small team of three to five departmental staff who are skilled at interpersonal relations and specifically trained on how to approach patients and visitors to collect their input in a pleasant, nonbusiness-like manner. This is a skill that eventually all staff will learn and use routinely.

Specially trained staff meet monthly with twelve to fifteen patients or more, depending on the volume of Customers and visitors served by the department. In a casual environment they talk about ideas for improving the department and their impressions of the total health care experience. No idea or comment is too simple, silly, or impossible to consider. Some of these sessions take place in the format of a focus group, but most occur in casual conversation. Some organizations incorporate this function as a part of the discharge process. *Warning:* If you choose to make this activity part of the discharge process, beware of rushing patients through these questions as you would other pieces of discharge information. The result will be disappointing, as patients are anxious to depart the hospital and will not necessarily give the kind of thought to the issue that they otherwise might have given.

A listing is made of all ideas and comments received. Ideas that can easily be implemented are immediately undertaken and assigned to someone. Those requiring more problem-solving effort are referred to the Do-It-Group (DIG) or other rapid problem-solving process that your organization uses. Repetitive ideas, which are the same idea offered by several people at different times, are noted as such because they represent the power of many Customers' voices and should be given higher priority.

Result: Each department in the organization is implementing a minimum of two new ideas or improvements per person annually for a cumulative impact of 1000 or more ideas implemented each year in an organization that employs 500 people. These are improvements that are important to your Customers, from whom the ideas or problems to be solved originated. As a special note, no new staff or work hours are added to carry out this Task. It is simply a new way of viewing each job; all Associates are now responsible for contributing ideas for improvement as a part of their job design.

Task 7. Analyze Associate Attitudes and Opinions. Associate Attitude and Opinion Surveys bring out the otherwise unspoken feelings and thoughts of the Associate population—knowledge of which is critical to effective executive leadership. Associate Satisfaction mirrors Customer Satisfaction. Without satisfied Associates there will be no satisfied Customers.

To get a handle on the level of Associate Satisfaction within your organization, review the results of your most recent Associate Attitude and Opinion Survey results. If the information is more than twelve months old, it is time to retake the organization's pulse. How satisfied are your Associates? Make no assumptions.

Attitude information that is less than twelve months old will probably still reveal the *hot spots,* or areas where Associate dissatisfaction is greatest, unless some remarkable changes have been made in the interim. These hot spots represent opportunities for significant, rapid, and positive change in Associate Satisfaction.

Where Associate Attitude and Opinion Surveys report some level of dissatisfaction in the organization, the question must be asked, "How significant is the dissatisfaction at your organization compared to the normal level of Associate dissatisfaction at comparable organizations on like topics?" The investment in the normative comparison data bank pays off right here. If the survey data being collected within your organization represent only internal organizational trends and show no comparative data, you have only half the picture. With half the information, assumptions must be made, and it is likely that errors in executive decisions will occur.

For example, no Associate population rates their compensation and benefits program as exceptional. With the help of a normative comparison you can judge whether your Associates are relatively more or less satisfied than most on this issue. The comparison puts your organization's responses into perspective, making it possible to make better executive decisions.

If your Associates are not entirely satisfied with the compensation and benefits program but they are more satisfied than Associates at comparable organizations, there is probably no need to invest great sums of money into those programs at this time. Some level of dissatisfaction on some issues will always be "normal." Without normative comparisons you cannot tell when the alarm bell should ring. Hence the value of comparable databases.

If a dramatically negative picture presents itself in the Attitude and Opinion Survey results, immediate work must be undertaken to resolve the causes of the agitation. Do not be surprised to find that what you thought was an acceptable Associate pulse is actually a rather nervous and somewhat agitated one. And do not underestimate the importance of negative Associate responses. You have given Associates an opportunity to speak. They have. Now you must listen and respond.

Great Customer Satisfaction comes only from happy Associates. It is important that the organization be involved continuously and actively in upgrading, updating, and improving Associate issues.

NOTES

1. Ron Kotulak and Jon Van. "Doctors', Nurses' Small Talk Can Be Bad Medicine." *Chicago Tribune*, August 12, 1995.
2. Physician Insurers Association. "Listen Doctors." Chicago Tribune, July 1, 1990.
3. "Teller Fee Backlash." *USA Today*, May 14, 1995.

Chapter
EIGHT

Building the Customer Satisfaction Team

If we can get all the imagination, creative ideas, observations, info feedback from Associates and patients and visitors to leadership, we will have all the answers we need to be the number-one rated organization in Customer Satisfaction.

—John Schwartz

Customers are not simply a source of ideas, they are the number one source of ideas. Think about it. How many managers do you have in your organization? Fifty or maybe 150? How many Associates do you have? Five hundred or maybe 5000? How many Customers will you serve in this one year alone? Five hundred or maybe 50,000 or more in inpatient, outpatient, and ER services.

The number of patients served is a large multiple of the number of Associates on payroll, and all those patients have family members and friends who also will experience your organization as they visit and call upon friends and family under your care. They all have ideas. Ideas that could help your organization.

New American Hospitals found that when they asked Associates for ideas, Associates would give them ideas to the tune of about one idea per person; 1100 Associates on payroll would generate about 1100 ideas each time a campaign for ideas was initiated. What would happen if you asked your Customers for ideas? What if there was a form in every waiting room with a message from the CEO on it stating the organizational quest for excellence and soliciting ideas on how to better improve the service provided?

Figure 8.1 demonstrates the power of ideation in Customer Satisfaction management and profitability. It is a graphic picture of the number of ideas generated and implemented at Holy Cross Hospital in the period of time between August 1993 and January 1996.

Notice that in a relatively short period, just thirty months, over 4500 ideas were implemented. These are not just ideas on a sheet of paper. They are ideas that were generated, processed, approved, and fully installed in the organization. With an Associate database of less than 1000 people, this translates to more than 4.5 ideas implemented per Associate in a period of thirty months, a little more than two implemented ideas per person each year.

ANALYSIS OF IDEATION: POINTS OF INTEREST

The situation at Holy Cross Hospital, which is similar to that of numerous other New American Health Care Organizations, represents a number of points of interest to executives.

Direct Relationships. Increased ideation equals increased Customer Satisfaction equals increased revenue and increased cost savings. There is a direct relationship between the number of Associate ideas implemented *and* the increase in Customer Satisfaction ratings *and* the increase in tangible savings generated for the organization. Notice that it took only several hundred implemented ideas in order to gain substantial improvement in Customer Satisfaction ratings. At the same time that these ideas were being implemented, any costs associated with implementation of the ideas were offset by the tangible return on investment on other ideas relating to improving system and work operations, reducing waste, and so on. As the number of ideas that are implemented increases, Customer Satisfaction increases, and tangible, bankable return on investment dollars increase.

Short Period of Time. It took a relatively short time, only seven months, from September 1993 to April 1994, to move the organization's

Figure 8.1. Impacts of Ideation at Holy Cross.

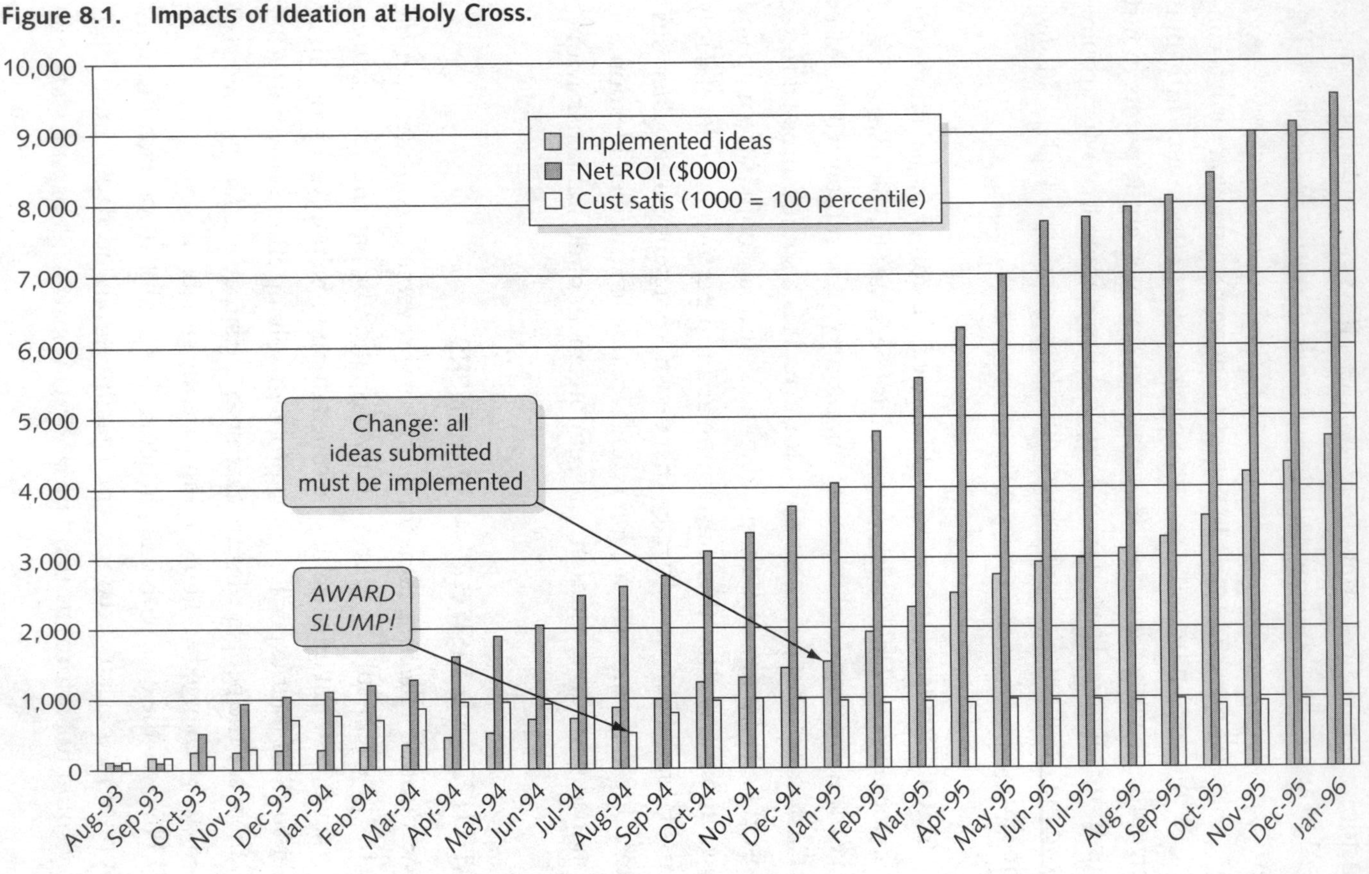

Customer Satisfaction ratings from the thirteenth percentile in September 1993 to approximately the seventieth percentile in April 1994. (Refer to Figure 8.1.)

In the following four-month period, Customer Satisfaction ratings continued to move up from the seventieth percentile to the ninety-fifth-plus percentile—another increase of over twenty-five percentile points in just four more months. These statistics support the opinion that when you remove the irritations, Customers will quickly respond with higher Satisfaction ratings.

Staying Power of Ideation. Top-rated Customer Satisfaction performance levels at Holy Cross Hospital have been sustainable over a period of years. It is not unusual for an organization to make substantial increases in Customer Satisfaction ratings. However, it is also not unusual to see those ratings dip significantly and demonstrate a sawtooth pattern up and down monthly rather than sustaining at a top performance level. Holy Cross Hospital has demonstrated that they have staying power. Their sustained top Customer Satisfaction ratings are due to sustained ideation and sustained reward, recognition, and reinforcement of desirable behaviors.

PATIENTS AND VISITORS AS PARTNERS

In addition to collecting ideas for service improvement, consider opening up the problem-solving process to participation by patients and visitors. Those who submit an idea may be called upon to help solve a problem or offer some of their expertise in the problem-solving effort. Why not? After all, these are the people who are closest to the situation. They know what needs to be changed and how to improve the situation.

This was the case with one particular hospital that was rich in values but poor in the bank account. Their facility surely needed painting, but they could not afford the paint or labor. Unknown to hospital staff, one visitor to the hospital was a paint contractor. While visiting his wife in the hospital he remarked to the staff, "You know, you need to paint this place."

The Associate handed the visitor a 3C card and kindly asked him to put that comment on the card in writing. "Maybe that will help get it painted," she said half-heartedly to the visitor.

Administration received the visitor's suggestion to paint the facility and responded with a note saying, "Thank you for your idea. You are surely correct, but we cannot afford to paint the building."

To make a long story short, the paint contractor wrote back to hospital administration, and in the ensuing interaction with the hospital, which was possible only because they were open to the idea of the Customer as a partner with the hospital, the entire hospital was painted by painting contractors and laborers, many of whom were thankful for what that hospital had done for them or their family members. Discontinued paint supplies were donated by the local painting contractors association, and the final product was a refurbished facility.

If you do not ask for creative answers to problems, you will not know whether there is a reasonable solution.

MAJOR LEAGUE PLAYERS

As in any major league event, there are specific role assignments and responsibilities to be carried out by each player if the team is to win the championship. So it goes with major league Customer Satisfaction management. There is a specific role for executives to fulfill, a different role for managers, and still a different role for Associates to play. Each role is equally important in winning Customer Satisfaction results.

Executive Role

Executive roles and managerial roles are frequently confused. Executives assume the work that managers should be responsible for, and in the meantime do not attend to what their executive duties truly are. This confusion is not entirely the fault of executives. For the most part they do not know what their executive role should be. They have been promoted from managerial ranks and see their responsibilities as those of a super manager. If we can clearly distinguish what the executives' role is in Customer Satisfaction management and leadership, and then hold them accountable for that role, managers will have a greater probability of fulfilling Customer needs.

Executive behavior centers around the following responsibilities.

Establish Big Hairy Audacious Goals (BHAGs). Executives are responsible for establishing organizational goals and breaking them down into department-specific, measurable goals that then become the responsibility of department leaders to meet or exceed. In the absence of organization goals, department leaders will operate goalless, and status quo performance levels are the likely result. Executives then wonder why they cannot get Customer Satisfaction levels to a more desirable level.

Barrier Busting. Executives have the position power, political power, and opportunity frequently needed to break down barriers getting in the way of a manager's best efforts to exceed goals. Some barriers take greater political clout and authority to bust than what a manager reasonably has to offer. Enter the executive—not to take over the work and do the manager's job, but to make it possible for the manager to succeed, to remove the barriers that are getting in the way of the manager's effort to make progress.

Executives—think of yourselves as the offensive line of the football team—keeping opponents out of the way of teammates rushing to make a touchdown or achieve an organization goal, smoothing political differences at the executive level that trickle down and generate factions among department leaders.

Reward, Recognize, and Reinforce. References to the 3Rs (reward, recognition, and reinforcement) have repeatedly been made throughout this book. So much so, that I am growing a bit tired of hearing about it myself. The point is that reward, recognition, and reinforcement are major keys to motivating and sustaining a new and different mode of behavior—a behavior that delivers exceptional Customer Satisfaction. Without the 3Rs there will be no change in Associate behavior.

In a recent telephone conference, a hospital executive invested several hours talking to me about the need to improve Customer Satisfaction at his organization. In his closing comments he said to me, "I think we already have a good Customer Satisfaction initiative under way." He went on to explain that they had requested that each Associate submit one idea for Customer Satisfaction improvement. These ideas were being routed through their Quality Management person, who was "overwhelmed," as he described her. This initiative was supposed to change their Customer Satisfaction ratings? I do not think so.

Although it was a novel approach for this particular organization and probably one that provided more structure than they were accustomed to, simply requiring one idea per Associate will bring little change unless the missing critical ingredients previously discussed in Chapter Seven are put into place. This organization had no operational Management Action Council (see further on in this chapter, under A System for Processing Massive Ideation) for ideation processing. No reward, recognition, and reinforcement component to motivate Associates. There were no tracking and accountability measures in place to see where ideas were being generated and where they were not. There was no infrastructure. This executive's request, or even command, for ideation is going to go nowhere.

If this sounds like your organization, pause and realize that the intention is honorable, but not all the pieces are in place. Reread earlier sections of this book, following the prescriptions precisely, then try implementing massive ideation. The results will be greater.

If you still are not getting great results, use the following performance improvement checklist in Exhibit 8.1 to be sure that you have all the pieces in place.

Exhibit 8.1. *Performance Improvement Checklist.*

- ☐ Are there specific guidelines on how to submit a DIG idea?
- ☐ Have all Associates been trained in how to use the DIG format?
- ☐ Has the MAC been thoroughly trained in how to manage the flow of ideas, trouble-shoot, communicate to submitters, communicate to executives, regulate the types of ideas generated, and so on?
- ☐ Is there a recognition, reward, and reinforcement program in place?
- ☐ Are there a Socialization Action Council and a Communication Action Council effectively in place?
- ☐ Do Associates have a common base of knowledge of what excellent Customer Satisfaction looks like? How to think in terms of excellent Customer Satisfaction? How to make decisions in terms of excellent Customer Satisfaction?
- ☐ Is there a means for tracking the return on investment of ideation and where ideation is being generated from?

Install Structure that Challenges Department Performance Levels. Establish protocols among departments that require the weaker performers to buddy with top performers to create action plans for competitive performance improvement. Make a game of it. A serious game.

Consistently poor performers might receive the "Pink Flamingo" award symbolizing their less than attractive performance. (Remember the pink plastic yard ornament flamingos?) Pink Flamingo awards are typically traveling awards. They go from department to department, residing with the poor performer for the given period. The beauty of such an award is that it makes a precise point—that the department's performance was not up to expected standards. At the same time, the negativism of highlighting poor performance is salvaged by the humor in the award. This idea is adapted from Domino's Pizza, the nation's largest retail pizza provider.

At Domino's Pizza Corporate Headquarters, there are several banks of elevators to carry staff up and down the many stories of brick and mortar in their high-rise corporate office building. Leadership at Domino's expressly programmed one elevator to be exceedingly slow. Associates know that this is the slowest elevator in existence. Rather than take this tortuously slow elevator, staff walk up and down stairwells. The point of the story is that each month the world's slowest elevator is named for the Domino's Pizza store with the poorest performance statistics—an unfortunate acknowledgment that is made companywide, but done so in a humorous way.

When less than great news has to be delivered, humor will help balance organization morale. Although poor performance is not a laughing matter, lightening up on how the message is delivered helps make it possible for staff to regroup and go forward.

Active Participation in Improving Customer Satisfaction. Executives who dictate that greater Customer Satisfaction performance results must be achieved but who personally remain remote, slightly involved, and somewhat distant, rarely see achievement of their goals. The reality is that active participation is easy to agree to, but more difficult to carry out. However, executives who are able to fulfill their commitment to participate actively at the levels prescribed in this book undoubtably experience the success that results from their investment of time and effort.

Manager's Role

The manager's role in Customer Satisfaction management is operationally focused. These are the people directly involved with selecting, training, and motivating the Associates who deliver the service to Customers. These are the people making needed changes in work systems to improve results. It is the responsibility of the managers to achieve organization goals that are assigned to them.

To be successful as a manager, the following skills and behaviors are required.

Assure that Departmental Goals Are Reasonably Achievable. Work to understand what performance levels executives want from your department, and then communicate, discuss, and help executives understand what is reasonable to expect. Do not agree to performance goals that are unrealistic to achieve. At the same time, open your ears and mind, and listen to why new, and perhaps previously unthinkable, goals must be established. Whatever the final goals are, regardless of your personal opinion, managers must, without exception, embrace them as their personal goals if they are to have any probability of achieving them.

"New thinkers" are valued managers who are open to learning, doing, changing, and constantly evolving. That is not to say that these "new thinkers" accept totally unreasonable objectives handed down from their supervisor, but rather that they are effective communicators and educators of the executives to whom they report.

Most important, the manager's role centers around problem solving. People who can and do find a solution to every situation are effectively managing their job, career, and goals.

Interpret Work Situations in Light of Customer Satisfaction Standards. Associates learn from managers who teach. And managers teach via words and deeds. Tough situations requiring management's interpretation present themselves daily. For example, when a patient complains of an unsatisfactory meal, what the manager does and says will be a teaching moment for observing Associates. As a manager, do you want to teach Associates to interpret the situation in purely economic terms—a substitute meal would mean additional costs, and because the organization is cost conscious, providing another meal would not be a good decision? Or, do you want to teach Associates to interpret the situation as an opportunity to create great Customer Satisfaction by replacing the meal with another one and not charging the patient for either meal, thus preserving and fortifying the Customer relationship?

Questionable situations that are consistently and favorably interpreted as Customer Satisfaction opportunities teach Associates how to view pri-

orities, and how they should think when making decisions. The more often managers can use daily situations to demonstrate the Customer Satisfaction priority, the more deeply rooted desirable Customer Satisfaction behaviors will become in Associate behaviors.

To teach a new way of thinking or prioritizing, one must demonstrate how to conduct the act. If the goal is to teach Customer Satisfaction thinking, one must *demonstrate* effective thinking as a way of helping others understand the situation and why the selected actions were undertaken. Teaching a new thinking process is most effectively done by sharing your own thinking process; that is, sharing what considerations you weighed while evaluating the situation—what options were considered, and why the decision was made as it was. It is a reality-based, informal learning process.

Sharing the thinking behind Customer Satisfaction decisions should become a routine part of conversations in every department. The more frequently staff are involved in dissecting the thinking process behind the manager's decision making, the more able they will be to make the decisions that you as manager want them to make.

Initiate and Support Ideation and Implementation. Top-performing organizations require participation of all Associates in ideation and implementation of improvements. Ideation is an expectation, not a request of staff. These organizations know that without the support and participation of Associates, efforts to become top-performing organizations cannot be achieved.

Reinforce Customer Satisfaction in Real-Time Behaviors. As a manager, when you see or hear staff making the right decisions, or behaving in an exceptional way, reinforce it—right then. Behaviors that are reinforced will be repeated. If you want the behavior to reoccur again and again, communicate your approval of the behavior to the Associate. Praise her publicly. Present her with a token award, make reference to her in a

meeting of peers or other Associates, note the situation in a story in the newsletter. Be creative in your efforts to recognize, reward, and reinforce the desirable behavior.

Participate in, Support, and Approve Routine Ideas for Customer Satisfaction Improvement. Recognition, reward, and reinforcement should not be for exceptional situations only. High Customer Satisfaction performance levels that are stabilized at top levels and continue to represent top Customer Satisfaction performance should not go unrecognized. Celebrate quarterly performance levels that remain exceptional. Let Associates know of your appreciation for the hard work invested in maintaining top performance levels. Do not take exceptional performance levels that have become new standards for granted.

Be a Role Model. Without exception, managers must personally behave in an exemplary manner with respect to Customer Satisfaction decisions and behaviors. "Do as I say and not as I do" buys no respect for a manager and generates no buy-in of desirable behaviors by Associates. What others see a manager doing speaks more loudly than any commands a manager could possibly issue.

Let Customer Satisfaction priorities drive all behaviors and decisions.

Coach the Team. Guide and redirect others who are performing at less than acceptable levels. Be kind yet firm and direct in your instruction. Tell Associates, show them, and then let them do as a means of learning. Be patient with most efforts to learn and intolerant of repetitiously unacceptable behavior.

The coaching style that you choose to use will be as individual as you are. However, all effective coaching styles include components of motivation, teaching, practice, discipline and reward.

Associate Role

Of the executive, manager, and Associate trio, Associate roles are most crucial in delivering top Customer Satisfaction, as Associates most frequently and directly interact with the greatest number of Customers. Effective Associate performance comes from effective management and leadership performance.

Associates of top-performing Customer Satisfaction organizations consistently perform in the following ways.

Naive, Active Listeners. Associates are tuned into the comments and questions of patients, physicians, and visitors. They are actively looking for Customer Satisfaction opportunities. Questions from patients and visitors serve as prompts. Staff should stop and think, "Why did they ask that?" when a visitor or family member poses a question. The answer to that question is a prompt to make a change or improvement that will eliminate that question or issue for the future.

Use Rapid Problem-Solving Processes. Top-performing organizations have an infrastructure in place for rapid problem solving by Associates. We recommend the Do-It-Group (DIG) process, but any rapid problem-solving process that reduces bureaucracy and elapsed time, supports organization values, and serves Customer needs will be effective.

Redirect Colleagues When They Stray Off Track. Customer Satisfaction is everyone's responsibility. The most effective retargeting of straying Associate performance comes from credible communicators among the Associate population. These are Associates who talk straight and true to co-workers and colleagues about redirecting poor performance. A colleague's empathy and call for corrective behavior is frequently more effective than directives issued from management.

Embrace Happy, Healthy, Positive Attitudes. Behaviors and language are contagious. Happy, healthy attitudes are the only ones acceptable at top-performing organizations. Problem solving is viewed as a constructive process to be undertaken with distinctive steps, roles, and positive expectations. Bad attitudes are counseled, rehabilitated, or eliminated from the organization. There is zero tolerance for good attitudes turned sour.

GENERATING IDEAS FOR PERFORMANCE IMPROVEMENT

Associates within your organization are the first-line resource for ideas for improving performance. Each day Associates struggle to perform their work fighting disease and death, hampered by bureaucracy and inefficient systems designed and developed by people who no longer use them. Out of these frustrations come the motivation to make change and the vision of what the change should look like. Each idea for improvement touches a piece of the work system that eventually has an impact on the patient.

Each Customer complaint that an Associate experiences is the potential source for a new idea or solution to an existing problem. The challenge is to collect and identify problems efficiently, then translate the problem into a solution—an improvement. Each time an Associate says, "I wish they would . . . ," an opportunity for the birth of an idea has been created or a solution to a problem has been identified. Each time an Associate says, "Wouldn't it be great if . . ." or "It would be so much better if . . ." another solution is identified. Take advantage of this valuable information. Collect it. Act on it.

A second source of ideas to improve work and the service system are patients, visitors, and physicians—the people rubbing up against and experiencing the system first-hand daily. Every Customer complaint is an opportunity to improve your service and system. But these opportunities must be captured in order to be processed.

The third source of ideas is something we fondly refer to as *Operation Bandit,* or the borrowing of the best ideas implemented by the competition and other excellently operated organizations. In some respects, all organizations experience many of the same challenges; for example, how to move information quickly through the organization, how to motivate workers, and how to reduce costs and improve quality. Do not waste time reinventing solutions to these issues. Use Operation Bandit to put solutions into place quickly, then move ahead to address more complex problems unique to your business.

For maximum effectiveness in identifying problems and solutions, department leaders need to learn the art of observation and adaption. Observe excellence in the world around you, and adapt concepts from other operations into your business world. Some call this benchmarking, but benchmarking is a formal approach to learning from other organizations. Operation Bandit is a way of consistently evaluating what you see around you, and actively applying it to your business—a real-time, highly active approach to ideation and performance improvement that occurs day after day in every aspect of living. For example, when you go to the grocery and see the retailer using bar-code technology contained on the plastic card of the Customer's key chain for purposes of rapidly identifying Customer banking information, credit limit, and types of approved payment, for starters, you might think, "Couldn't we use this same type of approach with a few small changes to capture and retrieve patient information upon admission to the hospital? Could we not use this same technology and approach to collect and retrieve basic patient contact data, health history, past test results, or even personal preferences while in the hospital?" Operation Bandit focuses on observing progress that is occurring all around you, and adapting those ideas to your organization.

Barrier Busting—Why People Do Not Offer Ideas

Why is it that some organizations successfully capture and use Associate ideas and intellectual capital, and others want to but are unsuccessful? To release the thousands of ideas held captive in the hearts and minds of Associates, two organizational dynamics must simultaneously be in place:

First, the organization must be free of fear, that is to say that Associates must feel comfortable submitting ideas for improvement. Many organizations are fear-filled, thus any potential for ideation and innovation are paralyzed. Second, there must be a reward system for those who participate in ideation generation and management.

Fearless Organization. To create a fearless organization, one must drive the present fear out of the organization. The fear referenced here is Associates' fear of rejection of their ideas or fear of retaliation and criticism from supervisors who may interpret Associate ideas as a criticism or threat.

To drive this fear out, routine and frequent communication from the CEO and management are required. The message must be consistent, "We value your ideas. We want your ideas, now." It is not enough for management to say that they want ideation. In a culture that has never supported this type of behavior, only a few brave souls would test such a new message. To build Associate trust and confidence in the message that "we want your ideas," management must actively support implementation of Associate recommendations for improvement, even when management feel that there is a different, better way of solving the problem.

As management learns how to loosen up control of ideation and implementation and share "how to's" with staff, fear within the organization will dissipate. Without aggressive implementation of 90 to 95 percent of Associate ideas, however, the new culture and behaviors surrounding ideation will not take hold.

A Reward System for Ideation Management

The 3Rs of recognition, reward, and reinforcement are essential for achieving and supporting Associates' participation in ideation for performance improvement. Without an incentive, few people will go the extra mile and take the risk of suggesting something different in operations. They are thinking, "What is in this for me? Why should I bother to go through this process just to be told, 'I don't think so.'" Recognition, reward, and reinforcement schemes bust through these historic barriers and make it worthwhile for Associates to try the new philosophy. The 3Rs scream, "It is worth it! Just once, give it a shot!"

Associates are thinking, "I have always thought this would be a good idea. Now, I will take the time to fill out the forms and tell someone who cares about the idea. At the same time, I will get a raffle entry to win that little TV. Yea, I think this is worth it."

However, to be effective, the 3Rs must be frequent, plentiful, sometimes formal, often casual and spontaneous, and provided by top management as well as by peers and department management. 3R schemes that lack any one of these characteristics are considerably weaker than those that include all of them. For more information on how to build a 3R program, see the *Recognition Action Guide* available through Management House.

Keeping Ideation Momentum High

The degree of Associate participation in ideation and implementation is predictable. Given the CEO's and top management's active support and attention, initially there will be a flood of hundreds of ideas from Associates. Following the initial flood of ideas, a lull in the quantity of Associate ideation typically occurs unless bold incentives are designed into the system. It is a direct relationship: The more you ask for ideas, the more ideas you will receive. The more you recognize, reward, and reinforce people for the new behavior, the more they will repeat it.

The following approaches have proven successful in maintaining a high ideation flow on Customer Satisfaction within the organization.

Integrate Ideation into the Compensation Structure. When individual changes in Associate performance are needed, the most rapid and effective way of motivating Associates is to tie new behaviors and performance levels to compensation.

It is not uncommon to find minimum standards of ideation required from all staff members at the most excellently managed organizations. For example, the Disney organization, among others, requires Associates to contribute a minimum number of ideas during each performance evaluation period in order to be eligible for pay increases. It is a basic requirement for additional pay consideration.

If ideation and problem-solving skills and behaviors are now expected from all Associates, minimum standards of ideation and implementation performance should be included in each job evaluation. A minimum of two ideas submitted per year for nonexempt Associates is suggested as an early standard of performance, with progressive increases in the number of ideas increasing gradually from two per Associate per year to twelve per Associate per year over the next three-year period. After all, is not ideation part of the intellectual capital that the organization is paying for? It is no longer good enough for Associates to simply possess standard technical competencies. Healthier organizations that will survive and thrive must also develop, nurture, and mine Associate intellectual capital.

Ideation standards for management and executive staff should be higher than for front-line Associates. Six ideas per manager per year is a minimum suggested standard in the first year. Twelve to fifteen ideas per manager per year is the recommended standard in the second and third year of progressive ideation management. Managers are exposed to multiple areas of the business and so have more fertile ground within which to observe and experience aspects of the organization that need improvement.

Further, executive compensation should be tied to the successful generation and implementation of ideation from all Associates under their wing. Performance tied to compensation is a matter of accountability, measurement, and management.

Install Performance Bonus Incentives. Some organizations award bonuses to Associates when the organization has had a surprisingly good fiscal performance period. Although the intent is good, return on investment for dollars spent is not necessarily maximized. An unexpected bonus check that is not directly tied to a particular behavior or performance does not modify, develop, or reinforce future behaviors. Consequently, an unexpected reward that is not tied to a specific behavior or achievement has little impact on the future of the organization but simply provides a short-lived day of pleasure for those receiving it.

For example, business was good this past year, so one hospital president awarded a $200 bonus to all full-time Associates. "Wow! An unexpected check! Manna from heaven," Associates were thinking. They were ecstatic for a day, or maybe a week. Then it was forgotten, the money was gone, and the conversation over coffee went something like this, "I wonder if we will ever get another one of those bonuses."

"I don't know," replies a colleague. "I guess it will depend on what the boss thinks and how business goes."

"Yea."

Contrast that approach to a planned bonus payout directly related to achievement of BHAGs (Big Hairy Audacious Goals), such as substantial Customer Satisfaction improvement ratings. The payout occurs only when the total organization achieves a predetermined BHAG level. Then the conversation over coffee might go something like this.

"That bonus sure came in handy."

" Yea. I wonder what the new goal will be and if we can make it. This goal was tough enough."

"Yea. It was close. I wasn't sure that we would be able to pull it through, but we did."

"Hmmm. Let's find out if there is going to be a new goal and bonus. I hope they don't wait too long to make the announcement. Heaven knows we will have to figure out some way of getting to those new numbers (goals)."

The beauty of the second approach is that it unifies people in their efforts to provide extraordinary service levels so everyone can earn the bonus. By tying a bonus to predetermined, measurable organization performance levels, everyone has a vivid picture of what needs to be done to claim the prize. Strong performers come to the aid of weaker performers, and weaker performers welcome assistance from stronger ones. Consistently poor performers will be made to feel uncomfortable by peer pressure, and over time they will eventually leave the organization if management has not already weeded them out.

When the moment of glory comes and the BHAG is achieved, the organization wins, staff win. There is a unity in celebration that will long be remembered. *Result:* the organization goal is achieved, the memory of the journey is fondly recalled, talked about, enjoyed, and relived for some time, and Associates are motivated to take on the next, higher target of performance.

Utilize "High-Light/Spot-Light" Meetings. The need to keep the spotlight on Customer Satisfaction is a lesson painfully learned by top-performing Holy Cross Hospital. After eleven consecutive months of skyrocketing Customer Satisfaction ratings, Holy Cross Hospital was awarded the prestigious Great Comebacks Award from the American Hospital Association.

During this period of celebration, staff egos rocketed, the organization swelled with pride, and during all the celebrations, they took their eye off the Customer Satisfaction ball. Just for a short while. Present success became a distraction from the work required to earn future success. As quickly as they rocketed to the top, they experienced a dramatic fall in satisfaction ratings. *Lesson:* Never, but never, stop monitoring and adjusting operations for improved Customer Satisfaction.

Following the brief but substantial dip in ratings, Holy Cross recovered to its position as a nationally rated, top Customer Satisfaction health care organization, with a new pledge and game plan to prevent such unfavorable situations from surprising them again. To keep their eye on the ever-moving Customer Satisfaction target, CEO Clement conducts monthly "high-light/spot-light" meetings with management. All department leaders attend.

During these meetings, Customer Satisfaction ratings and weekly performance trends are the sole agenda items. The meeting objective is to "high-light" top-rated departments in Customer Satisfaction—provide them with recognition, reward, and reinforcement for their outstanding performance, and within the same meeting, "spot-light" departments with the worst Customer Satisfaction ratings. An action plan for poorer performing departments is created during the meeting; all department managers contribute ideas and assistance.

"High-lighting" top performers, and "spot-lighting" lesser performers creates several interesting and somewhat opposing dynamics that generate a final energy force that moves department performance in the right direction. First, there is an immediate pulling together of the organization into a unified team attitude. Everyone is ready to support and assist poor performers. At the same time, a second dynamic of a growing intolerance for consistently poor performers is occurring.

Peer pressure stems from the compensation structure that requires the total organization to achieve a predefined BHAG level before a bonus will be paid. It is an all-or-none plan. If all departments meet the organization goal, all Associates get a bonus. If anyone misses the goal, no one gets a bonus. In an all-or-none bonus structure, those who know how to fix Customer Satisfaction problems are energized and motivated to help those without a clue because there is a direct personal payoff for their investment.

Victory Scoreboard. Think of the scoreboard at your local ball park. The scoreboard is there for one primary reason: to broadcast the current standing of the team. It tells observers and players whether their team is winning or losing and by how much, and how much time is left in the game. The Victory Scoreboard for Customer Satisfaction serves the same purpose. It is a source of information on how well the team is performing in Customer Satisfaction management at this particular point in time, and how much time is left in the game or performance period.

Associates of your organization are like members of one big team. When they know what the score is, they know how much more or less they have to invest in order to "win" the game. Customer Satisfaction ratings and supporting details are posted weekly on the Victory Scoreboard as an easy reference for Associates to see how well their department and the organization are performing in the game of Customer Satisfaction management.

The idea of a Victory Scoreboard was first introduced in Dr. Clay Sherman's book, *Creating the New American Hospital: A Time for Greatness* (Jossey-Bass). In summary, a large scoreboard is located in the cafeteria or other routinely used area of the organization. On the scoreboard Associates can see the organization's Customer Satisfaction performance ratings as compared to organization goals. The Victory Scoreboard represents a quick source of easy-to-read information and serves as a conversation-starter and rallying point for action planning by Associates.

Internal Competition. Most people like a good challenge, especially if it is made to be fun and there are payoffs for the winners. One design for effective internal competition is pairing best-performing departments against each other for percentage increases in Customer Satisfaction results. Using percentage increase points as a measurement levels the competitive field among two top performers, and provides an incentive for even greater performance levels.

Each time the Olympics occur, we see new Olympic and world champions. New world records and greater and greater performances in the same fields of sports are achieved. Why is it that new and greater performance records are continuously being set, and who are the people setting these new records?

It is not uncommon for current world record holders to break their own records and establish new performance levels during Olympic events. Why? Because they have trained specifically for the Olympic events and their specific field of competition. They are competing against the best performers in the world, and competition among the best of the best will typically produce greater results than individual competitors have previously achieved. Great performance by one athlete drives greater performance by other athletes, and so on. A self-perpetuating synergy is created. Strong competition is its own motivator.

The same synergistic dynamic will occur when you pair top-performing departments against other top-performing departments and establish a worthy prize for the winner. Great performance by one department or team of departments will drive greater performance by another department or team of departments, and the positive energy from one success feeding upon the other continues as new performance levels for the organization are created.

An Alternative Competitive Structure. An alternative approach to achieving creative competition among top performers is to form teams combining top-performing departments with lesser performers in an effort to achieve a balance within each team. All teams would be structured about the same way in order to achieve initial balance in talent and drag.

This structure creates teamwork and support within each unit as stronger managers and performers move to aggressively assist weaker or poorer performers in the interest of the entire team. The talent and energy of the top-performers might also "rub off" on the lesser performers and help increase overall quality too.

In any competitive environment there must be a prize, a purse, some payoff for the winner. This should come in the form of recognition, reward, and reinforcement by the CEO, one of the most highly valued payoffs, followed by dollars, time off, special awards that participants wear on their uniform, invitations to award programs presented by the CEO, and so on. You can go on and on with creative ideas for recognition, reward, and reinforcement. Be generous. The 3Rs keep the competition for goal achievement hot, and a top Customer Satisfaction rating is worthy of the cost.

Trinity Hospital in Chicago awards a blue ribbon to departments with the highest Customer Satisfaction ratings. This award includes a banner large enough to hang over the entrance to the department. The blue-ribbon team is awarded a reserved table in the cafeteria for the month, along with other perks. Now, what does all that cost? Nearly nothing. What does it do for staff? It instills the pride of achievement and a motivation to do more and do better.

A SYSTEM FOR PROCESSING MASSIVE IDEATION

Ideation is valuable only when ideas are translated into actions that improve performance. Consequently, processing and implementing ideas are equally important as generating them.

Do-It-Groups (DIGS)

DIGs are a standardized and systematic structure for processing Customer Satisfaction improvement ideas and solving problems. The standardized and systematic structure makes the DIG process easy to communicate to Associates, thus creating a common Associate knowledge base of what to expect when an idea is generated. The DIG process is a multidisciplinary, time-bound, problem-solving approach that keeps DIG groups focused, paced, and accountable for implementation and results.

Each DIG has about thirty days to solve its assigned problem. The structure calls for weekly, one-hour meetings for a period of four or five weeks. The four defined steps of the process are

D = Define the problem—what it is and what it is not

O = Outline options or solutions to the problem

I = Implement solutions

T = Track results

DIGs are not only responsible for creating a solution but also for implementing approved recommendations and tracking results to assure that expected results do materialize.

Just-Do-Its (JDIs)

JDIs are work or business improvements that can be implemented by an identified person or job position in the organization without the assistance of a problem-solving process like a DIG. What needs to happen is clear, and the assignment to "Just Do It" is given to the person whose job description is responsible for the core content of whatever the JDI involves.

For example, the construction site at one particular hospital was causing traffic congestion and parking confusion for visitors. It was decided that the addition of specific signage would help the situation. The obvious solution was identified by someone other than the facility management staff, who ultimately would be assigned the JDI to install the signage where needed.

Because the idea was generated by someone other than facility management staff, it was put onto a DIG/JDI form and sent to the Management Action Council (MAC, a central ideation clearing house; see below). The idea did not require further problem-solving work and was acceptable to the organization, so the MAC issued a Just-Do-It to the facility management department, and the recommendation was then implemented. They "Just Did It." See Figure 8.2 for a flow chart of the DIG/JDI processes.

Beware of taking the simple logic of DIGs and JDIs as described in this book and applying it broadly without understanding further administrative details. Tracking, communication, and recommendation guidelines are essential to assuring that the DIG and JDI process will bring desirable results. Extensive discussion on how DIG and JDI processes are implemented organizationwide are available in the *DIG Guide* from Management House.

Figure 8.2. Do-It-Groups and Just-Do-Its: A Flow Chart.

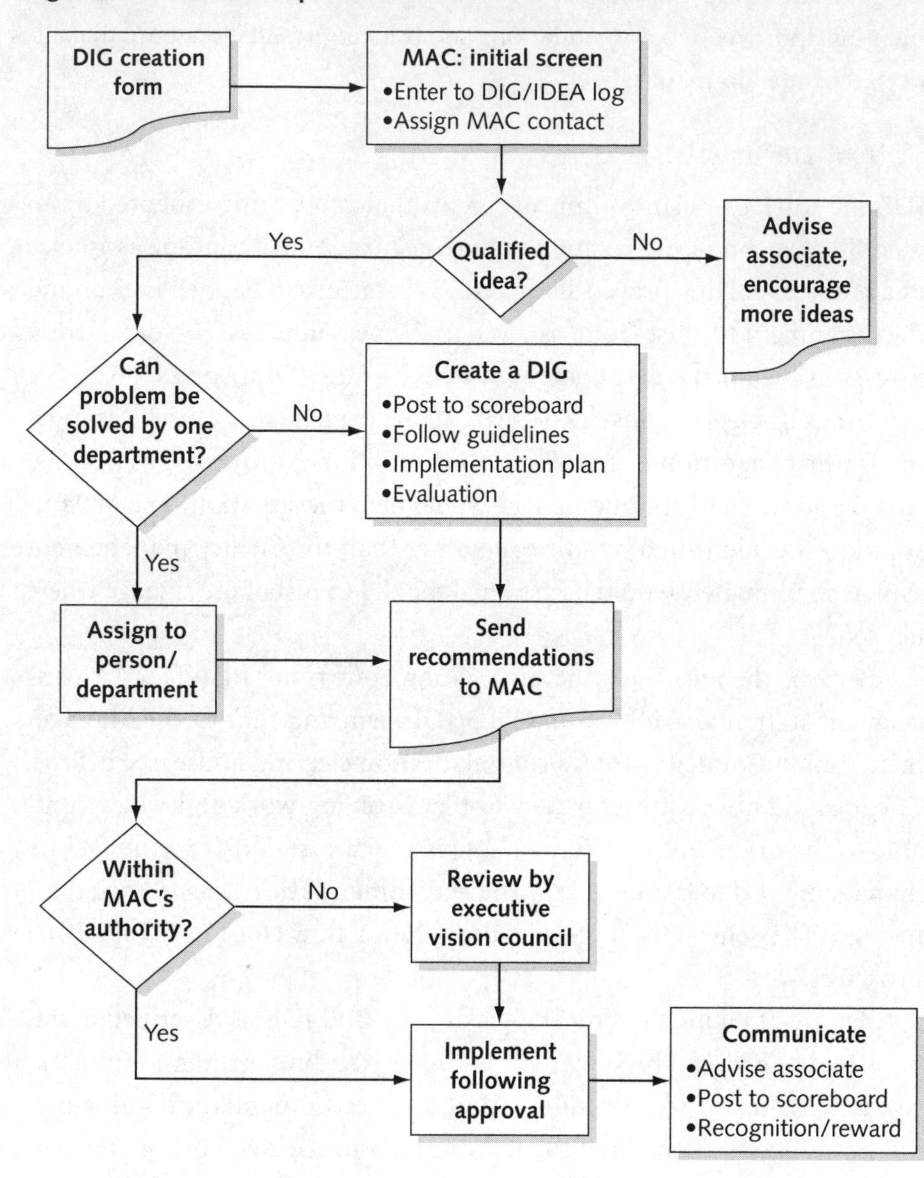

Management Action Council (MAC)

MAC is a central processing unit for organizationwide ideation and implementation. Ideas that relate to operations outside of an Associate's assigned department are submitted to the MAC for processing.

At first glance the MAC might appear to be an additional layer of bureaucracy. It is not. It is a structure necessary to assure the efficiency and effective management of massive ideation. MAC members do not represent additional people to the payroll, or new overhead expenses. They are top-performing department leaders—the cream of the management crop at your organization. Typically, managers assigned to the MAC are people who are thought to be too busy to take on additional responsibilities because you have already overloaded them with extra projects. Knowing that, these are the managers you can count on to get important project work completed on time and in a quality manner. They represent a select few of the management team.

Responsibilities of the MAC are as follows:

Avoid duplicity of work. Assure that no effort is expended on ideas that are duplicates of one another.

Assure proper representation. DIGs that are approved for processing must include representatives from all departments affected by the submitted idea. This is a quality assurance component of the DIG/JDI process, and avoids the dumping of unwanted solutions from department to department.

Manage accountability. Specific roles, such as the DIG Chairperson, are held accountable for management of the DIG process and follow-through of approved implementation plans. Some DIG Chairs are by nature more accountable than others. The MAC is responsible for tracking and reporting the accountability of DIG Chair and DIG member activities. The results of this tracking translate into accountability reports that are shared with respective executives and the CEO. Executives take appropriate coaching and disciplinary action with managers and Associates who are not performing at prescribed levels.

The MAC is not responsible for administering disciplinary activities. It is responsible for tracking performance improvement information, analyzing data, and making recommendations for action to the executive group.

Track ideation and return on investment. If ideation does not generate payoff in the organization, there is no reason to continue supporting it. And if there is payoff, as we know there is, tracking where the return on investment is coming from and to what degree it is growing within the organization is important executive information.

Executives will want to know which people and departments are contributing the most to the return on investment, and in what business areas the greatest number of ideas are being implemented. The tracking function provides this information.

Maintain ideation as a priority in the organization. There are an ever-growing number of priorities tearing at executive shirttails. Maintaining ideation as a priority is a newly learned behavior for executives and managers. Hence, it is easy to slip back into old behaviors and allow ideation to get lost among the many other priorities pressing for attention. It is the responsibility of the MAC to assure that ideation and executive support for it remain in clear view and among top executive concerns.

Communication Action Council (CAC)

Individual behavior is modified by information. Timely, accurate information made available to Associates will generate one level of organizational behavior and performance, whereas lack of information will produce another level of organizational behavior. Staff need frequent and varied types of communication on Customer Satisfaction performance, both for the organization as a whole and for their respective department or subunit.

The primary responsibility of the CAC is to maintain Customer Satisfaction information on the Victory Scoreboard and provide numerous other means of Associate communication on Customer Satisfaction issues. The most effective CACs approach Customer Satisfaction with a wide brush, thus keeping the topic fresh and prominently presented in every aspect of organization living. It is the wide scope of Customer Satisfaction issues that need to be routinely communicated. The CAC can do this through various means.

Promoting Customer Satisfaction stories. Stories of everyday heroes delivering exceptional Customer service need to be promoted as well as stories of extraordinary Customer service events. Unfortunately, the extraordinary stories usually get all the publicity. Be contrarian—recognize everyday heroes as well as extraordinary heroes in Customer Satisfaction stories. Keep the support and reward, recognition, and reinforcement high.

Reporting satisfaction performance goals and current performance levels. Via the Victory Scoreboard, the organization's newsletter, special reports, visuals, graphics, and any other channels of communication you want to add, inform Associates of the status of the organization's progress toward goals. Individual departments' performances in addition to organization-wide performances should be included in the communication. Associates need to know who is doing the work well and leading the pack—the "A" performers—and which departments are pulling down overall organization performance with less-than-goal-breaking achievements.

Information is one source of motivation. When Associates see the scorecard of departmental and organization performances they will make the changes necessary to move the organization in the right direction, provided management and leadership are appropriately performing their roles.

Reporting DIG/JDI topics and status. When hundreds of ideas or improvements are swirling around the organization, it is not uncommon for Associates to think, "I wonder if anyone is working on this particular problem?" A central posting area, which usually coincides with the Victory Scoreboard area, and a DIG/JDI hotline are two means for providing specific DIG/JDI information. Posted information should include the DIG/JDI identification number, brief description of the problem to be solved, chairperson's name and contact information, whether additional DIG members are needed, and names and contact information of current DIG members.

The best Victory Scoreboards categorize the DIGs by Key Business Result (KRA) areas. All Customer Satisfaction DIGs are grouped together, all Economic DIGs are grouped together, and so on, thus presenting a picture of where the greatest number of changes are occurring. Associates can easily reference the Victory Scoreboard to see whether anyone is working on a particular problem, who the chairperson is, and whether additional DIG membership is needed. If the DIG idea they had in mind does not appear on the Victory Scoreboard, they can complete a DIG creation form and forward it to the MAC for processing.

The DIG hotline is an internal telephone line, either automated or manned, and easily accessible by Associates inquiring as to the status of a particular DIG/JDI. Automated systems include a menu of items for accessing various types of data. Use of the DIG/JDI identification is the most direct route for locating a particular DIG/JDI. If the DIG/JDI identification number is unknown, access can be gained via a Key Result Area (KRA) or department.

A last resort for locating a particular DIG/JDI is to contact a MAC member to help locate the information needed, or request a listing of all DIGs/JDIs and corresponding information. All of this information can be accessed via the DIG/JDI hotline.

Presenting words from the source. The single most important accolade that a work improvement can earn is the good word and support of Customers who have sampled the new and improved experience. Testimonials and endorsements from happy Customers say it all.

Many CACs provide video and written endorsements from satisfied Customers as a reinforcement of the value of the process and work being done. An easy-to-do and highly effective format for endorsements is a videotaped discussion with a patient or physician talking about how a particular DIG idea positively affected patient satisfaction, or an Associate endorsing a change in how the material management department processes requests, and the positive impact it has had on Associate work processes or the nursing units.

Think of this communication channel as your in-house cable news network. Keep it amateur yet respectable in quality. The casualness of an amateur approach will make it more entertaining to watch, thereby retaining the attention of more Associate viewers. Play the testimonial videos on a closed-loop basis in the cafeteria where Associates and visitors waiting in food lines can see the vignette. Keep the stories new and refreshed. Reruns lose their panache after two or three presentations to the same audience.

Providing motivational, inspirational, and practical Customer Satisfaction tips. Using the words of your own staff, or perky satisfaction tips from other sources, keep pumping Customer Satisfaction information through the organization. Insert an occasional quote in each piece of executive correspondence to Associates. Include Customer Satisfaction tips on the cover sheet of satisfaction ratings reports, in newsletters, e-mails, screen savers (see below), and other frequently viewed sources.

Small books of inspirational quotes have been top sellers in recent years. People are receptive, even seeking out wisdom, simplicity, and inspiration. Help feed that inner human desire to do good through internal organization communication.

Keeping CAC communication channels open. Various media and channels of communication are needed to get the message across to a diverse Associate population. Notices in newsletters and periodic paycheck stuffers are inadequate for this Task. Customer Satisfaction messages and information need to be delivered to Associates and Customers through various communication channels and with great frequency in order to gain and retain Associates' attention. The following approaches have been blended successfully. Use these and add more of your own. You cannot overcommunicate.

- Customer Satisfaction newsletter column. The Customer Satisfaction column should appear in a prominent place in each edition of the organization's weekly newsletter. It should be authored by an executive to give position credibility to the topic and content. Augment the executive message with articles and stories from contributing Associate authors. Topics can be current satisfaction ratings, tales of star and dog department performers, updates on changes in progress, comments from Customers, and stories of goals successfully achieved or failed (including why). Keep the column newsworthy if you want high readership. Let your passion show.

- Flags and banners representing Customer Satisfaction messages. Colorful banners with simple messages of one, two, or three words representing the mission, values, or goals of the organization can double as esthetic decoration for the facility and Associate reminders of values and mission. Such banners are usually made of silk, have vibrant colors, and are hung within the halls of the organization or Associate work areas. Sometimes the core message of each corporate value is placed on a different colored banner as a way of keeping organization values in front of Associates and visitors. Sometimes the message is a simple work of inspiration or emotion. These banners add color and energy to the otherwise conservative, and often dull facility, while simultaneously providing a constant reminder of what the organization stands for.
- Neighborhood news. When good things happen, and satisfaction ratings are up, use local newspapers to headline the story and provide free marketing. Stories of high Customer Satisfaction send a positive, powerful marketing message to the community, and reinforce Associates for the good work they have done.
- Screen savers. Computer screens are common in every department. Most of them sport screen savers with little flying toasters or neon fish swimming around. Change the message. Seize the opportunity to communicate and remind Associates of Customer Satisfaction tips in a colorful, artistic, and interesting screen saver design. See your Information Services department for assistance in designing custom screen savers that reinforce the priority of Customer Satisfaction.

- Marketing materials. If your organization has achieved substantial Customer Satisfaction goals, and perhaps has received awards for those performance levels, use these recognitions to promote your organization. Include tag lines representing these achievements on marketing and information brochures, in patient information packets, and as headers and trailers on the in-house television channels that patients can access. For example, if your organization is in the top 5 percent of all organizations of your type in Customer Satisfaction ratings, then add that piece of information to marketing and communication materials, including your letterhead. Spread the good news. Send messages reinforcing Customers who have chosen your organization for services by telling of your high Customer Satisfaction ratings, and encourage other would-be Customers to elect your facility the next time they need health care assistance. This approach also reinforces high levels of Associate performance and standardizes expectations for more behavior of the same or greater levels.

Physician Action Council (PAC)

The objective of the PAC is to integrate the physician constituency into the Customer Satisfaction tactical plan. Connecting with physicians is not as difficult as many suggest. The following attitudes and activities will help you to better integrate physicians into your Customer Satisfaction initiatives.

View physicians as Customers. Consider what physicians would like to see changed in the organization. As a primary Customer constituency, physician satisfaction levels need to be as important as patient satisfaction levels in the scheme of Total Customer Satisfaction. If you link the concepts of physician and patient satisfaction together, then prioritize a select number of physicians' irritations as top-priority items for resolution, physicians will encounter an initial positive experience with your organizationwide Customer Satisfaction initiative. This then becomes the starting point for further physician involvement in Customer Satisfaction initiatives in which physician cooperation is needed.

Share information. Provide physicians with your hospital Customer Satisfaction ratings. Share your progress and upward trends as well as the occasional downward dips. Use the information, both good and bad, to motivate and drive changes in physician behavior.

Information and data influence individual perceptions and attitudes. Business improvement statistics such as improved Customer Satisfaction ratings are attention-grabbing statistics for physicians. When physicians see that your organization is serious about making Customer Satisfaction improvements they will be more likely to invest their time, effort, and support in additional initiatives.

If your Customer Satisfaction ratings are rising, physicians are probably noticing and experiencing a number of the improvements first-hand. However, quantifying the amount of improvement and the level of sustained improvement can substantially influence their perception of the organization and therefore the manner in which they are willing to partner with you. Substantially improved Customer Satisfaction could easily translate to more admissions or more cooperation and involvement with the organization. Both are winners.

Act as a sounding board. As the hospital is undertaking hundreds of new ideas for improvement, some of these ideas will fall into themes that could or would directly have an impact upon physicians. For example, visiting hours or privileges represent one area where Customer Satisfaction improvements are routinely suggested, and where changes in policy might generate a significant response from physicians. In such a case, the PAC can provide hospital management with an idea of how physicians might respond to proposed new policies and why. Such feedback can help solidify an administrative decision or reopen it for modification.

Influence politics. If the PAC has a number of physician leaders, politically well-connected within the medical constituency, then they may, on occasion, be helpful in communicating a particular administrative point of view to the balance of the physician population. Or they may be instrumental in helping shape and influence the opinion of the larger medical group on an important topic. In some rare cases, they may even choose to exert peer pressure on physician colleagues who are behaving outside professionally accepted norms.

Plugging the Black Hole

The great black hole, as described by Associates, is the void into which ideas go and are never heard from again. Forever lost and unrecognized ideas are the number one correctable and controllable factor defeating Customer Satisfaction efforts. Associates who invest time to submit an idea for improvement deserve the common courtesy of a response.

We recommended that the MAC plug the black hole of lost ideas and return a timely communication to each person submitting an idea. Thirty days is the maximum recommended timeframe within which an acknowledgment should be delivered to the idea submitter. For those Associates participating in ideation, timeliness of communication is equated with effectiveness of the process.

The content of the communication would include acknowledgment of receipt of the idea, what the next steps and timing will be, a thank you for participating, and a message of reinforcement for continued ideation. Remember the manners that Mother taught you. "Please" and "thank you" go a long way in making people feel respected and valued.

ACTION PLAN FOR TOTAL CUSTOMER SATISFACTION

Task 1. Review Roles and Responsibilities that the MAC, CAC, and PAC Will Have in Your Customer Satisfaction Initiative. Are you comfortable with the roles and responsibilities of each council? Are the reporting relationships of each council clear? Who among the executive team will be the official champion of these councils—the one to whom they report? This will mean a secondary reporting relationship for some council members, as not all members of all councils are likely to have a natural reporting relationship to the same executive. Are executive relationships strong enough to handle secondary reporting relationships of managers? Document the roles, responsibilities, and limits of each council to reduce innocent, but unfortunate mistakes.

Task 2. Select and Orient Your MAC, CAC, and PAC Membership. Specific qualifications for membership on each respective council are peppered throughout this chapter. Be selective in choosing your members. It is easy to see the positive characteristics of individuals and why they would make a good council member. At the same time, there are a few, specific personal characteristics that, if possessed by a council member, will adversely limit the effectiveness of that individual and possibly the entire council.

The following characteristics should be avoided at all costs. Even if an individual appears to have everything that you desire in a council member, if they possess any one of the following qualities to any degree, do not include them in your selection process.

1. Is insensitive to political realities in the organization.
2. Has a dominating conversation/discussion style. (Don't confuse a dominating style with an assertive style.)
3. Doesn't "walk the talk."
4. Has a temper, or pouts when decisions don't go his or her way.
5. Is too busy to invest the time needed.
6. Has biased attitudes of any nature.
7. Possesses questionable honesty and truthfulness.

The orientation of council members to their purpose, role, and responsibilities should be thorough and well prepared. Include information on how to carry out their roles. Include the expected challenges for each position, and how to manage those challenges. Finally, be clear as to what the expected results of the council are, how councils should relate to executives, Associates, and other managers, and what interim reporting will be required.

For more information on how to select and orient council members and examples of expected results from each council, order the *Change Management Driver* from Management House, Inc.

Task 3. With the Executive Team, Establish the Ideation BHAG (Big, Hairy, Audacious Goal) for Your Organization. Ideation is the single most potent source of rapid performance improvement that any organization has to offer. How large will your ideation BHAG be? We recommend that you set it at one idea per Associate for the first year. Do not publish the ideation BHAG until the system for processing and managing DIGs and JDIs has been put in place. Set a timeframe for achievement of the BHAG. Incentivize the goal. Make it fun. Keep it visible. Track the results.

Task 4. Review the Do-It-Group and Just-Do-It Processes and Adapt Them as Needed for Use Within Your Organization. Use the flow chart in this chapter (Figure 8.2) as a firm guide for the flow of ideation processing. Do not deviate from the proposed flow until you have had experience in managing massive ideation. This proposed process is tried and true. You may wish to make modifications to the process after your organization has had some experience using the system, and you more clearly understand the multiple dynamics that are generated in and around it.

Task 5. Design and Deliver Do-It-Group and Just-Do-It Training Sessions. An easy-to-use formula for immediate problem solving and performance improvement is needed for all Associates to use. Create customized DIG/JDI training for your organization and schedule training for just-in-time Associate applications.

Just before an Associate is ready to participate on a DIG/JDI, they must attend DIG training to learn how the process works, what the roles of each participant are, the powers and limitations of DIGs, and what the expected results are. Effective training on these topics generally includes a take-away packet for easy future reference summarizing the teaching points and roles and responsibilities of participants.

Task 6. Design and Deliver DIG Chairperson Training. Skills required to chair a problem-solving group like a DIG are different from skills needed to be a DIG participant. Chairpeople must know how to manage group dynamics, what to do when a DIG member acts in an inappropriate manner, how to handle participants who are not accountable for the assignments given them as a DIG member, and how to manage group decision making, as well as have other group management skills.

Most Associates, regardless of job title, are fully capable of handling DIG Chair responsibilities provided they receive a training program. Even those Associates who routinely lead business meetings should attend DIG Chairperson training to learn what is being taught to Associates and to pick up professional tips on managing group dynamics.

Training for DIG Chairs should be made available on a just-in-time basis. Training that occurs too soon before the skills are to be used is lost training. Train, use, and reinforce.

Task 7. Create a DIG/JDI Tracking Database. Tracking of ideation management is essential. This task is concerned with the creation of a database that will track, at a minimum, the following fields of information.

- Who submitted the idea
- When the idea was submitted
- When acknowledgment correspondence was sent
- Who the Chairperson is, along with job title and telephone extension
- Who DIG members are and their contact information
- Whether the idea is a duplicate or otherwise not usable, and if so, a note as to why

- What the DIG recommendations are and if they were approved
- What the expected return on investment will be
- When the recommendations were implemented
- What follow-up communication has been made with the idea submitter

In addition to using the computer to track ideation management, you will also want to use it to generate customized correspondence to idea submitters and DIG members. A number of form letters with fields to customize the correspondence should be designed for frequent use. You will need correspondence that serves the following purposes:

- Advises that the idea has been received and where it is in the process of evaluation
- Gives an update on the status of the idea
- Serves as a reminder to DIG Chairs that the interim DIG report or final DIG recommendations are due
- Thanks idea submitters and encourages more ideas
- Thanks DIG members for their hard work and contribution
- Keeps communication to the idea generator timely

Task 8. Use Adopt-a-Patient Program to Instill a Renewed, Expanded, and Heightened Passion for Patient Satisfaction in All Associates, Regardless of Position. No one is exempt from this effort—not executives, not housekeepers, not anyone. In order to instill a renewed and enlightened understanding of what it feels like to be a patient or what it will take to provide exemplary Customer Satisfaction, we recommend the Adopt-a-Patient Program. The Adopt-a-Patient Program is an excellent means of achieving on-going organizationwide involvement in Customer Satisfaction management while effectively managing Customer needs. This is what is involved in the Adopt-a-Patient Program:

Participants: All Associates in the organization regardless of location or position are participants. No one is exempt. And every patient who is served by your organization is a potential participant. Obviously not all patients need to be involved. Start first with inpatients, then expand the program to outpatient services, and then to ER services until all patient populations are involved in the process.

Objectives:

1. To provide outstanding Customer service to every patient through the usual patient management channels as well as through a personal Customer service contact who is assigned a specific patient and made personally responsible for assuring that patient satisfaction for that individual is at an exceptional level.
2. To actively engage each Associate in providing personal Customer service in a one-on-one patient environment, and become more aware of patient needs, problems in the work systems, and what is required to deliver "Wow!" Customer service.

Process: The following sequential steps are used to build and install an effective Adopt-a-Patient program.

1. Gain executive commitment to the process and objectives. This is more than a one-time or one-year effort. It is a commitment for the long haul.
2. Differentiate between the Adopt-a-Patient program and services conducted by an Ombudsman or Customer Satisfaction manager. There should be no overlap in workload, but rather a complimenting and integration of efforts. For example, if the staff Patient Ombudsman routinely visits patients, this is one function that will no longer be centralized under the Patient Ombudsman job description but will be decentralized to every Associate in the organization on an organized basis. Consequently, the amount of time the Ombudsman previously spent visiting with patients becomes free time for other duties. Addi-

tional or new duties for the Ombudsman might include providing patient satisfaction skills and management classes, closely analyzing satisfaction measurement results, and implementing action plans for advancement of results. The Patient Ombudsman job is not necessarily dissolved. Rather, it evolves into a more sophisticated leadership and problem-solving role.

3. Develop just-in-time training curriculum for Associates ready to participate in the Adopt-a-Patient program. No need to train far in advance, as training that is not practiced soon after learning is quickly forgotten. Curriculum for the training includes the following components:

   - When and how to introduce yourself and your purpose to the patient. Introductions should be made within two hours of inpatient admission, and within fifteen minutes of outpatient or ER patient registration. For the ER, one or two staff should be assigned to Adopt-a-Patient for all patients in the ER for the period of one full day rather than having a separate Associate relationship for each patient.
   - Welcome statement.
   - Associate's name.
   - Why they are there—to serve as a personal representative during the patient's hospital visit, assuring that patient needs are met on a timely basis. (This should be a scripted, standardized statement for each Associate.)
   - How patients can easily reach their assigned satisfaction representative. The key is that communication from patient to assigned representative must be easy and occur immediately upon request. Cumbersome communication systems or delays in communication discredit the program.
   - What to expect when patients do contact you; that is, that you will work to meet their request in the most timely way possible, that you

will personally check in with them daily to see how they are doing but they should feel free to contact you at any time.

4. Train all employees on how the Adopt-a-Patient process works, what roles patient representatives are to play, and how that role works together with primary caregivers and technicians. It must be made clear that the primary responsibility for patient satisfaction belongs to each person coming into the patient's room.
5. Establish Customer Satisfaction standards of performance for all patient situations. Proposed standards include
   - Call lights to be answered within three minutes and acknowledged within thirty seconds.
   - Each patient visited every thirty to forty-five minutes.
   - Telephones answered within five rings.
   - Patient-oriented problems resolved within sixty to ninety minutes.
   - On-hold telephone status not to exceed thirty seconds.

You can add more standards for patient satisfaction to this list, then publish the standards and train Associates on how each component is to be handled. Do not assume that all Associates will know what to say when they enter the patient's room every thirty to forty-five minutes. They must be trained in what to say and how to say it. For example, you might want them to say, "Mrs. X, I wanted to see how you were doing. Is there anything that I might get for you?" on their first visit. On the second visit, they would say, "I thought I would stop in to see how you were doing. How are you feeling now?"

If Associates are not trained on what to say with each visit, or if they are given latitude to say just about anything, the resulting dynamic will be more of an annoyance to patients than an assistance, and the variability in performance will be a deterrent to Customer Satisfaction efforts. Associates will come bopping into the patient's room, with statements like, "How are you doing now?" over and over again.

Chapter
NINE

Designing Your Customer Service Strategy

To be really great with little details is a quality so rare as to be worthy of our highest regard.

Within each of the previous chapters we shared aspects of the philosophy of Customer Satisfaction management, examples of how these particular aspects play out in the most excellently managed organizations, how to adapt the philosophy and actionable items into everyday living in a health care organization, and specific work Tasks to assist your organization in processing and implementing additional work of a similar nature.

In this chapter we focus on seven specific themes that provide the basis for the balance of your Total Customer Satisfaction Strategy. Each of the seven areas addresses a major component of work to be done in order to create an organization prepared to deliver extraordinary Customer Satisfaction within a dynamic and complex environment.

Each Task contains a set of clear objectives and a specific approach to achieve the objectives. Consider the Tasks as open-ended work to be done. Expand the scope of each Task as you see fit to enhance your organization. Examples provided are a starting point.

Beware of making too many modifications to the Tasks provided, however, for fear of distorting their original intention. Each aspect of each Task has been tested and implemented in hundreds of organizations.

Organizations that have innocently modified the Tasks too greatly have lost the effectiveness and objectives of the work.

IMPLEMENTATION STRATEGY

There are two ways of approaching this work. One way is with a small group of assigned people methodically working through each Task, one or two at a time, until all are completed. This approach is tedious, time-consuming, and highly controlled, and improved Customer Satisfaction results are long in coming. The results will come, but not in a sudden blast, as will be the case with a more rapid implementation approach.

The second approach involves a more rapid implementation schedule. The speed of implementation is directly related to the number of people involved. This approach is a coordinated, decentralized approach to getting the Customer Satisfaction strategy rapidly designed and in place. Another difference between the first, more time-consuming approach and the second, more rapid approach is the number of people involved in the process.

Those involved in the more rapid process include eight Customer Satisfaction Council members, numerous DIG participants, all department leaders, and most Associates. The number of people involved in the tightly controlled process is about eight: only the Customer Satisfaction Council members. Occasionally a few extra people may be drafted to help with a Task. The process is the same. The difference is in the deployment of people.

Choosing the Right Approach for Your Organization

If your Customer Satisfaction ratings are dramatically lower than you want them to be, you might be a candidate for the rapid implementation approach. The dynamics of organization and management for the rapid implementation approach differ from the more tightly controlled, conservative approach. Before embarking on a rapid track to progress, be sure that as the leader you are comfortable with these dynamics. The dynamics are described below.

Powered-Up Associates and Diluted Executive Direct Decision Making. Executives who feel that they must be involved in all decisions regarding change and improvement in the organization will not be comfortable with rapid and massive change. They will be more comfortable with incremental, controlled, slower change processes, and therefore should use the Total Customer Satisfaction strategy but employ a small group of managers to do most of the work. If you are comfortable with powering up Associates to make decisions and implement changes that are in direct relationship to organizational values and improved Customer Satisfaction, you will be comfortable with the rapid implementation approach. Of course, financial limitations are imposed on Associate decision making, and a reporting or monitoring of these improvements is tracked through the Management Action Council (MAC) (see Chapter Eight).

We recommend establishment of a financial limitation of $100 for Associate decision making related to Customer Satisfaction goals. In other words, any Associate may make a decision valued up to $100 to correct an otherwise unsatisfactory Customer experience. For example, if the meal that is delivered to a patient is found by the patient to be unacceptable, the meal server can decide, on the spot, that the meal will be replaced and at no charge to the patient. Bam! The Customer's problem is resolved on the spot, by the Associate's making the same decision that the supervisor would have made, but without taking time out of the supervisor's day. The financial threshold for Associate decision making may be modified by your organization, but the principle is the same—a powering up of Associates, and a breaking down of bureaucracy.

Massive, Simultaneous Performance Improvements. Initially, the Total Customer Satisfaction Strategy will feel well organized and coordinated. It will feel as though everything is tightly controlled. However, as departmental Customer Satisfaction teams get under way, hundreds of improvements will simultaneously be made throughout the organization without necessarily being reported through supervisory channels. There are simply too many changes and improvements to be made in too short a time to allow the bureaucratic process of supervisory review and approval. Besides, it would be an unnecessary exercise, as Associates and DIGs are limited to making recommendations within a prescribed set of boundaries. Hence, supervision of the process should remain supervision of the process, not active involvement in the review portion of each DIG.

Associates will operate within a uniform, core understanding of the priority that Customer Satisfaction plays in overall organization performance, how Customer Satisfaction is defined, and the limits within which they can operate. Consequently, numerous improvements are going to be made that may not necessarily employ the same approach that you as leader would have used. If this makes you uncomfortable—if you are an "all knowing executive," meaning that you must know all that is happening within the organization at all times—employing the more conservative approach would better fit your style. But it would also slow down the speed of progress considerably.

Choose the approach that best fits your executive style— rapid performance improvement or incremental performance improvement—and follow the same steps in this book to create a customized Total Customer Satisfaction Strategy for your organization.

ORGANIZING THE TOTAL CUSTOMER SATISFACTION STRATEGY

There are two components to organizing the Total Customer Satisfaction Strategy: the operational structure of the strategy, or how the work will get done, and the Total Customer Satisfaction Strategy document design. This document is a consolidated listing of all Tasks to be completed to improve Customer Satisfaction ratings, with corresponding information on who is assigned each Task, during what part of the fiscal year each Task will be worked on, and when each Task is due to be completed.

The operational structure centers around the Customer Satisfaction Council. The Customer Satisfaction Council is made up of eight of the organization's top-performing department leaders. One of the eight leaders is assigned the role of Customer Satisfaction Council Chairperson and is responsible for creating, coordinating, and implementing the Total Customer Satisfaction Strategy. Each of the remaining seven department leaders are assigned one of the seven focuses of the strategy. It is their responsibility to assure that the Tasks assigned to each of them is completed on time.

Total Customer Satisfaction Strategy Design

Seven specific areas of focus for Customer Improvement are headlined in the Total Customer Satisfaction Strategy.

1. Targeting and Managing Customers
2. Customer Communication and Orientation for Results
3. Making Service Work—Removing Irritations
4. Making Service Work—Adding Value
5. Meeting and Exceeding Customer Expectations (Customer Satisfaction Measurement)
6. Linking Associate Performance to Customer Needs (Human Resources Connection)
7. First and Last Impressions

Within each of the seven areas of focus, a number of specific Tasks are provided that will boost Customer Satisfaction at your organization. Tasks previously presented in this book were largely led by management staff or conducted by patient satisfaction staff. The Tasks in this chapter involve ideas directly generated and implemented by the Associate population of your organization.

The end result will be a major "to do" list of improvements in Customer Satisfaction to be made at prescribed times and led by assigned individuals. Most of the work will involve nonmanagement staff.

Size of the Total Customer Satisfaction Strategy

The most effective Total Customer Satisfaction Strategies involve a large number of improvements. It is not uncommon to find that as many as 400 to 500 ideas were included in the best-laid plans. Shorter Total Customer Satisfaction Strategies yield fewer results, and for obvious reasons. They are doing less. Fewer irritations are being removed, fewer components of value-added are occurring, and so on.

Sometimes the argument is proposed that smaller organizations should have shorter Total Customer Satisfaction Strategies. No. Smaller organizations have as many problems to resolve as do larger organizations, although the nature of the problems can be somewhat different. There is no correlation between the number of improvement items in a Total Customer Satisfaction Strategy and the size of the health care organization.

GETTING STARTED ON YOUR TOTAL CUSTOMER SATISFACTION STRATEGY

Focus 1. Targeting and Managing Customers

In Chapter One department managers identify who their specific Customers are, and what it will take to earn exceptional satisfaction ratings from each Customer. The following Tasks build upon the work done in Chapter One by profiling specific Customer complaints and problems, creating schedules, and assigning parties for problem solving and building the business.

Task 1. Profile Customer Problems and Complaints. The common problems and complaints of Customers are no secret to staff. They know what the complaints are regardless of whether they see their validity. The objective of this Task is to identify the problems and complaints that each Customer group expresses, respectively, and to create and implement an action plan to improve satisfaction levels. This Task can be organized and directed by taking the following steps.

1. Revisit the Customer identification list created in Chapter One. Next to each Customer, list common problems and complaints that have been reported. Make no judgment as to the legitimacy of the complaint. Simply brainstorm with staff, and make a common list of all the problems and complaints. For patient populations, use the generic label of "patients" or a descriptor of a specific type of patient if the complaint is commonly heard from a particular type of patient. For example, "C-section patients" may have a commonly voiced complaint that is unique only to that patient population. The best way to do this is to create a chart using the following format:

Customer Name	***Complaint/Request Frequency***
____________________	____________________
____________________	____________________
____________________	____________________

2. Prioritize problem-solving efforts for each Customer. Use the following prioritized list (most important first) as a starting point for identifying which problems to work on first. Include staff in determining priorities.

- Problems that represent a legal or health care hazard.
- Problems most frequently sited or reported by the greatest number of Customers
- Problems irritating Customers that bring you the greatest volume of business, or Customers that represent repeat business or a source of numerous referrals

3. Create a calendar for problem solving each of the listed complaints. Use DIG/JDI processes for internal problem solving and implementation. Note special participants or talents needed to help with some of the more unique situations. Add a date for when each problem will be addressed, and stick to your schedule.

4. Plan a celebration when each DIG/JDI is completed and a complaint is resolved.

Task 2. Build Your Physician Customer Base. A primary source of increased patient volume is physician and patient referrals. Given the powerhouse of influence that physician referrals represent, it is good business to assure that the physician Customer base is well managed in terms of providing a highly satisfactory work and patient experience at your facility.

In addition, the future of your organization depends on a well-rounded physician base with a depth of expertise in numerous medical specialties that you are prepared to offer patients. Too often organizations become dependent upon one large medical practice to provide the majority of patients—a dangerous situation in which to be. More than one health care organization has undergone traumatic difficulties as the result of losing part of, or the entire base of, physicians from a particular medical practice. A diverse and well-balanced source of admissions represents stability for the organization.

The objective of this Task is to analyze where your organization is strongly represented in terms of physician specialties and patient census, and where it is weakly represented. Bolster business by gaining a greater percentage of each physician's admissions referred to your organization, and by recruiting new physicians to your facility. One way of making this a reality is through improved patient and physician satisfaction with how the facility is operated, and through improved physician relationships. Take the following steps to help organize this work:

1. Identify which physician groups, specialties, and medical practices are presently well represented at your organization, and which are needed to build the business. For physician groups currently represented, go to work to remove known work-system irritations directly affecting these physicians and their patients. These people represent your bread and butter and are essential to the continued existence of the organization. Treat them with intense interest.

The objective is to solidify their view of your organization as one that provides exceptional service—the best place to practice medicine and the best place to be a patient. This is an offensive move designed to increase Customer loyalty and ward off competitors who by now, or at some time in the near future, will be courting your physicians to their competing organization.

2. Target physician practices and referring organizations that would enhance services to your organization. Assign skilled physician account managers to discover and explore what these physician and referral centers find most appealing about their current situations, and what they find most irritating. This information will help you position your organization in a way that is attractive to these potential future business partners. *Warning:* It is possible that the conversation surrounding what they find appealing at their host hospital will include some aspect of financial support. Note this one aspect of the conversation, then widen the discussion to include other aspects of the business relationship that contribute to physician success. Tell them about your superior system efficiencies that allow surgeons to perform more surgeries within the same amount of time, or to see more patients within the same allotment of time. Be sure to tell them about the extraordinary patient satisfaction that your skilled and friendly staff provide, among other conveniences provided by your organization.

Task 3. Manage Physician Accounts. Think of the template for Customer management that the banking industry has provided in the past few years. As a vendor, banks have prioritized various types of Customers and created various levels of service for each type of Customer. Premier Customers, people or organizations with large bank accounts or those who represent substantial cash flow through the bank, are assigned a "personal banker" to handle problems and serve as a resource to "make things happen" when needed.

As a primary source of business, physicians should be treated as premier Customers with a personal account representative assigned to resolve problems quickly, and "make things happen" when needed. The beauty of the physician account representative model is that a relationship among the physician, physician office staff, and the physician account rep develops. There is a special comfort level for physicians in knowing that they do not need to spend time and effort working through the bureaucracy of the organization for every little problem. Their personal account rep will be on hand to resolve those issues quickly and easily. A sense of power and ego are reinforced in knowing that they are highly regarded by the administration of the organization and will receive prompt attention to any matter that develops.

This arrangement is a mutual win for your organization, for the physician, and for their office staff. Increased physician satisfaction contributes to increased organization loyalty, and perhaps more business from professional referrals along with an extraordinary reputation for service.

The objective of this Task is to create a physician account management system and use it to enhance referrals, build physician loyalty, and boost physician and patient satisfaction ratings. The following steps provide direction on how to accomplish this goal:

1. Identify physicians on staff and the number of admissions or patients and business dollars that each represents for each of the past three years. Look for trends within each physician and physician group. Which groups have growing numbers of admissions and greater revenue contri-

butions to the organization? Which have flattened performance levels? Which have declining statistics?

2. Group physicians by type of practice. All Ob/Gyn physicians together, all oncology physicians together, and so on.

3. Identify possible physician account representatives. Give substantial consideration to professionals who already have a positive relationship with a particular group or type of medical practice. For example, the head nurse on the pediatric unit may have a wonderful relationship with pediatric physicians at your facility.

Existing positive relationships should be among the primary initial screening criteria for selection of physician account representatives. *Warning:* Some CEOs and COOs who are accustomed to being the primary connection with physicians may feel uncomfortable with the idea of physician account representatives. To soothe the discomfort, assure executives that they will remain in the direct chain of physician communication, and that physician account representatives will keep them abreast of significant issues or problems as they arise that would more appropriately be handled by the COO/CEO. However, executives must realize that their limited access and lack of desire to be involved in solving daily operating issues is presently a great dissatisfier for physicians.

Due to the political nature of this position, leadership in the organization must be comfortable with the quality of decision making and the communication skills of assigned physician account representatives. Other considerations for selection of account representatives include the following:

- Degree of service orientation. The sole purpose of physician account representatives is to provide increased service to doctors and their office staff. Account reps must have an extraordinary sense of service excellence and how to deliver it.

- Dedication to the function. The start-up phase for this Task usually requires more time commitment than the maintenance phase of the Task.

Physician reps need to have time to service accounts as a part of their regular job function. The amount of time required to serve this function properly depends on the level of dissatisfaction and existing problems currently existing between the hospital and assigned physician practices. If your organization is operating reasonably smoothly, the estimated amount of time a physician account rep will invest is approximately three to five hours per week. Facilities where physicians are beleaguered by operating problems will require a substantially greater time investment for account management and problem solving.

- Clustering of practices and medical specialties. The fewer the number of physician account representatives, the better. Three to five reps is the recommended number for medium-large-sized organizations. To keep the number of reps reasonably small, cluster several types of medical practices together under one account representative who possesses exceptional interpersonal skills. Clustering should prove to be an asset, because it is likely that problems or frustrations expressed by one physician are also being experienced by other physicians. For example, delays in lab reports are not unique to one medical practice. Therefore, correcting the problem for one physician is a benefit for all physicians. Clustered physician practices also keep the communication web among the entire physician constituency and hospital management tighter, an asset for both parties.

4. Sort out physician account rep authority and accountability. Account reps must have power to be effective. Powerless account reps are nothing more than added bureaucracy, an effect opposite that intended for this Task. The following authority levels are recommended for physician representatives:

- Account reps are to have financial authority to approve expenditures up to $1000 for physician satisfaction purposes without additional authorization. Such financial expenditures must be budgeted.

- Account representatives have access to vice presidents, the COO, and the CEO within one business day of a request for authorization beyond their approved levels. Executives commit to provide approval of over 90 percent of requests made by physician account reps.

5. Provide physician account reps training. Training will be needed in the following areas:

- Managing frustrated, angry, or otherwise upset physicians
- Addressing unreasonable physician requests
- Promoting good work, problems solved, and successes achieved by the organization
- Coordinating interdisciplinary problem-solving groups for rapid solutions and implementation
- Managing relationships
- Effectively listening to what is being communicated

Task 4. Conduct Customer Contract Reviews. Managed care providers, large employers, and employer consortiums represent another segment of important Customers warranting Customer Satisfaction management for maintaining long-term relationships. The objective of this Task is to develop expanded relationships with current and potential Customers to cement current relationships and foster new business relationships in the future. The following steps are recommended for organizing this work:

1. Identify present contractual Customers, the present means of communication with key contact people at the Customer location, and dates for contract renewal. Look for current frustrations and irritations within your present contractual relationship, Customer-specific needs and desires, and clues for value-added services that, if fulfilled, would win renewed and/or expanded contracts.

The goal is to correct problems before they become barriers to future business and to make desired improvements in your relationship and services that will positively position your organization for renewed and expanded contractual services.

2. Identify potential contractual Customers, any recent communication with them, and known opportunities for your organization to reenter negotiations for services with them. Mobilize the problem-solving team and break down barriers to qualifying for the business. Then add value until you have exceeded expectations and become the provider of choice.

3. Assess the skills and effectiveness of staff presently assigned to negotiate on behalf of your organization. Aside from negotiating skills, are they skilled at developing and nurturing professional and organizational relationships? If currently assigned staff are short in either of these areas you may wish to augment the team by adding someone who compliments the present shortcomings.

4. Assign account representatives to each present and potential contractual account. The responsibility of the account rep is to develop and nurture organizational relationships. This includes uncovering irritations the Customer is experiencing and quickly correcting them, anticipating Customers' needs, and providing more than what is expected in terms of patient satisfaction as well as account satisfaction.

5. Train account representatives in how to manage exceptionally challenging situations. The goal is to win the contract in a manner that is a win for all parties. Frequently this requires creative thinking, problem solving, and education—skills that current account reps may not necessarily possess.

Task 5. Target Employer and Coalition Customers. Customer Satisfaction ratings have taken on an expanded role as a report card of performance. These report cards are used by large employers and employer coalitions, who receive feedback from Associates on satisfaction with health care providers to whom they pay handsome insurance premiums.

Building your business requires new sources of patients. Large employers and employer coalitions are continuously seeking the best combination of high quality, low cost, and high Customer Satisfaction packages provided by health care organizations.

The objective of this Task is to build your business by targeting new employer and employer coalition Customers. Use the added dimension of exceptional Customer Satisfaction ratings and your commitment to provide exceptional Customer Satisfaction as the determining factors in acquiring a contract for services. Do not count yourself out of the competition simply because your organization does not offer the full spectrum of services that a competing facility might offer, or because your organization is not a teaching facility like the one with which you are competing.

In summary, if your organization can offer exceptional Customer Satisfaction (or a plan and commitment to provide Customer Satisfaction such as the one developed in this book) in a cost effective manner, and with a respectable level of quality augmented by a rapid problem-solving system, you are in a highly competitive position as viewed by employers. To develop this market use the following steps to assist you:

1. Implement the DIG/JDI processes in your organization for rapid, problem-solving situations.
2. Get a handle on your current Customer Satisfaction ratings and create a Total Customer Satisfaction Strategy document to organize the work or improvements to be made.
3. Identify potential employer and employer coalition organizations for new or renewed contract opportunities.
4. Identify frustrations and irritations that employers and employer coalitions are currently experiencing. If you are presently engaged in a contract with an employer or coalition, make immediate improvements to relieve frustrations. Irritations that are not corrected may evolve into barriers to a renewed or new contract.

5. Identify an account representative responsible for developing an organizational relationship with the employer or coalition. Account reps are also responsible for barrier busting, problem solving, and all-around good business practices to make the current or proposed relationship valuable to all parties involved.

Focus 2. Customer Communication and Orientation for Results

The objective of communication is to transfer information from one source to another, one person to another, a person to a machine or data center, a data center to a person, and other combinations. Inadequate or nonexistent information creates anxiety in people, mistakes in judgment, and wasted time and effort.

The difference between an average health care experience and an exceptional one depends largely on the extent of comprehensive and effective communication occurring among and between various parties. Communication among physician, staff, and patients relieves patient anxieties, develops greater mutual understanding of each party's respective situation, and arguably increases the quality of clinical outcomes through increased patient follow-through on posthospital care instructions. Communication among staff members results in fewer clinical mistakes and errors in judgment, again affecting patient outcomes.

Communication in and around the facility is first and foremost an indication of consideration for Customers. How easy have we made it for people to navigate through the complex facility? Second, it shows the messages that we think are most important to send to our Customers. Those are the messages we see posted on walls, floors and doors.

The objective of this Task is to enhance staff understanding of the patient's experience, open up channels for Customers' communication of complaints and the organization's rapid resolutions of them, and improve facility communication and messages.

Task 6. Implement Customer-for-a-Day Assignment. The best recommendations for Customer Satisfaction improvements come from people who see things from the Customer's perspective. And there is no better way to see things from the Customer's perspective than to be one: *a Customer for a Day.*

Notice: This assignment is to be a *Customer,* not necessarily a *patient,* for a day. Certainly patients are the primary Customer for many departments, but some departments have other internal departments as Customers as well. Do not assume that Customer universally means patient for this assignment.

The following information and steps help organize and direct the Customer-for-a-Day program.

1. Each department in the organization is responsible for implementing the Customer-for-a-Day program at least once weekly until all Associates have experienced the process. The process is repeated annually for departments with less than fifty-two Associates, and repeated on a cyclical basis for departments with more than fifty-two Associates. The on-going nature of the process allows each department to fix and correct Customer problems continually as they are identified, before they become major problems.

While playing the role of Customer-for-a-Day and experiencing all that goes with being a Customer, Associates are to make a list of things they experience or observe that adversely impact Customers. In the Customer-for-a-Day role, Associates are empowered to correct as many of the difficulties as possible while in their role and to create DIGs for resolving the rest.

2. For departments that serve patients directly, the role is Patient-for-a-day. Obviously, staff do not actually become patients. They select a patient and accompany that patient throughout the entire day, a twelve- to fifteen-hour experience, noting comments about their feelings about the experience and identifying opportunities for improvements that the patient had not noticed or commented on. For example:

- Waiting times longer than five to seven minutes
- Inappropriate staff comments
- Noisiness
- Inconveniences of any nature
- Broken equipment
- Work to be redone
- Duplicate clinical and paper work
- Cleanliness issues
- Completeness of work issues
- Attitude issues

The value of this assignment is that

- It brings staff closer to the realities that patients/Customers experience. Everyone gets to experience the front line—where the Customer rubs up against the organization.
- Multiple problems are quickly identified and resolved each week.
- The creative brain power of every Associate is employed. What one does not see, another will catch. A common base of knowledge and understanding is built among all staff.

Task 7. Create Customer Hotline. When patients have a problem and need a solution but no one seems to understand, when "helpless" is the common quality among staff, a Customer Hotline committed to solving the problem is a welcome solution. Customer Hotlines are intended for nonmedical complaints regarding visitation policies, cleanliness of room, food quality, creature comforts, and so on. Ideally, they include around-the-clock staffing and a telephone number for patients and visitors to call when they cannot seem to get a solution to their problem.

When the caller places a complaint, the Hotline immediately follows up by contacting the appropriate resource to assure that immediate attention is paid to the problem. As soon as a reasonable solution has been identified, Hotline staff recontact the caller to assure them that the problem has been satisfactorily resolved from the Customer's perspective. If no one has solved the problem as promised, the administrator on call or house supervisor is contacted and expected to give rapid closure to the situation.

Calls to the Hotline should be tracked by type of problem reported and location of problem. On a regular basis these data are analyzed for trends and trouble spots; that is, similar types of problems representing a systemic problem, or routine problems in the same department representing a management problem. Use the data to further identify where root problems exist.

To be effective, the Customer Hotline requires active promotion. People need to know it exists if they are to use it. Consider using a red Patient Hotline sticker, with telephone number, to be placed on the phone equipment in each patient room and throughout the hospital. Include a brief explanation of the Hotline in the patient information brochure, on closed-circuit television in patient rooms and waiting areas, and as part of the Adopt-a-Patient introductory information.

Typical information collected for each caller would include the patient's name, room number, date, time, type of complaint, to whom the complaint was referred for resolution, call-back results, and whether referral to the administrator on call was needed.

A couple of variations on this idea have been tried with great success. One New American Health Care Organization assigned managers to field Hotline calls in rotation; managers who did not meet housewide minimum Customer Satisfaction standards staffed the Hotline two or three times more often than peers who had met service standards. This variation had the effect of rewarding managers with excellent Customer Satisfaction ratings, and increasing the awareness of managers with operations in need of improvement. The calls were routed to a portable phone so managers were available at all times to respond to calls.

Task 8. Solve Customer Navigation Problems. Most of the hospitals and medical center buildings, including physician office buildings, leave much to be desired in terms of ease of navigation around the facility. Generally, if you can find someone to ask, you might get lucky and talk to a person who knows how to get to where you want to go, but after the directions are provided, a feeling of confusion overwhelms you and you can hardly recall them. A worthless effort.

The objective of this Task is to improve the ease of navigation around your facility. Some New American Hospitals have adapted a method used commonly throughout the United States in another context, a system with which people are readily familiar, that of naming streets. Halls and floors are named for medical legends, such as Florence Nightingale, or pleasant thoughts, such as the Sunflower Floor. Maps with hall names are published at hall intersections and elevator exits. Telephone operators have a master map available to them so callers can dial 0 for the operator and get directions to navigate from their present location to their desired destination. Customer-friendly maps are also available for visitors to navigate their way.

Lastly, Associates are trained to escort visitors personally to their destination if the visitor has questions about how to get there or seems disoriented in the facility. *Training* is the operative word. Staff must know their way around the facility in order to direct others. Too frequently volunteers are planted at the reception desk to answer questions and give directions without the necessary familiarity with the facility. If volunteer staff are to be used in this capacity, invest in their training as well as support tools, or they will create dissatisfaction and ill will rather than providing a desirable service.

Testing signage. To test the effectiveness of organization navigation systems, we suggest employing a teenage student to maneuver through the organization by using the maps and support services provided by the organization. If teenage students can find their way to desired destinations, you probably have a pretty good system.

As a second tier of testing, ask your mother or father to call the hospital's main telephone number and ask for directions to the hospital. If your mother or father can understand the directions and use the directions to navigate their way to the hospital, you surely have a winning system. If, however, either of these small tests are challenged, see the message for what it is: Further improvement in facility navigation is needed. Beware of the tendency to rationalize any difficulties experienced in the trials. The student is *not* too young or inexperienced to handle the assignment, and your parents are *not* learning disabled. The system has to be designed so that anyone can use it.

Test the system several times. Use a patient focus group or local school to help you assess your facility's navigation friendliness. Do not hire a signage consultant. The costs are too high and results are frequently disappointing.

Task 9. Implement the 3C Card: Compliments, Comments, and Criticisms. Chapter Two introduces the concept of a centralized card for patients, visitors, and staff to use for rapid and easy communication of ideas, comments, and compliments, and provides a sample design. Your responsibility is to assure that the 3C card concept is implemented in your organization.

Distribution points would include waiting areas of all facility locations on the main campus as well as outlaying buildings and offices. Information and promotional campaigns for the 3C card will increase use of the organization. The goal is to generate use of the 3C card.

Some people have mistakenly interpreted little or no use of the card to mean that there are no problems in the organization or that Customers and visitors have nothing to say. In fact, little or no utilization means that there is no communication occurring; this is an unhealthy organizational situation.

Track use of the 3C card. Expect three to five cards per week for smaller organizations, and as many as ten to twenty cards per week for larger organizations. High levels of use are a plus. It means that interaction among patients, visitors, and your organization is occurring—a healthy situation.

Focus 3. Making Service Work—Removing Irritations

A large percentage of the reasons Customers downrate your service is rooted in little irritations that they constantly encounter. Navigation directions were inadequate, or parking was full. Equipment was missing or broken. Medications were unavailable when needed. The call light was not promptly answered, and so on. No one irritation alone is a big problem, but add them up and the total experience becomes one of dissatisfaction.

It seems that most people can handle one or two small irritations without feeling that the entire experience was less than exceptional, particularly when some aspects of the encounter were truly exceptional. But when the same irritations occur over and over again, or when there is an apparent endless stream of agitating arrangements, satisfaction ratings will reflect the agitation, and Customer behavior will change as prior Customers begin looking elsewhere for a different service provider.

The objective of this Task is to focus on removing the numerous, small irritations that exist within the facility and work systems, and to create an emotionally calm, truly healing environment.

Task 10. Remove Customer Irritations. Patients entering the hospital experiencing pain, discomfort, or anxiety do not understand why the admitting process has to take so long. They are making a judgment about the organization. When the call light goes on, the patient judgment process begins. Rightly or wrongly, patients begin judging the whole organization based on the fragments that they experience.

If staff respond rapidly and pleasantly to the call light, patients think, "This a nice hospital, with nice people who take good care of me." If there are delays in response times, or staff are uninvolved with patients, staff will be judged as noncaring, and the facility will be labeled as a not-so-good place to go. It is that simple.

Every time the Customer, patient, or physician rubs up against a policy, protocol, or encounter in your facility, a Moment of Truth occurs. That Moment of Truth will either be a positive and reinforcing experience, or it will be an agitating and irritating one.

The objective of this Task is to identify and remove all Customer irritations. This includes patient, physician, and internal Customer irritations. To keep balance and perspective in this assignment, it should be noted that not all irritations can be totally eliminated. Financial, clinical, or physical limitations may make total elimination of some problems impossible. However, in every case, some improvement should be possible for the Customer.

To orchestrate this Task effectively, department managers should conduct a staff meeting to compile a list of all known Customer irritations. Make this a brainstorming session, using the same communication rules that apply in brainstorming. Don't make judgments or discuss items during the session. Just list the problems as staff see them.

When the brainstorming session starts to slow down and ideas dry up, use the eight dimensions of health care quality shown in Exhibit 9.1, adapted from the work of David Garvin and the article, "Competing on the Eight Dimensions of Quality," *Harvard Business Review,* November–December 1987, to help prompt further thinking about Customers' judgment of the health care experience. Studies indicate that Customers rate some dimensions as more critical than others, and of course the evaluation of the importance of each dimension will differ from Customer to Customer.

Task 11. Create a Healing Environment. All hospitals, health systems, medical practices, and clinics are not created equal. Some create a truly healing environment while others are mechanic shops where people

Exhibit 9.1. *Eight Dimensions of Health Care Quality.*

1. *Performance.* Performance refers to the primary operating characteristics and measurable attributes of the service provided. Do people actually get well? Is the work done correctly, or is there a need to redo tests and procedures until it is finally done right? Where can primary patient care outcomes be improved? Where can we make it easier for the departmental Customer to do their work? Think through these questions to prompt further points of Customer irritation.
2. *Features.* The secondary aspects of "performance," which supplement the basic functions of what we do, are the features. Features are the little "extras" that make dealing with your organization more pleasant or acceptable. Do we nickel and dime people for TV, parking, and incidentals that should be included in a package price? These are features that can turn into irritations before your very eyes. They need to be changed or discarded. As irritations are identified, seek out alternative ways to turn the irritation into a valued feature.

   For example, hospitals usually have a pharmacy on-site, but they rarely offer to fill prescriptions prior to discharge. I never understood this. There we are, patients who can also be pharmaceutical Customers. Why is it that prescriptions cannot be filled before we leave the facility? Why isn't there an option offered: You can pick your prescription up in our hospital pharmacy before you leave, or we can call it into your local neighborhood pharmacy for an easy pick-up on the way home. What is wrong with a paper prescription given to the patient at discharge? The patient is ready to go home. He has been released from the hospital, and probably he is not feeling all that well. Instead of taking his filled prescription home with him, he has to stop at his neighborhood pharmacy to drop off the prescription and make a return trip later to pick it up. Two trips rather than one or none; this is how Customer irritation is created and revenue lost by the hospital.

   Customers will not choose to use all the features and options offered by your organization, but having a choice leads them to viewing your organization as a quality provider, one who has thought through every aspect of the Customer experience.
3. *Reliability.* This means that the products and services provided will not fail over time or be wrong. This measure applies more to durable products such as equipment than to services, but some element of the idea is applicable to services. When lab tests need to be done over, or there are complications in a procedure that lead to a redo or worse condition, these are reliability issues.

   Where does work in the organization have to be redone, causing Customer irritations? For example, when a second or third blood sample must be drawn in order to redo lab tests that were not properly conducted the first time, this translates to patient inconvenience as additional needle sticks are made and additional waiting time is incurred while the test is rerun. In worst-case scenarios, test results are inaccurate and the wrong diagnosis occurs—these are reliability issues.

Where do Customers complain of waiting times, wrong results, work redos? These are opportunities for improvement in reliability.

4. *Durability.* Similar to reliability, durability poses the question of whether there is enough usage received from the product or service before it has to be replaced or discarded. Did it last, or did it deteriorate?

   Where are we producing services that are not worthy of the cost charged for them as viewed by the Customer? Could these services be done for fewer dollars or inconvenience to make their value to the Customer greater?

5. *Conformance.* This dimension of quality addresses the ability of your organization's services and products to meet established standards. The Joint Commission on Accreditation of Healthcare Organizations (JCAHO) standards are one set of standards that may be important to hospital staff but have no direct meaning to patients. However, there is a long list of socially established standards such as short waiting times, pleasant common courtesy, and tidiness that patients and physicians have become accustomed to in society but do not necessarily occur within all health care organizations.

   A non-fit of societal experiences with your organization's performance creates a feeling of nonconformance. When patients and physicians rub up against these nonconforming elements, they become irritated and disenchanted with the organization. Where does your organization not conform to socially expected standards or to clinically required standards?

6. *Serviceability.* This is a dimension defined as the speed, courtesy, competence, and ease with which services are conducted. How easy is it to deal with your staff? How cumbersome is the system that the patient or physician must use in order to access the service? How quickly do staff get to the work of servicing the Customer? How quickly will Customers see results?

   Irritations occur when the serviceability of your organization is less than that of other social or local institutions that the Customer comes into contact with, as when it takes too long to get lab results, attention from the call light, or answers to medical or processing questions. We are on the verge of the instant information age. Are your services up to speed with the rest of society? Or will your organization appear even more lackluster as society advances serviceability and your health care organization cannot keep up?

7. *Esthetics.* This dimension deals with the way the product, service, or facility looks, feels, smells, or tastes. Although this is clearly a subjective evaluation, there are patterns of what Customers prefer. For example, tidy housekeeping is a universal societal expectation. What housekeeping practices are in need of adjustment at your facility?

   In addition to the visual dimension of esthetics, there is the sensual dimension of how things feel. A calm, quiet, restful environment is what is expected in a health care setting. Unfortunately, that is a sometimes a rare find, even when inpatient census is lower than normal. Without fail there are the hallway conversations of staff that can be heard in any of the neighboring three patient rooms, the loud voice down the hall reminding a colleague not to forget so and so, and my favorite, the Christmas carolers. Who approved that idea? Someone thought Christmas carolers would be a nice thing to do, so other hospitals thought, "Well, we can do that, too. A nice holiday touch." But what are they thinking? Patients in the hospital do not care to hear "Jingle Bells" when they are combating a migraine headache, postoperative recovery, or a host of other conditions. Peace and quiet is what they want. Can I say that any louder?

Meal preparation has several esthetic elements related to it. The color, aroma, and presentation of the food are good starters. Then there is the always desirable flavorful quality. If flavor is not always possible, can we at least arrange to make the mealtime tray attractive, or does it have to look like institutional food?

Finally, what most people think of when we talk about esthetic is the decor. Is there something of interest on the hallway walls, or are they blank and beige? Have you looked at the esthetic of the facility and asked where improvements can be made in a low-cost/no-cost manner? Open up the issue, within prescribed guidelines, to a DIG for ideas of how a particular esthetic dimension might be improved. You will be amazed at the results.

8. *Perceived quality.* This dimension represents the reputation or brand names that come from a history of dealing with an organization. Customers often cannot judge the inner workings of a product, so they judge the product or service by the intangibles that they come to know. For example, we cannot see the inner workings of the Maytag washing machine, so we judge the quality of the product by the reputation for serviceability and long durability—the intangibles that we come to know of.

   What perceptions do people have as they approach your organization or department? Are they thinking "This is the best medical facility in the area, and I am glad to be able to get health care assistance here." Or, are they thinking something less positive?

   What perceptions do people have as they depart from your department? Was the experience as good as or better than expected? Or was the Customer somehow disappointed? Perceptions upon arrival may be very different from perceptions upon departure. If they are, what were the incidents contributing to the change in perception? What irritations are detracting from a better reputation?

go for bodily fix-ups, and the true healing occurs at home or elsewhere. The environment that surrounds the patient while at your organization has a significant influence on their ability to heal and their rate of recovery.

The objective of this Task is to transform your organization into a true healing environment. Begin by auditing each patient healing environment within the organization. These are the areas where patients spend any length of time greater than a few hours. Begin with the inpatient areas and work your way toward outpatient areas. Conduct an unbiased review of the facility. Take into account the physical room or area patients reside in, and the factors that interact with the patient while they are in that location. For starters, look at the following items:

1. *Lighting in the room.* Is the overhead lighting harsh and cold fluorescent, or are there options for more homey, bed-side lamp-like lighting? Are the window coverings adequate to keep out unwanted daylight as well as to permit desired sunlight? Are window dressings easy for the patient to manipulate from the bed, or must a nurse or aid be called to adjust the window coverings? Lighting options are relatively inexpensive options to add and have an immense impact on how the patient feels.

2. *Noise.* Are the only sounds that a patient hears those of a caretaker environment: the rattling of equipment, conversations of staff, dead quiet? Or, do patients have the option to be exposed to sounds of soft, restful music or natural sounds? Such natural sounds are soothing and restful, and are available on cassettes for individual patient use.

Soothing audio sounds can be augmented with visual aids of the ocean surf, aquarium fish swimming, or fireplaces burning that are available for use with a VCR and television, equipment that is already wired to and available in the patient room. The objective is to provide additional stress relief during the stay at your facility.

3. *Educational information.* Are there adequate patient and family education materials easily accessible by patients and family members?

Because patient education has largely been relegated to caregivers who are already pressured with a heavy load of clinical work, the amount and quality of patient education is not what either the patient or caregiver would like it to be. With the help of easily accessible patient education information, patient and family members can do some self-educating in preparation for the few minutes of formal patient education that they will receive. Consequently, they will be better prepared to ask pertinent information of the hospital and medical staff.

4. *Comfort and company.* How often do patients have the opportunity to interact with other people? Some patients have nearby family members and therefore have regular opportunities to interact and receive the comfort of others. Others are alone during one of the most desperate and unsettling times of their life, hospitalization or outpatient surgery. The only words of care and concern that these patients might receive are the kind words from your staff.

What opportunities can be provided for personal interaction, comfort, and company for those that need it? Some organizations use pastoral care staff to assist in this function. Others train volunteers to be effective companions. Still other facilities like those in England allow some patients to arrange to have companionship from carefully screened pets while they are in long-term care facilities. The goal is to provide some sense of personal interest to counteract the loneliness that some patients experience.

When pastoral care, volunteer, and paid staff options have been exhausted, there is one additional means for providing some sense of companionship. That is the level of interaction that hospital staff provide as they enter and leave the patient room for various reasons. Are staff entering and exiting quietly with no interaction? Or is there some small level of brief conversation that occurs when patients are awake and the situation is appropriate? Train staff in the common pleasantries of light conversation for appropriate times.

5. *Room redesign and amenities.* The physical design of rooms in typical health care facilities is far from convenient and efficient for either pa-

tient or caregiver. In retrospect, health care facilities have undergone architectural changes and modifications over the years without consideration for the future and how health care delivery might evolve. Consequently, a great many health care facilities are handicapped by their layout. Immobile walls, permanently placed equipment, and an unfortunate physical design are the challenges that yesterday's decisions present to us today.

However, you can start to make changes now. Work around these challenges. Plan to make the environment of all patient service areas more home-like, residential, and comforting rather than institutional. Use wallpapers, wall colors, linens, and dressing gowns that reflect softness and a residential feeling rather than accepting the stiff, economical products that vendors typically push. Consider floral and soft landscape wall coverings, colored tissues. It costs no more to buy soft toilet papers than sandpaper-tough ones. It does not cost more to select colored tissues or bath towels instead of white ones. It does not cost more to choose a warm color of paint for the walls rather than the institutional and aged colors so frequently found. Floral dressing gowns are not more costly than hospital green-colored ones. In short, camouflage the institutional nature of the health care environment.

Women's health care centers were among the first to reflect the new, residential design in the Birthing Center concept. This was then carried over to the Women's Services Center. However, the trend seems to have stopped there—perhaps because no one has championed the concept hospitalwide.

Focus 4. Making Service Work—Adding Value

Adding value and removing irritations are frequently closely related. What first appears to be an irritation may be an opportunity to provide Customers with a value-added service, or vice versa. What management sees as a value-added service may actually turn out to be an irritation. For example, from management's point of view, automated telephone menus are supposed to provide efficiency and a more direct connection for the caller. From the Customer's point of view, they are often viewed as an annoyance, either because of hearing difficulties, mental processing difficulties, plain confusion, or just annoyance with having to deal with something other than a real, live person.

When an organization becomes aware of Customers' irritations, action to remove the irritation or make a positive change in the process results in fewer irritations, hence more satisfaction, and possibly a value-added component—all of which translates into greater Customer Satisfaction. The concept of "value adding" is to provide something extra, something different and helpful from a Customer perspective that was not previously available or that is unavailable from competitors. Once a value-added component becomes common among all providers, it is no longer considered value-added, but is viewed by Customers as a standard expectation.

Task 12. Add Value to Each Service, Product, or Experience that the Customer Encounters. I was sharing the value-added concept with an audience of hospital department leaders recently. Upon conclusion of the presentation, the director of radiology came up to talk with me. He said, "I understand what you are saying about adding value, and for little or no cost, but how does one add value to a radiology test?"

"Good question," I replied. "I do not have all the answers, but I believe your staff might have some good ideas."

He went back to his department, shared the objective of adding value with staff, and asked them to think of ways to add value to the radiology experience. The result was amazing. A few weeks later a letter arrived at my office from this director of radiology. In the letter he explained with a sense of delight how they were able to add value to the radiology experience.

He went on to explain. Do you know what happens when you put the patient on a large, stainless steel radiology examination table? They shudder and wince, "Ooooooh!" from the cold of the steel. Well, staff thought that if they could warm up that table, it would be a lot more comfortable for the patient—value-added. Yes! So they looked at the possibilities of warming lights like those used in restaurants to keep food warm. They looked at an electric heater as a possibility. Finally, they decided that if they placed an electric blanket on the table prior to the arrival of the patient, and then whisked that blanket off just before the patient was placed on the table, the desired result would be achieved. And they were right.

Rather than an, "Ooooooh!" from the patient, they received an "Ahh-hhh!" Much more comforting to the patient—value-added. And for what cost? The cost of an electric blanket. Here is the kicker. Because patients were more at ease when they were placed on the table, it was easier for radiology technicians to place the body and limbs properly in position for the best quality of test results. A double win!

Your Task is to identify low-cost and no-cost value-adding ideas for each department in the organization. The Task is orchestrated and coordinated by a small group of people. However, the value-adding ideas are to be created and implemented by each department.

Begin by training department managers in the concept of no-cost and low-cost value-adding. Then assign a timeframe of about thirty to forty-five days for managers to work with department staff to identify at least five ways of adding value to the services or products they provide. If more than five ideas are created, terrific! Department managers are to prioritize each value-added idea and assign an approximate cost for implementation. These ideas are then forwarded to the Total Customer Satisfaction Strategy Council for a brief review by the MAC before they are included in the Total Customer Satisfaction Strategy for the organization.

To help with your idea generation, the following is a brief listing of value-added ideas that others have created.

General Health Care and Patient Care Category

- Home visits for people living alone (this is a variation of home health)
- Special dietary meals available for purchase from the hospital (fee-for-purchase basis)
- No charge cholesterol and blood pressure screening

involvement. Some services should be provided to all patients, and some made available on a pay-for-service basis. The point is, your organization is doing many more little things, value-added, to make the health care visit as pleasant as possible.

Focus 5. Meeting and Exceeding Customer Expectations

In order to achieve top Customer Satisfaction ratings you must meet or exceed Customer expectations. Some people would argue that this is not entirely possible. I propose that it is.

What we have learned from the previous chapters in this book and the research you have conducted at your own facility under the direction of specific Tasks in this book, is that there are really only a handful of things that Customers expect. There are a few core expectations that if performed extraordinarily well will boost Customer Satisfaction ratings. In summary, they are as follows:

- Treat the patient with respect, kindness, and care.
- Create work systems that are efficient and invisible to the patient.
- Provide a quality service or product—help the patient heal.
- Remove irritations in the environment.

Anything else that you can do for the patient beyond these four core items is value-added from the patient's perspective. It is an unexpected bonus, a pleasant surprise, a "Wow!" experience. It makes the Customer say, "Wow!" when they encounter the service or product because what they are experiencing is far beyond what they had expected to encounter—an experience that exceeds expectations.

These four items are not rocket-science formulas. They are the same formulas that excellent organizations use in creating Customer Satisfaction and loyalty. They are formulas for success that are created and delivered by the Associates of your organization.

Task 13. Identify Opportunities to Create "Wow!" Service in Each Department. The coordinating group for this Task is responsible for training management and staff on what constitutes a "Wow!" experience. Following this training, department managers are to work with Associates to identify and implement at least five changes that are aimed at providing a "Wow!" experience for Customers.

The changes may be as simple and straightforward as pharmacy prescriptions from the hospital delivered to the patient's home or provided to the patient before she leaves for home. Or it may be something along the lines of hand-held video games for children waiting in the ER, a distraction from their illness or boredom while waiting for medical attention. Creative attention given to generating "Wow!" experiences should be wide open, boundaryless. Think freely.

Many of the "Wow!" services are a mutual win for the organization and the Customer. For example, providing carry-out pharmaceutical prescriptions is a revenue generator for the organization and a service to the patient.

"Wow!" suggestions are to be submitted to the MAC for review. The MAC will review the ideas for consistency with organizational values, their cost implications, political or legal implications, and so on. Upon approval by the MAC, "Wow!" improvement ideas will be added to the Total Customer Satisfaction Strategy for implementation, and the department manager will be advised to go forward with implementation on a defined and coordinated schedule that will take place within the next twelve months.

Notice that this Task assigns quantities of work to be done, that is, five "Wow!" improvements per department, and implementation within a defined and scheduled period. Specifying the quantity and timeliness of work to be done establishes structure. Managers that cannot or will not operate within the prescribed structure should be reevaluated for effectiveness in and suitability for a managerial role.

Focus 6. Linking Associate Performance to Customer Needs

There are only two components needed to achieve top satisfaction ratings. One is Associate understanding of what is needed to deliver top Customer Satisfaction. The second is Associate motivation to perform in such a manner. If Associates do not have a universal and clear understanding of what is meant by Total Customer Satisfaction, they will not be able to achieve top satisfaction results regardless of how heavily the initiative is incentivized. And if there is no reason to change their behavior, no personal incentive, then Associate performance will remain status quo.

The following four Tasks are aimed at improving Associate understanding of Customer needs, and tying individual performance levels to compensation and rewards.

Task 14. Staff Swapping. Temporarily assign back-room staff (those who have little direct exposure to patients and physicians) to front-line positions where they can hear, see, and feel Customer anxiety and frustration. This would mean temporarily assigning finance department staff, for example, to patient-floor clerical positions, front-line food service positions, the central reception area, or clerical positions within patient-care departments. Administrative support functions would be swapped with basic clerical or service-patient-care functions, and vice versa. In most situations, swapped staff will not be able to conduct the full range of responsibilities of the swapped position. Frequently they may need to be assigned basic work functions such as clerical duties and low-level patient care duties. The level of work performed is not essential. What is essential is the learning that occurs when swapping occurs.

Because there is a real limit to the work that can be performed in swapped positions, the duration of the swapping should be relatively short. Perhaps two or three days for most positions. On occasion, more extensive swapping could be beneficial. One organization swapped a manager from the business office with the director of the ER for a period of ninety days.

Business aspects of the ER performance, including profitability, made dramatic improvements during that period. Swapping of staff accomplishes a number of goals.

1. It provides real-time insight into how the Customer is feeling about the organization and service provided.
2. It provides an orientation to what the workload is like in another department, a department that deals directly with the primary function of the organization—healing patients.
3. It creates greater understanding among departments and staff, thus breaking down barriers to progress and building new, valued relationships.

As leaders of this Task your responsibility is to coordinate and schedule staff swapping throughout the organization. This does not mean that you personally work with individual department schedules. It means that you work with department leaders to identify which positions within their department can be swapped with other positions outside the department, and on what schedule the swapping should occur.

A checklist of objectives that swapped staff are to achieve during their time away from the home department should be created. After all, this is not paid vacation time. Swapped staff should be accomplishing something. A sample of objectives to achieve might look something like the following:

1. What is it that their home department can do better that will benefit the department you are visiting, or the Customer that is being served?
2. How can better relationships among departments be built?
3. What new information did the swapped Associate learn about Customer management and service delivery?

Staff swapping is often used extensively in large corporations where Associates are being groomed for top management positions, or as a management development opportunity. At McDonald's, every new Associate at the corporate headquarters spends their first month working at a hamburger stand, doing all the jobs they are to do at a hamburger stand: serving Customers, making fries, cleaning floors, unloading trucks. This is performed by corporate attorneys, secretaries, clerical staff, management—anyone joining the organization. The thinking is that if you do not know what it is like at the point where the Customer meets the product, then you cannot be effective in your corporate position in supporting those who deliver the service to the ultimate Customer. The same is true for health care organizations.

The more Associates understand how their individual work affects the work of others, the more effective they can be in identifying ways to improve the overall product or service. Why not have every Associate scheduled to work on a patient care unit for two or three days sometime during their first six months of employment?

Task 15. Tie Customer Satisfaction Performance to Compensation. When compensation is tied to Customer Satisfaction ratings, Associates will get more serious about meeting and exceeding expectations. There are three primary ways of structuring a compensation system that supports Customer Satisfaction performance.

1. Organizational performance bonus—all or none.
2. Department manager's individual performance level for Customer Satisfaction.
3. Spot rewards.

Organizational performance bonus—all or none. The easiest way to create a pay-for-Customer-Satisfaction performance system is to establish an all-or-none organization bonus for achievement of predetermined Customer Satisfaction ratings. In other words, if the organization achieves its predetermined Customer Satisfaction rating objective, all Associates will receive a $100 check, or some predetermined payout. Womp! Look out now! The dynamics within the organization will change within a blink of the eye. Smiles will be plastered on Associates' faces. Staff will ooze with kindness, and the ratings will be a highly anticipated reporting event. When you make the goal, egos will soar! Morale will build! Teams will gel.

If the goal is not achieved, it is an opportune time to analyze why, to point out the weak performers in the organization, and to establish the infrastructures discussed earlier in this book, that is, high-light/spot-light meetings, managerial assessments, and Customer SWAT teams. Then set another goal, higher than the last one. *Word of warning:* Never reduce the performance goal for Customer Satisfaction. You may have to make periodic adjustments in financial goals due to external pressures and unanticipated or uncontrollable events, but there is no reason ever to modify the Customer Satisfaction goal downward. To modify the Customer Satisfaction goal downward would be like saying, "We thought you could serve the Customer at this higher level, but I guess you can't reach that high"—an offending gesture to anyone with pride.

Department manager's individual performance level. In addition to organizationwide Customer Satisfaction performance levels, individual managers may be evaluated on their personal and departmental Customer Satisfaction ratings. These ratings are then weighted and used to calculate individual merit increases for a given period.

Weighting segments of the performance evaluation tool for Customer Satisfaction will have a substantial impact on managers who have historically received lower Customer Satisfaction ratings. They will see that if their ratings do not meet goals, they personally will not receive a merit raise. It does not get any simpler or clearer than that.

Spot rewards. Spot rewards are not necessarily tied to any predetermined level of performance or a particular event. They are awarded when an extraordinary Customer Satisfaction event occurs. The spot reward is presented to an individual or team of individuals involved in the event.

An excellent means of providing reward, recognition, and reinforcement, spot rewards are generally smaller in value and impact on the future performance of the organization, as they are given spontaneously and not attached to a particular goal achievement.

Your Task is to evaluate which of these three means of compensation, or any combination thereof, would be most effective for your organization at this time. Be aware that commitment to any one design is a commitment only on a trial basis and your choice can be changed, improved, or deleted at the conclusion of the trial period.

Typically, we find that it is most fiscally conservative to build the incentive for goal achievement into individual manager performance evaluations. With this design, the organization is not paying out any more dollars in compensation and reward than it normally would. However, individual performance is more directed and focused on achieving Customer Satisfaction goals.

On the other hand, the approach that will garner the most excitement within the organization, and build the greatest sense of teamwork and camaraderie, is the organizationwide bonus involving all Associates. In fact, if the Customer Satisfaction goals are set high enough, the achievement of such goals should pay off handsomely in Customer referrals, making the financial payout affordable.

The best arrangement is a combination of both organization bonus and individual merit incentives for achievement of satisfaction goals. For greater detail on how to construct a compensation plan that is integrated with other organizational goals and objectives, contact Management House, Inc.

Focus 7. First and Last Impressions

First and last impressions are the lasting impressions. That is why the best talent in entertainment is scheduled at the start of the show and at the conclusion of the show for a lasting impression.

Think back on the last family gathering or social event that you attended. Although not everything about the event was as exceptional in your assessment as if you had hosted the event, nonetheless if the start and finish were good, you were likely to give the overall event a rather high rating. That is because the first and last impressions are the ones that we tend to remember most easily. They stick in your mind, and the overall perception of the event is influenced by those recollections.

The same dynamic is operating in your organization. The first impression of the organization and the last impression of the organization significantly shape the overall perception of the organization.

If the entrance to the facility is easy to navigate. If it is clean and neat and professional appearing, people will think, this is a nice place.

If the entrance is littered with cigarette butts, gummed up dirty sidewalks, dirty windows, and so on, visitors or Customers will think, "Oh, I'm so sure this is where I want to go."

If the admissions process is smooth and easy and Customer friendly, people will think, "This is not so bad." Or, "This is a very well organized operation."

If the admissions process is delayed, cumbersome or unfriendly, people might think, "Why don't they see that it would be better if . . ." Or, "I wonder why they do it that way when anyone can see that it would be better if . . ." and an unfavorable initial impression is created.

The same is true of the Customer's last impressions. Were the last encounters with the organization pleasant, helpful and easy to manage? Or, were they difficult, frustrating, and anxiety-creating? Were people saying, "Gee, I'm glad that is over!" Or, on a more positive note are they saying, "It's amazing how well they . . ."

Task 16. Managing First and Last Impressions. Impressions are 50 percent reality. They become reality to those who hold them. The good news is that impressions are manageable. Because you know that first and last impressions generate most of the overall impression of the product, service, or experience, these are the places to focus your attention for improvement.

The objective of this Task is to evaluate and improve the first and last impressions in all aspects of the organization. Begin by identifying the various ways in which a Customer can enter the organization. That would include entry points such as preregistration, on-site registration such as in the ER, and outpatient registration. It would also include telephone reception and other reception points. Think beyond the traditional entry point of doorways.

At each point the Customer encounters the organization for the first time, look at the following elements:

Physical plant. Is it clean, tidy, well maintained, and appropriately equipped? These are elements that are not capital-intensive but do have a significant impact on the Customer's first impression.

While on a recent trip out of town, I had occasion to use a walk-in medical clinic in a city that I was totally unfamiliar with. Looking in the Yellow Pages Directory I found a community walk-in clinic affiliated with the larger medical center in the region. I was feeling pretty good about the clinic at that moment. "Affiliated with a major medical center," I thought, "This clinic is probably as good as it gets."

Upon arrival at the facility I found the parking lot to be littered with paper, the front door covered with old decals, the windows in need of washing, and the carpet at the entrance torn and tattered. I did not go any farther. I did not even go in. My thinking went like this, "If this is as good as they can do on the entry, I am in trouble." They lost my business before they had a chance to even present themselves. Their first impression was devastating.

Will your physical plant pass the test?

Preparedness. Are you ready to serve the Customer's needs? Is the prerequisite paperwork as simple and straightforward as possible? Are supplies and equipment easily within reach, or do staff have to run back and forth sharing equipment among patient care sites, offices, or desk tops? Are you waiting for supplies to arrive? Are staff available to serve the Customer, or is there another waiting period?

To the extent that you are prepared to serve, the first impression will be favorable. If everything else is in place but staff are not ready to provide the service in a smooth, seamless fashion, the impression will be one of chaos, even if it is organized chaos to which staff are accustomed.

Staff accustomed to "making do" and "doing without" become callous to the negative impression that such functioning has upon the Customer.

Early messages. What are the very first messages the Customer receives? Are they warm, welcoming messages that reinforce the Customer's choice of health care providers? Or do you get right down to business, asking for their name, address, and health insurance card?

Take a clue from the best-managed businesses, and market your organization at every opportunity, starting with the very first message delivered. Drivers for transportation vans that pick up patients and visitors in the parking lot and transport them to the hospital front lobby should extend a welcoming message and reinforcing message. Such a message might be, "Welcome to Our Lady of the Wallet Hospital. Your comfort and satisfaction are our primary concern. As one of America's top rated hospitals in Customer Satisfaction, we are constantly working to meet and exceed your expectations. Please feel free to call upon any of our Associates for assistance at any time. It is our goal to provide you with the best health care experience possible."

Look at the first messages sent to patients as they encounter your organization for the first time. Consider each point of entry to the organization. Make the first messages delivered to patients ones that create a genuine feeling of welcome and reinforce the Customer's choice of your organization as a health care provider. Do not rely on the CEO's welcome letter. Although that CEO's welcome letter is a valuable piece of communication, it is but one piece and it is delivered after the first impression has already been made.

Make the very first message to the Customer that you are about to care for come from a living, breathing, warm person. Think through this assignment and include evaluations of the telephone point of entry to your organization and whether it is meeting your objectives. Few hospitals have a Customer-friendly telephone system. Most of them have moved like lemmings to a complex set of automated menus that seldom take the caller to their desired destination without much unnecessary time and frustration. In short, the system is not working. Ask your teenager, mother, or father to test the system. If older adults cannot navigate the system, you are losing a great portion of your patient population. I know that I rarely am successful navigating the telephone system of any hospital that I call.

Chapter
TEN

Prescriptions for Sustaining Top Customer Satisfaction Ratings

The essence of Total Customer Satisfaction is understanding and believing that the Customer-Associate relationship is at the core of your business, and that sustaining effective Customer Satisfaction management is based on the prerequisites of a value-driven organization, led by hands-on, participative executives with a passion for Customer Satisfaction who advocate powered-up Associates, and promote the need to change and improve work systems, among other things, as a way of raising Customer Satisfaction. It is an organizational culture that permeates all aspects of how business is conducted. It is a way of being.

Up to this point in the book we have focused on the details of "how to" boost Customer Satisfaction ratings. Once satisfaction ratings are at the desired level, the next challenge is sustaining them at exceptional levels.

It is not uncommon for organizations to place great emphasis on a Customer Satisfaction initiative that includes training, Associate reminders, and little messages promoting the initiative, the results of which are a temporary boost in satisfaction ratings. However, few organizations are able to sustain top Customer Satisfaction ratings from week to week and year to year. What is frequently found is that there is a sawtooth effect, an up and down and up and down of ratings from period to period rather than a smooth, consistent top-rated performance.

It is possible to sustain a top-rated Customer Satisfaction organization. To create this type of organization, executives must understand the integrated nature of the five primary components of the organization (see Figure 10.1):

Figure 10.1. The New American Hospital.

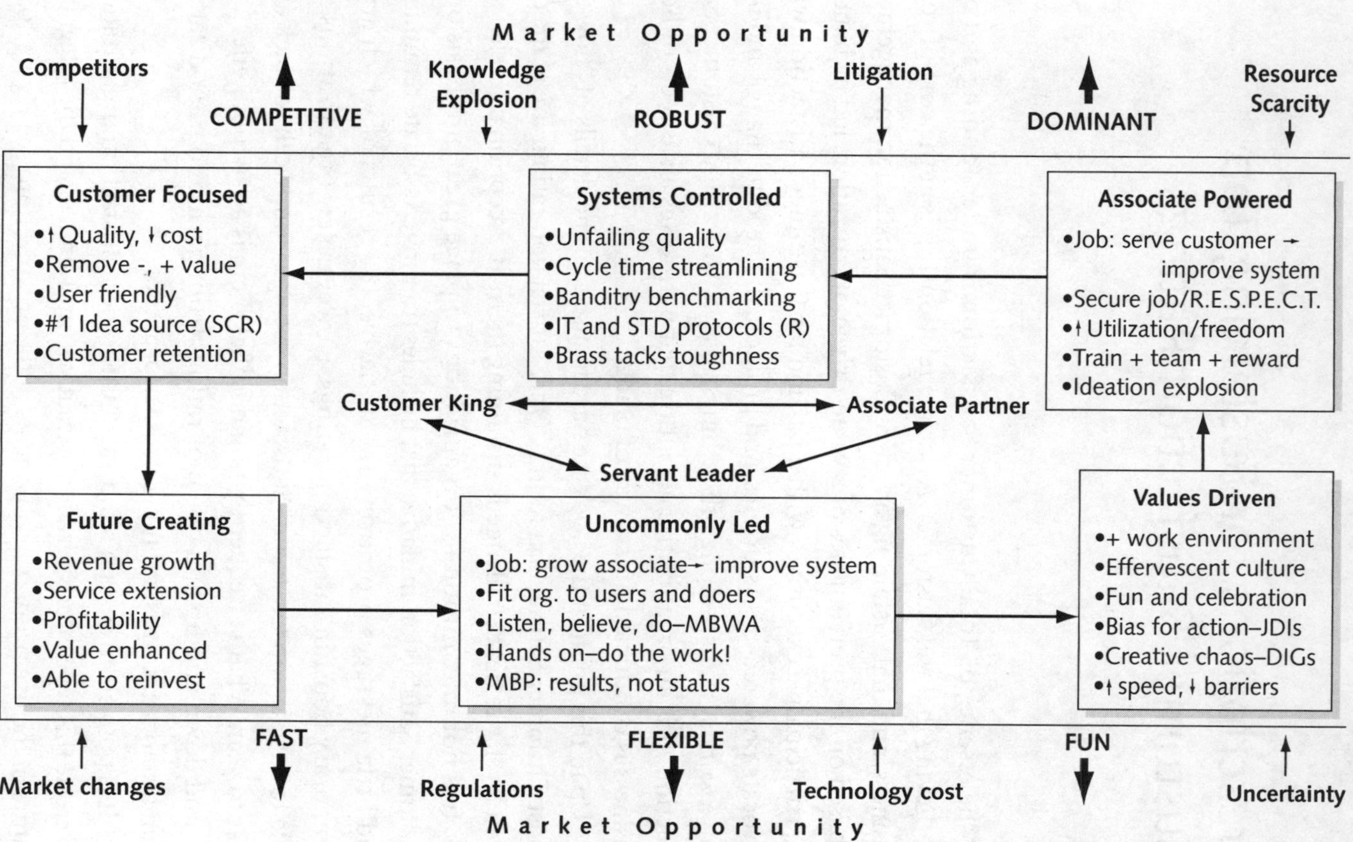

- Values-driven management
- Uncommon leadership
- Powered-up Associates
- Improved work systems
- Customer focused

In Figure 10.1 we see that the only reason for an organization to exist is to serve the Customer. The Customer-Associate relationship is the primary focus. In order to create an organization that supports, nurtures, rewards, and recognizes performance that exceeds Customer expectations, leaders of the organization must understand the intricate underpinnings, or structural support, that allows such organizational performance to occur. When this support structure, philosophy, and operating infrastructure are in place, sustained top satisfaction ratings are a matter of daily performance, not an occasional incident. All five components must be operating at a level of excellence in order to provide consistent, sustainable top Customer Satisfaction ratings. Let's talk in greater depth about these five components.

VALUES-DRIVEN MANAGEMENT

Top-performing organizations start with a values-driven culture. Although many organizations have a mission statement espousing their purpose, not all organizations have articulated organizational values or even a simple listing of how leadership intends to operate the business. What is important is *the way* in which organizations conduct their business.

Values driven organizations are consistent in their behaviors and decision making. Their values drive their actions and decisions. In such organizations, where Customer Satisfaction is a stated value of the organization, there is a bias for action that will deliver and improve Customer Satisfaction. There is a bias for speed in problem solving. There is an ease with which decisions are made—centered around the Customer and other articulated values.

These organizations integrate their values into every aspect of the way in which they do business. Their values are a part of the compensation structure, the reward and recognition structure, and a part of daily employment. There are rewards for living the values, and severe penalties for ignoring them. Associates are taught how to live the values, how to make individual decisions that are in keeping with the values, how to behave in a way that reflects the values. The entire value-centered system of management should support Customer Satisfaction initiatives.

When an organization culture is created that values Customer Satisfaction, among other things, and anything less is unacceptable, sustaining top satisfaction levels becomes a way of life, not a short-term goal.

UNCOMMON LEADERSHIP

Uncommon leaders are willing to do what others are not. They actually do what others talk about. They are participative, highly structured, considerate, demanding, in touch with Associates and Customers, and willing to do whatever it takes to develop Associates and light their motivational fires.

Expectations of leaders and accountability for results are high, as are the rewards for achievement. Decisions are consistently based on the values of the organization. Work becomes a challenge and fun. Associates want to follow their lead. They believe. They sacrifice. They achieve. They are rare.

POWERED-UP ASSOCIATES

Powered-up Associates are trained to contribute and implement ideas, make changes and improvements, and solve problems. Bureaucracy is carved out of the organization and in its place are expectations, training, and alternatives designed and implemented by Associates around the articulated values of the organization.

There are, of course, limitations to Associates' power. There is a maximum financial authorization level, and there are particular areas where Associates may not make decisions, such as employment areas or financial decisions beyond an authorized level. However, powered-up Associates do have the authority to serve the Customer in whatever way they deem to be appropriate within the articulated organizational values and newly established authorization levels.

CUSTOMER FOCUSED

When all Associates of the organization understand that the sole purpose for being is to serve the Customer, and the goal is to provide exceptional Customer Satisfaction, there should be little or no conflict within the organization. After all, everyone is aiming for the same target—Total Customer Satisfaction. So what is there to debate? Only how best to get there. Rather than debate endlessly, Customer-focused organizations with powered-up Associates allow Associates to determine first-hand how to satisfy each individual Customer when the situation presents itself.

IMPROVED WORK SYSTEMS

Work systems are the means within which the work of the organization takes place. Without work systems nothing can happen. Efficient and effective work systems are a cornerstone to delivering exceptional service. An organization with all other aspects of the New American Health Care Organization, but without controlled systems, can never achieve desired Customer service levels.

It never ceases to amaze me to hear executives talking about the Customer Satisfaction training that they are installing in their organization.

When I ask what the components of the training include, without fail, they talk about giving appropriate directions to visitors, smiling Associates, and valet parking. Granted, some of these ideas do add to Customer Satisfaction. However, executives are largely missing an essential component to delivering top Customer Satisfaction: improvement in the efficiency of work systems.

When work systems are highly efficient and long wait times and wasted resources are no more, the Customer is not inconvenienced with waiting, and the cost of the service is less. Why do people miss this obvious and essential component to creating excellent Customer Satisfaction?

Use the checklist in Exhibit 10.1 to test the level of work system efficiency in your department or organization.

Exhibit 10.1. *Self-Audit Test for Work System Effectiveness.*

	Often	Sometimes	Never
1. Patients frequently wait for 10 minutes for services to be rendered.	☐	☐	☐
2. Patients frequently wait for 10+ minutes for results to become available.	☐	☐	☐
3. Processes or steps in the work process are redone.	☐	☐	☐
4. As an Associate, I can see at least one way to improve the current work systems.	☐	☐	☐
5. Patients or physicians complain about some aspect of the work our department does. Timeliness, quality, quantity.	☐	☐	☐
6. Work flows smoothly through the process. There are never bottlenecks, backlogs. or uneven flows of work.	☐	☐	☐

If you answer "sometimes" or "often" to more than one question, there is a serious need for work system improvement in your operation.

True Story

While on vacation, a member of our family had occasion to use the hospital for a number of unexpected outpatient lab tests. The physician in charge had ordered the lab tests "stat," and there were a series of three of the very same tests to be conducted on three separate specimens, each to be conducted on a sequential day.

On the first visit, we arrived in the Outpatient Registration Department of a large, modern-looking medical center. Even though the lab order said "stat" we were instructed to wait in line with the other twenty patients in Outpatient Registration. Finally, it was our turn. The registration clerk was pleasant enough, but the work systems were unwieldy. An investment of about thirty minutes was required to provide her with personal contact information, insurance data, and other pertinent information. Most of this time was spent waiting for the computer system to respond, and watching the clerk walk back and forth down the hall to make copies first of the insurance card, then the driver's license, and so on—nonproductive motions and wasted time.

At the end of the first experience, I said to the receptionist, "We'll be back again tomorrow and the day after for the same test, only with a different specimen. Can we have a coupon or something so that we can just drop off the specimen and not have to wait in line again and go through this very same process?"

She responded, "I'm sorry but that won't be possible. We have to go through the same steps each time that you come in."

"Wow!" I thought. Ninety minutes of clerical time and three sets of repetitive work motions, most of which are unproductive, plus ninety minutes of my time and three separate trips to the hospital were consumed when it should only have taken thirty minutes and one encounter. Wasted time and inconvenienced Customers. Was I satisfied? I don't think so. Not when I can go to the local grocery store or car repair center and get a better history and computerization support than I get at the hospital—the place where I really want to feel that they are on top of things.

Work systems affect Customer Satisfaction ratings directly (and often massively).

CEO TIPS FOR SUSTAINING TOP PERFORMANCE

Boosting organization performance from low or mediocre performance levels to top performance levels requires one set of leadership skills. Maintaining or boosting organization performance in an already top-performing organization requires a somewhat different set of skills.

From CEO Mark Clement of Holy Cross Hospital in Chicago, a top-rated Customer Satisfaction hospital for years running, and CEO John Schwartz of Trinity Hospital in Chicago, an up-and-coming challenger to America's top-rated Customer Satisfaction organizations, comes wise, insightful advice on how to sustain top Customer Satisfaction performance.

Do Not Believe Your Own Good Press

Reports Mark Clement:

> *You are only as good as your last Customer encounter, and things can change on a dime. Success is garnered one Customer at a time.*

He would know. Having built a performance record of consistently achieving national top-rated Customer Satisfaction, Holy Cross leadership and staff diverted time and attention away from the Customer focus as they celebrated success. They had arrived. They had achieved. Egos were soaring and celebrations were happening, and attention to Customer Satisfaction management was diluted. Consequently, their ratings fell dramatically. Refer back to Figure 8.1, specifically the month of August 1994.

To recover to a top-rated position, they had to reinstall and reenergize the support systems, priorities, ideation management, and previous attention given to Customer Satisfaction management. What they learned was the intense and direct correlation between the amount of proper time and attention given to Customer Satisfaction management, and the corresponding results. Fortunately or not, time and attention to Customer Satisfaction support systems and correlating satisfaction ratings is a one-on-one relationship. You get what you give. Unfortunately, there is no grace period. When you give up on the one aspect, time and attention to Customer Satisfaction management, you also give up the results. It is immediate. Fortunately, the converse is also true. As soon as you invest time and attention in the appropriate support systems and priorities, Customer Satisfaction ratings will immediately reflect the results.

Expect a Lot from People

Mark Clement says with a smile:

Push Associates hard, then love them hard and reward them greatly.

Equal parts of high levels of structure, tough standards on performance, deadlines for achievements, a nonwavering commitment to the goal, and high consideration for Associates are essential in leadership positions. When you expect a lot, Associates will give you a lot. Then, you have to love them a lot. Reinforce them a lot for their achievement and effort. Make them feel valued and respected, and they will perform magnificently again.

Expecting a lot from people is easy to do but difficult to achieve without supporting systems that make it possible for Associates to perform at higher levels. Simply stating, "I expect a lot more from you," will not bring greater performance results. Along with great expectations must come great executive support for change and improvement in the work systems that create the results. A standardized system like the DIG/JDI system promoted in this book is needed for Associates to make rapid and widespread change.

In addition to a systematic way for making rapid improvements, powering-up of Associates must occur. Each individual Associate must have the power to do what is needed to satisfy the Customer—now. Satisfaction delayed is satisfaction denied. And it is expected that Associates will use their power in a way that supports and enforces the articulated values of the organization, of which Customer Satisfaction is one.

Finally, much love, admiration, respect, and appreciation from executive to Associates must be displayed. This comes in various forms of reward, recognition, and reinforcement.

A great number of health care organizations have unbalanced structure and consideration elements within their management profile. Health care management teams as a whole typically fit high-consideration profiles, meaning that they make decisions based on caring, consideration, and softness in their approach to Associates. It is part of the nature of the health care business to be soft, considerate, and caring. After all, these are the qualities necessary for effective patient care. However, high consideration alone will not deliver high Customer Satisfaction ratings. A considerate behavior balanced with high structure is also needed.

High structure represents a standardized management system supported by management by objectives, including specific timeframes, budget limits, and expected results. High structure also means defined and standardized protocols and expected behaviors. It is a way of reducing the amount of variance in the management practices within the organization.

The Better the Organization Performs, the More Difficult It Is to Make Additional Progress

It is often the case that Associates and executives see a substantial improvement in Customer Satisfaction ratings and then think that the improvement they have made is "good enough," and they settle. The better the organization performs, the more difficult it is to motivate people to do more, achieve more.

Do not settle for high Customer Satisfaction ratings. Set your sights on the top spot. Shoot for the moon—to be the number-one-rated organization in Customer Satisfaction! There is nothing newsworthy in being a runner-up. Silver and Bronze Olympic winners do not get the press. They do not get commercial endorsements. Gold Medal winners get the glory and press.

Would you like to put a sign on the front lawn of your organization that says, "We are the number-ten-rated organization in the country in Customer Satisfaction." Passers-by would think to themselves, "Well, I wonder who numbers one through nine are." Or would you rather hoist a flag that says, "We are the number-one-rated organization in Customer Satisfaction in the country." With number one ratings come free publicity—publicity the likes of which you could not afford to pay: national news stories in top-shelf business publications, prominent news stories in local and national newspapers. *Remember:* There is danger in the comfort zone. Top satisfaction ratings can disappear overnight, as the team at Holy Cross Hospital will attest.

Be Visible and Accessible to All Employees and Customers

CEOs, roll up your sleeves and get involved. Top CEOs lead by example. Herb Kelleher of Southwest Airlines hoists luggage on "Black Wednesday," the day before Thanksgiving, the busiest air travel day of the year.

CEO Rich Reif of Doylestown Hospital said there wasn't a job in his organization that he would ask someone to do that he would not do himself. To demonstrate his statement, Rich was photographed cleaning toilets at the Doylestown Hospital. Surely a publicity move, but one with a message. Get the point?

When CEOs get involved with the people and the front-line work, they learn more about the business—more about the irritations in the work system that need correcting. They hear first-hand what Customers are saying.

Visibility is one aspect of CEO involvement in the organization. A second aspect, of equal importance, is Associate and Customer access to the CEO. Break down the barriers to mahogany row. Routinely reserve time on your calendar for private and public meetings with Associates and Customers. Establish written channels of communication whereby Associates and Customers can write directly to the CEO without fear of recourse from their supervisor, and a timely response from the CEO will result.

Keep numerous channels of direct communication to the CEO open and easy to use. It is the only way leadership will really get to know what is going on in the organization.

Give Credit to Others

It is easy for the CEO to stand in the spotlight as awards are given for top Customer Satisfaction, or celebrations are held for substantial progress toward Customer Satisfaction goals. After all, the CEO's office is where broadcasters go to request interviews, where benchmarking organizations call to find out how your organization achieved what they achieved, etcetera. And it feels good, as CEO, to receive recognition.

However, if you wish to sustain organizational performance at these top levels, the wisdom of the ages will tell you to share the spotlight, and I will tell you to shed the spotlight. Divert attention, praise, and honor from the CEO's office to the staff and Associates who did the work to earn the recognition for the organization.

Associates are the people delivering service, and managers are the people orchestrating work systems. If you want people to continue to deliver outstanding performance levels, praise the work and behaviors that you wish to see repeated.

In the course of eighteen months following their rise to top-rated hospital status in Customer Satisfaction, Holy Cross Hospital was inundated with calls from other health care organizations requesting a speaker to visit their organization and share the secrets of their success, or requesting a site visit to Holy Cross to learn how to do what Holy Cross had learned to do so well. Rather than absorb those opportunities personally, CEO Mark Clement assigned various managers and Associates to conduct the speaking engagements and manage the site visits. He deflected the spotlight from his office to those who earned the recognition for the organization. It was a stroke of genius and a high level of recognition, reward, and reinforcement that continued to fuel the interest and motivation of staff and management to do more of this good work.

Align Customer Service to Your Vision, Mission, and Business Strategy

Do not forget the purpose and roots of your organization, its mission and vision. Within the mission and vision the voice of Customer service should be clear. Connect the dots between mission, vision, Customer service, and business strategy so every employee can clearly understand how the four elements are integrated and work together. Even for-profit organizations are operating in a not-for-profit industry, and they must act accordingly, realizing that the first priority of business is to achieve its mission—to deliver quality health care to those in need—not to put profits ahead of mission.

True Story

Tim Bidell, a veteran housekeeping supervisor of eighteen years with Holy Cross Hospital, commented in a newsletter story,

> *Holy Cross Hospital has become a not-for-profit hospital again. I know it has always had the status of a not-for-profit hospital, but now it is acting more like a not-for-profit hospital by talking about how to take care of patients and not about finances.*
>
> CEO Clement says,
>
> *We are obviously mindful of economics, but the real emphasis must be on caring for patients—improving quality, service, and cost.*

When leadership can connect vision, mission, and Customer Satisfaction in a way that is meaningful to Associates, then you have something.

Create a Culture that Values People

Service is delivered by people, and people must feel valued if they are to interact with physicians and patients in a manner that makes the Customer feel valued and special.

Powering up Associates is one way of making them feel like valuable, trusted members of the team. Reward, recognition, and reinforcement are other means of demonstrating how much you value the people of the organization. But it goes farther than that. Consider the Human Resources management of Associates of your organization. Is your organization providing adequate training and development for changing health care occupations? Are there channels of communication in which Associate ideation can be channeled and ideas heard, recognized, and implemented? Are communications regarding organizational operations, changes, and news shared on a timely basis with Associates, or do they learn of what's happening on the 6:00 P.M. television news?

There are many and various ways in which leadership can and should make Associates feel important.

Another True Story

Two hundred jobs were planned for elimination or redesign at Holy Cross Hospital. With advanced planning, voiced commitment to the people of the organization, and a sharing of the plan for change, the 200 job changes were implemented without layoffs or terminations—a demonstration of leadership's valuing of each and every Associate.

In some cases, Associates were assigned temporary responsibilities until their new position was ready to accept them. In other cases, there was a smoother transition from one job to another. In every case, the value and respect of each Associate was made clear.

Most remarkable are the results of an anonymous survey taken prior to the job redesign initiative. In that survey, 100 percent of the

Associates on payroll, including the 200 people who knew their jobs were in some type of jeopardy, agreed that the direction of change in the organization, including changes in job structure and roles, was good for the organization even though these same Associates knew that it would mean uncertainty for them, in terms of what their new job assignment would be and how happy they might be in that new job. Associates trusted leadership because they were made to feel valued in the organization.

Reports Mark Clement:

Success depends on a roll-out of communication that is straightforward, frequent, and complete.

Never Declare Victory

Victory is a daily battle that is won one Customer at a time. Today you may be winning. Tomorrow you could be losing. Rather than declaring victory, declare an eternal battle for excellence, which is an ever-moving target.

Keep Your Ideas Fresh

Routine behaviors or programs generate routine results, not exceptional results. Fresh ideas for Associate recognition keep ideation alive. Ideas for value-added and improved service and product delivery keep the organization on a competitive edge and keep staff fresh.

The focus is always the same—Customer Satisfaction—but the way in which motivation of Associates occurs must be ever-changing. The goal is the same—top customer satisfaction ratings—but the game of how the organization motivates, recognizes, and rewards achievement of the goal must be refreshed frequently to retain Associate attention. To keep ideation alive within the Associate population, there needs to be something in it for the Associate. So, in addition to adding ideation to the performance evaluation system, make it fun and a challenge, and entice Associates with rewards for participation.

I like to think of ideation management much the same as the chef at my favorite Mexican restaurant views his menu management. Ingredients in most Mexican meals are largely the same. Refried beans, rice, tortilla, tomatoes, lettuce, cheese, and a shredded meat. Only the name of dish and how the ingredients are assembled change, yet each time they shuffle the ingredients a little and put a new name of it, it feels like a new recipe. Really each dish has basically the same ingredients, just rearranged differently. The same is true for ideation management. Ingredients for success are the same. Reward, recognition, and reinforcement for targeted ideas. To keep it fresh and interesting, just vary how the rewards, recognition, and reinforcement are put together and put a new name on the incentive.

Maintain Constancy of Purpose

There are many distractions pulling and pushing for executive and managerial attention. Do not let distractions sway you from the primary purposes of the organization's existence—to serve the Customer. Keep the priority of the organization first and foremost in executive and managerial decision making and attention.

As crisis situations and important issues present themselves, interpret each situation in the light of Customer Satisfaction by asking yourself, "How will this decision, or how will this change, benefit our Customers?" If the answer is, "not at all," you know that the so-called crisis is a low priority. If the answer is, "Yes, this will enhance the Customers . . ." then it is a situation worthy of your time. Or, it is a decision that should be implemented.

Do Not Take Anything for Granted

The danger of being good at something is that you think you have the situation under control, that you have all the answers and know how to do it best. It is when you are successful that you are most vulnerable and need to be taking aggressive action for further improvement. Success is fleeting. Do not take it for granted. Continue to build upon past success and strive for the number one spot.

Do Not Let Others Convince You That You Are Good

Humility is an attractive quality.

Require Disciplined Executive Leadership

Effective executive leadership teams share uniform management systems, operating systems, and philosophy, plus a shared commitment to performance results. Free-wheeling executive approaches that in theory are supposed to compliment one another and represent a sense of diversity actually represent chaos, unnecessary overhead, and a bogged down organizational structure—one that is difficult to compete with.

When all executives and managers are operating off the same song sheet, the orchestration of efforts results in greater achievement, as no time is spent on coordination efforts. Coordination is built into the synchronized system. Organizational priorities are standardized across all departments and communicated to all Associates. Team dynamics replace discord. For a standardized management system for executives and managers, contact Management House for the MANSYS System.

Invest in Training

You have hired the brightest and best people to work in your organization, now protect that investment with training and further development—not just any training, but a strategic training and development plan with the specific goal of building a common knowledge base among all Associates in important areas, such as Customer Satisfaction management, innovation management and implementation, and problem solving.

Do not overestimate the management knowledge base of your department head team. Most department leaders advanced from technical positions to their management job with little or no management training. They are managing in the dark, hence the hodgepodge of management techniques and the disconnect between and among managers and executives. Invest in a management development effort that synchronizes thinking along lines of clearly articulated values, and the entire team will stop stepping on each other's toes.

CONCLUSION

Over and over again we prove that organizations that truly desire to serve the Customer are willing to invest in what it takes:

- Training for people.
- A system to communicate and implement massive ideation.
- Executives and managers committed to leading with a passion.
- Information on what Customers want, and a system for installing rapid change.
- The ability to integrate and balance leadership, systems improvements, Associate Satisfaction, and Customer Satisfaction.

Customer Satisfaction is not a sometimes thing. It is an everyday commitment.

ACTION PLAN FOR TOTAL CUSTOMER SATISFACTION

Task 1. Conduct a Self-Audit Using the CEO Tips for Sustained Success, Exhibit 10.2, as a Guide. With the executive team discuss which, if any, of the fourteen CEO Tips for Sustained Success your organization embraces and which it does not necessarily agree with. If you discover that there are a number of these CEO Tips for Sustained Success that are not embraced by your leadership, discuss whether a change in behavior is appropriate, and how that change will occur. If no change in leadership behavior is agreed upon, identify as a group what the risks of sustaining current behaviors will be.

Excellently led organizations embrace each of the fourteen CEO Tips for Sustained Success. The choice is yours to make.

Exhibit 10.2. *Self-Audit CEO Tips for Sustained Success.*

	Agree	Disagree	To Do	Done
1. Don't believe your own good press.	☐	☐	☐	☐
2. Expect a lot from people.	☐	☐	☐	☐
3. The better the organization performs, the more difficult it is to make more progress.	☐	☐	☐	☐
4. Be visible and accessible to all employees and Customers.	☐	☐	☐	☐
5. Give credit to others.	☐	☐	☐	☐
6. Align Customer Service to your vision, mission, and business strategy.	☐	☐	☐	☐
7. Create a culture that values people.	☐	☐	☐	☐
8. Never declare victory.	☐	☐	☐	☐
9. Keep your ideas fresh.	☐	☐	☐	☐
10. Maintain constancy of purpose.	☐	☐	☐	☐
11. Don't take anything for granted.	☐	☐	☐	☐
12. Don't let others convince you that you are good.	☐	☐	☐	☐
13. Require disciplined executive leadership.	☐	☐	☐	☐
14. Invest in training.	☐	☐	☐	☐

Recommended Readings

Albrecht, Karl. *At America's Service.* Homewood, Ill.: Business One Irwin, 1988.

Belandi, Deanna. "Consumers First." *Modern Health Care,* January 26, 1998, 30, 32.

Bell, Chip R. *Customers as Partners: Building Relationships that Last.* San Francisco: Berrett-Koehler, 1994.

"Beyond May I Help You." *Business Week/Quality,* 1991, 100–103.

Billington, Jim. "Five Keys to Keeping Your Best Customers." *Harvard Business Review Newsletter,* 1996, *1*(2), 1–4.

Blumberg, D. F. *Managing Service as a Strategic Profit Center.* New York: McGraw-Hill, 1991.

"Bringing Sears into the World." *Fortune,* Oct. 13, 1997, 183–184.

Garvin, David, A. "Competing on the Eight Dimensions of Quality." *Harvard Business Review,* Nov.–Dec. 1987, 101–109.

Glen, P. *It's Not My Department.* New York: William Morrow, 1990.

Gonzalez, William, G. *Reason for Being: Measuring and Improving Patient Satisfaction, Hospital Administration,* Feb. 1990, 62–64.

Hammonds, Keith H. "Where Did They Go Wrong." *Business Week/Quality,* 1991, 34–38.

Hart, Christopher, and Heskett, James, L. "The Profitable Art of Service Recovery." *Harvard Busi-ness Review,* July–Aug., 1990, 148–156.

"The Healing Touch of a Cold, Wet Nose." *Country Life,* January 29, 1998, 38–39.

Jacob, Rahul. "Thriving in a Lame Economy." *Fortune,* Oct. 5, 1992, 44–54.

"Learning How to Serve Well." *Houston Chronicle,* August 23, 1990.

Liswood, L. A. *Serving Them Right.* New York: HarperCollins, 1990.

Machan, Dyan. "Great Hash Browns, But Watch Those Biscuits." *Forbes,* Sept. 19, 1988, 192–196.

Mescon, Michael H., Mescon, Timothy S. "Smart Customers, Smarter Managers." *Sky,* Oct. 1989, 148–150.

Morgan, Rebecca L. *Calming Upset Customers.* Los Altos, Calif.: Crisp Publications, 1989.

Reichheld, Frederick, F. "Learning from Customer Defections." *Harvard Business Review,* March–April, 1996, 56–69.

Reichheld, Frederick F., and Sasser, Earl W., Jr. "Customer Defection: Quality Comes to Services." *Harvard Business Review,* Sept.–Oct. 1990, 105–111.

Schlesinger, Leonard A., and Heskett, James L. "The Service Driven Service Company." *Harvard Business Review,* Sept.–Oct. 1991, 71–82.

Sellers, Patricia. "Getting Customers to Love You." *Fortune,* March 13, 1989, 38–49.

Sherman, Clayton V. *Creating the New American Hospital: A Time for Greatness.* San Francisco: Jossey-Bass, 1993.

Steward, Thomas A. "GE Keeps Those Ideas Coming." *Fortune,* Aug. 12, 1991, 41–49.

Stewart, Thomas A. "A Satisfied Customer Isn't Enough." *Fortune,* July 21, 1997, 112–116.

Zmeke, Ron. *The Service Edge: 101 Companies that Profit from Customer Care.* New York: New American Library, 1989.

Index

A

Account representatives: for contractual Customers, 305–306; for employers and coalitions, 308; for physicians, 303–305

Accountability: of Do-It-Groups, 277–278; of physician account representatives, 304–305

Action Plans: for Customer Satisfaction Strategy, 212–219; for Total Customer Satisfaction, 19–22, 66–85, 117–137, 152–154, 176–180, 240–249, 285–292, 354–355

Admissions process: first impressions and, 333; in-room, 324; time of, 182

Adopt-a-Patient programs, 32, 75, 289–292; objectives of, 290; ombudsman and Customer Satisfaction manager services versus, 290–291; participants in, 290; process of, 290–292

Age variable, in patient satisfaction scores, 112–116

Alignment, 349

Amenities, room, 320–321. *See also* Rooms

American Association of Retired Persons, 206

American Express, 168–170

American Hospital Association, 270

Anderson's "Enterprise Award for Customer Satisfaction," 17

Anxiety relief skills, 78

Appointment scheduling, in medical practices, 111

Associate Attitude and Opinion Surveys: resolving dissatisfaction and, 248–249; review of, 78–79, 248–249

Associate performance: improvement of, 251–292; linking, to compensation, 330–332; linking, to Customer needs, 328–332; rewarding, recognizing, and reinforcing, 48–49; uniform standards for, 51–54. *See also* Customer Satisfaction improvement; Reward, recognition, and reinforcement; Standards

Associate Satisfaction: collecting feedback on, 214–217, 248–249; as driver of Customer Satisfaction, 39–44, 79–80, 210, 337; factors of, 43; productivity and, 229–233; protecting, 44, 79–82, 231–233; review of, 78–80, 248–249; sample survey form for evaluating, 215–216

Associates: collecting feedback from, 214–217; communication of, 226–227, 240–241; crediting, for top Customer Satisfaction, 348–349; Customer-for-a-Day programs for, 178–180; dissatisfied, 45–46; Do-It-Group process for, 60, 179; employer obligations and, 10–11; empowerment of, 56–57, 194–197, 218, 245–246; evaluating service potential of, 200–201, 202; generating awareness in, 211; high expectations for, 345–346; ideation

of, 251–254, 264–274; job swapping of, 328–330; positive, happy, healthy attitudes of, 264; powered-up, 295, 340–341, 345–346, 350; respect for, 231–232, 348–349; retention of, 39–40, 45–46, 79–80, 229–233; roles and responsibilities of, 263–264; sustaining motivation of, 351–352; traits of good service staff and, 198–199; turnover of, 45–46, 78–80, 229–230; valuing, 350–351. *See also* Reward, recognition, and reinforcement; Training
Awards: Associate, 49; for Customer Satisfaction, 17; internal, 274–275

B

Baby boomers, Customer Satisfaction ratings of, 18–19
Banking industry, Customer management in, 301–302
Banners and flags, 282
Barrier busting, 256, 265–267
Barrier, J., 165
Bell Federal Savings, 224
Bellandi, D., 219
Benchmarking: Associate turnover rates, 80; Customer Satisfaction, 55–56, 184–185; Customer Satisfaction ratings, 123–124, 126–128; departmental satisfaction ratings, 131–132; informal, for ideas, 265; with national databases, 126–128, 145–146
Bidell, T., 349
Big D (major dissatisfaction), 33–34, 76
Big, Hairy, Audacious Goals (BHAGs): bonus payouts for achieving, 269–270, 271, 330–331; committing to, 34–37; executive establishment of, 256, 287; managers' responsibility for, 259–260
Birthday cards, 207
Birthing Center concept, 321
Black hole of lost ideas, 285
"Black Wednesday," 347
Black-eyed Pea Restaurants, 234
Blue Cross, 7
Bonus incentives, 268–270, 271, 273–274, 330–331
Bowen, D., 42
Brandon, D., 11
British Airways, 51, 77
Broadcasting, negative, 161–164, 166–167
Buffalo State University, 199–200
Bureaucracy, 56–57, 75, 195, 198, 211, 218, 246
Business indicators, as indicators of Customer Satisfaction, 144
Business results, balancing the seven key areas of, 49–50, 82
Business strategy, 349

C

Calendar for problem solving, 300
Call light answer time, 129, 131, 314–315
Calming Upset Customers (Morgan), 161
Campbell Soup Company, 208
Capacity, excess, 6
Career "shadow days," 206
Carey, R., 116, 137*n*.2
Carl's Corner, 237–240
Celebration, 300
Center for Bio Ethics, University of Pennsylvania, 226
Center for Studies in Creativity, 199–200
CEO Welcome Letter, 69, 71–72, 335
Chairpersons, Do-It-Group, 277, 288
Change: in Customer Satisfaction ratings, 344–345, 351, 352; and frequency of feedback, 133–134; initiating rapid, 294–296, 345–346
Change Management Driver, 287
Cheerfulness, 226–229, 236–237

Chief executive officers (CEOs): Big D of, 33–34, 76; communication of, 68–69, 71–72, 74, 347–348; crediting Associates versus, 348–349; Customer access to, 347–348; Customer Satisfaction communication with, 30; physician relationships and, 303; self-audit for, 355; tips for, for sustaining top performance, 344–355; visible involvement of, 347–348. *See also* Top executives
Chief operating officer (COO), physician relationships and, 303
Child care, 208, 324
Children: listening to, 234–235; value-added services for, 324–325
Christmas carolers, 318
Civility, 236–237
Clark, K. F., 22*n*.1
Clas Forney International Group, 39–42
Cleanliness, 237, 317, 333, 334
Clement, M., 11, 16, 270–271, 344, 345, 348, 349, 351
Clinics, freestanding: Customer Satisfaction measurement for, 135. *See also* Medical practices
Coaching, 262
Comfort and company, 320
Comfort zone, danger of, 346–347
Comments: listening to Customers', 176–177, 180, 207; negative, 226–227, 228, 241, 246; overheard in hospital elevator, 226–227; overheard in preoperative preparation room, 176–177
Communication: of Associates, 226–229, 228, 240–241; to calm anxious patients, 67–68, 78, 183–184; of chief executive officer, 68–69, 71–72, 74, 347–348; with Customers, 31–33, 38–39, 69, 71–73, 308–314, 335–336; example circumstances of, 244–245; about idea action, 285, 289; negative, 226–227, 228, 241, 246; within organizations about Customer Satisfaction, 29–31, 68–74, 124–126, 278–283; of patients about bad experiences, 161–164; with patients about their needs, 184; with patients' families, 243; with physicians about Customer Satisfaction ratings, 284; positive, 227–229, 236–237, 240–241; strategy for, 308–314; training in, 78, 199, 240–245; about waiting times, 122–123. *See also* Listening to Customers
Communication Action Council (CAC), 278–283; activities of, 279–283; media and channels of, 281–283; member selection and orientation for, 286–287; responsibilities of, 278–279, 285–286
Community involvement, 201–202, 204–209, 218; active, 218; value-added services and, 325–326
Community newspapers, 282
Community of patients, 207–209
Company, for patients, 320
Compensation, 43, 210, 248–249, 267–268, 330–332. *See also* Reward, recognition and reinforcement
"Competing on the Eight Dimensions of Quality," 315
Competition: borrowing ideas from, 264–265; departmental, 131–132, 258–259, 272–274
Competitive advantage: cheerful climate as, 229, 236–237; Customer Satisfaction as, 3, 6, 62; service quality as, 236–237
Complaints: converting, to problem statements, 200; Customer Hotlines for, 310–312; as learning opportunities, 32; letters of, 144–145; percentage of patients who don't share, 155; profiling, 298–300; reasons for patients' reluctance to share, 155–160; as sources of ideas, 264. *See also* Dissatisfied Customers; Irritations

Compliment letters, 144–145
Computer screen savers, 282
Conformance, as dimension of health care quality, 317
Construction disruption, 47
Consumer choice, 4, 62
Continuous improvement, of departmental internal Customer Satisfaction, 216–217
Continuum of care, patient irritation and, 136
Contract reviews, Customer, 305–306
Cornelius, C., 237–240
Cost: of one lost Customer, 166–170, 178; quality and, 12, 64
Counterfeit patient, 177–178
Creating the New American Hospital: A Time for Greatness (Sherman), 57, 81, 226, 228, 272
Customer annoyances. *See* Complaints; Irritations
Customer contract reviews, 305–306
Customer defection, 170–176; competition and, 6; control of, 61, 68, 164–166, 179, 180, 194–197; detection of, training on, 66–68; economic cost of, 166–170, 178; feedback from, 206, 207, 219; physician relationships and, 21–22; reasons for, 26–29, 161; service recovery and, 164–166, 193–199. *See also* Complaints; Dissatisfied Customers
Customer expectations: education and, 192–193; meeting and exceeding, 326–327; versus reality, 191–192. *See also* Customer needs and wants
Customer Hotline, 32, 310–312
Customer incentives, 206, 235–236
Customer influence, 1–2; contemporary trends and, 3–12
"The Customer is always right" philosophy, 221–225
Customer loyalty: Customer Satisfaction ratings and, 64–65; profitability of, 201–204; realities of, 187–191; relationships and, 183–185, 207–208; satisfaction guarantees and, 181–183; strategies for gaining and maintaining, 204–209; winning and retaining, 181–220; zones of satisfaction and, 188–191
Customer needs and wants, 90–92, 161; Associate performance linked to, 328–332; change in, 133–134; in emergency room services, 100–103; in hospital services, 92–100; identifying, 213; in medical practices, 107–109. *See also* Customer expectations; Special needs
Customer Satisfaction: Action Plans for Total, 19–22, 66–85, 117–137, 152–154, 176–180, 240–249, 285–292, 354–355; alignment of, to vision, mission, and business strategy, 349; Associate satisfaction and, 39–44, 79–80, 210; baby boomers and, 18–19; changes contributing to power of, 3–12; comprehensive nature of, 29; Eighteen Commandments of, 23–59; evangelizing, at every organizational level, 29–31; factors in, 87–137; importance of, 1–2; irrational nature of, 221–249; lackluster, 24; maintaining constancy of, 352; most important factor of, for organizations, 105–106; most important factor of, for patients, 106–107; Nine Realities of, 59–66; obsession with right to, 6–7; versus other business indicators, 2–3; patient education and, 192–193, 205–206; priority of, versus other improvements, 65–66; proactive actions for, in case example, 47; profitability and, 41–42, 201–204; subjective nature of, 105–106; Success Cycle of, 8–10, 42; unexpected benefits of, 12–18

Customer Satisfaction Competencies Checklist, 202
Customer Satisfaction Council, 120; composition of, 297
Customer Satisfaction improvement: areas of focus for, 297; checklist for, 258; departmental competition for, 258–259, 272–274; departmental plans for, 246–248; difficulty of sustaining, 346–347; in emergency rooms, 103–104; executive role in, 255–259; in hospitals, 99–100; incremental versus rapid, 294–296; massive, 295–296; in medical practices, 109–112; prioritizing areas of, 118–122; strategy for, 293–336; to-do list for, 298. *See also* Action Plans; Customer Satisfaction strategy; Ideas; Ideation; Implementation of ideas
Customer Satisfaction management, 19–22; Eighteen Commandments of, 23–59; Nine Realities of, 59–66
Customer Satisfaction measurement: alternative approaches to, 140–146; areas of, 132–133; break outs for, 128–133; of distinct patient populations, 117; for free-standing clinics, 135; frequency of, 25, 133–135; of internal Customers, 214–217; meaningful, 139–146; methods of, 74–75, 140–146; methods of, assessing current, 74–75, 154; methods of, selecting, 146–152; monthly, 134; for physician practices, 135–136; purposes of, 139–140; quarterly, 133–134; through Customer contact, 31–33; validity of, 63–64; vendor versus do-it-yourself approaches to, 64, 118, 120; volume of, 133–135; weekly, 134–135. *See also* Customer Satisfaction ratings; Customer Satisfaction surveys; Data collection
Customer Satisfaction measurement vendors, 120; added value with, 153; "can do" attitude of, 148–149; checklist for evaluating, 152; cooperative and flexible, 150; versus do-it-yourself approaches, 64, 118; forward thinking orientation of, 149–150; on-site support provided by, 149; for postdischarge survey administration, 141; pricing, 151; qualities required of, 146; research ability of, 148–149; selection and evaluation of, 146–153; timeliness of data from, 150–151, 153; training and development provided by, 152; weekly feedback and, 135
Customer Satisfaction Pledge, 69, 71–72
Customer Satisfaction ratings: age variables in, 112–116; analysis of, 137; breaking out, by departments, 128–129, 130–132; breaking out, by key performance areas, 129–132; Customer loyalty and, 64–65; gender variables in, 112–116; ideation and, 252–254; interpretation of, 37–38, 76–77, 105–106; justification of poor, 46–48; mandates for, 11–18; mean of, 118; national databases of, 11–12; need for excellent, 188–191, 346–347; organizational communication about, 29–31; as performance report cards, 306–307; posting, in departments, 124–126, 127; saw-tooth effect in, 337; sharing, with physicians, 284; subjective nature of, 105–106; sustaining top, 337–355; timeliness of, 150–151, 153; zones of, 188–191
Customer Satisfaction statistics, charting trends in, 212–213
Customer Satisfaction stories, publicizing, 279, 280–281
Customer Satisfaction strategy: Action Plan for, 212–219; Associate-performance-linked-to-Customer-needs focus of, 328–332; components of,

296–297; Customer communication/orientation-for-results focus of, 308–314; designing, 293–336; document design of, 296; first-and-last-impressions focus of, 332–336; incremental versus rapid improvement and, 294–296; meeting/exceeding-Customer-expectations focus of, 326–327; operational structure of, 296, 297; service improvement/adding-value focus of, 321–326; service improvement/irritation-removal focus of, 314–321; size of, 298; targeting/managing Customers focus in, 298–308

Customer Satisfaction surveys: assessment of, 74–75; correlation of, to likelihood to recommend, 117–120, 119, 148; departmental, 154; frequency of, 25; versus informal feedback, 31; internal Customer Satisfaction, 215–216, 217; mandates for, 11–12; postdischarge mailed, 141–142; postdischarge telephone, 142–143; return rates of, 143–144; statistical correlation of, 143–144, 147–148; at time of discharge, 142; validity of, 63–64. *See also* Customer Satisfaction measurement; Data collection

Customer Satisfaction team: Associate roles and responsibilities in, 263–264; building, 251–292; coaching, 262; Communication Action Council and, 278–283; Do-It-Groups/Just-Do-It-Groups and, 274–276; executive roles and responsibilities in, 255–259; ideation of, 264–274; Management Action Council and, 277–278; manager roles and responsibilities in, 259–262; Physician Action Council and, 283–285; roles and responsibilities in, 255–264

Customer Service Tip of the Week, 126; sample, 125

Customer share, 58; analysis of, 85

Customer SWAT teams, 331

Customer-Associate relationship, 337–339. *See also* Associate satisfaction; Associates; Customer Satisfaction; Customers

Customer-focused organization, 341

Customer-for-a-Day program, 178–180, 309–310

Customer/patient profile, 245

Customers: communication with, 31–33, 38–39; concept of, 87–90; contractual, 305–306; defined, 87–90; dissatisfied, 155–180; identifying, 213, 298, 299; overserving, 245–246; as partners, 254–255; patients as ultimate, 7–8; physicians as, 283; profiling problems and complaints of, 298–300; provider selection by, 191–192; as source of ideas, 232–236, 237–240, 242–244; special needs of, 38–39, 62–63; staying close to, 210–212; targeting and managing, 298–308. *See also* Dissatisfied Customers; Patient *headings;* Physician *headings*

Customization of service, 88, 90

D

Data collection: from defectors, 207–208; by distinct patient populations, 117; informal methods of, 176–180; from internal Customers, 214–217; methods of, 74–75, 140–146, 154; for Service Excellence improvement plans, 246–247. *See also* Customer Satisfaction measurement; Customer Satisfaction measurement vendors; Customer Satisfaction surveys

Databases: benchmarking to, 126–128, 145–146; mandates for, 11–12; national, 120; participation in, 126–128; vendors of, 146–147

Decision making: financial limitation on, 295, 341; implementation strategy and, 295
Decor, 318, 320–321
Delivery system services, 209
Departments: competition among, 131–132, 258–259, 272–274; creating Customer "Wow!" experiences in, 327; Customer-for-a-Day programs in, 309–310; feedback loops and, 187; internal Customer Satisfaction measurement in, 214–217; management development for, 353–354; mini-focus-type groups in, 176–177; performance improvement of, 258–259; satisfaction ratings by, 128–129, 130–132; Service Excellence improvement plans for, 246–248; surveys of Customer Satisfaction measurement in, 154; team meetings of, 29–30; testing responsiveness of, 177–178
Dietary services, 208, 323
Digital Equipment Corporation, 222
DIG/JDI Hotline, 279, 280
DIG/JDI process flow chart, 276. *See also* Do-It-Groups; Just-Do-It Groups
Discharge surveys, 142, 247
Disney Corporation, 54, 226, 227–228, 268
Dissatisfaction: Associate, 45–46, 248–249; costs of, 166–170, 178; major, 33–34, 76; payer, 167; physician, 167. *See also* Complaints; Customer defection; Irritations; Physician satisfaction
Dissatisfied Customers, 155–180, 188–189; economic costs of, 166–170, 178; Moments of Truth and, 169, 170–176; negative broadcasting of, to potential Customers, 161–164, 166–167; recovery of, 164–166; rules of dealing with, 195. *See also* Complaints; Customer defection
Distribution chain, listening to everyone in, 211
Dixie Rock Restaurants, 234
Do-It-Group (DIG) Guide, 57, 60, 75, 275
Do-It-Groups (DIGs): accountability of, 277–278; Chairpersons of, 277, 288; Communication Action Council and, 278–283; flow chart of, 276; Management Action Council and, 277–278; Physician Action Council and, 283–285; for problem solving, 60, 179, 180, 228, 247, 263, 274–275, 300; process of, 274–275, 276, 287; reporting topics and status of, 279–280; review of, 287; training for, 287–288
Domino's Pizza, 210, 258–259
Doylestown Hospital, 347
Dressing gowns, 321
Dressing rooms, 174–175
Duplicity of work, 277
Durability, as dimension of health care quality, 317
Durable medical equipment, 208–209

E

Eastwood, C., 162
Education, patient, 192–193, 205–206, 319–320
Efficiency, 341–344
Electronic industry organizations, 80
Elevator, comments overhead in, 226–227
Emergency rooms (ERs): Adopt-a-Patient program in, 291; Customer defections from, 61; Customer Satisfaction improvement in, case example of, 36–37; Customer Satisfaction ratings of, sample report, 119; friendliness and sensitivity factors in, 101–103; job swapping in, 328–329; patients' likelihood to recommend, factors in, 100–103; priority index for improvement of, 103–104; waiting times in, 26–29

Employee performance evaluation, 268
Employees. *See* Associate *headings*
Employer coalitions, 205, 306–308
Employers: Customer Satisfaction and, 10–11; involvement with, 205; targeting and marketing to, 306–308
Empowerment, 56–57, 194–197, 218, 245–246. *See also* Powered-up Associates
Endorsements, Customer, 280–281
Entrance area, 333
Esthetics, as dimension of health care quality, 317–318
Executives. *See* Chief executive officer; Top executives
Experts, Customers as, 232–233
External report card, 139–140

F

Families: communication with, 243; educational materials for, 319–320; value-added services for, 324–325
Fayette Memorial Hospital, 10–11
Fear: of mistakes, 198, 266; in organizations, 266; of patients to complain, 156; of patients undergoing medical treatment, 183–184, 213
Features, as dimension of health care quality, 316
Federal Express, 56
Feedback. *See* Customer Satisfaction measurement; Customer Satisfaction ratings; Data collection
Feedback loops, 185–187
Fields, Marshall, 232–233
Financial authority: of Associates, 295, 341; of physician account representatives, 304–305
First Chicago Bank, 224–225
First impressions, 332–336; dynamics of, 332–333; managing, 333–336
Flags and banners, 282
Florida Power and Light, 50
Focus groups, 75, 143, 176–177
Food service: esthetics of, 318; in hospitals, 94, 95, 97, 148, 318; for special diets, 208; value-added, 325
Fortune, 7, 17
Four Seasons Hotels, 51, 196, 223, 226, 245

G

Galvin, R., 212
Ganey, R. F., 92, 94
Garvin, D., 315
Gender variable, in patient satisfaction scores, 112–116
General Electric, 226
General Motors, 163
Goals. *See* Big Hairy Audacious Goals
Great Comebacks Award, 270
Guarantees, 181–182; in health care, 182–183
Guardians, 89

H

Harris Bank, 224
Harvard Business Review, 315
Harvard Business School, 222
Hawaii Advertiser, 236
Hays Medical Center, 48
Healing environment, 315, 317–318, 319–321
Health care facilities: first impressions of, 333, 334; healing environment in, 315, 317–318, 319–321; health plan providers and, 8–10; navigation aids in, 312–313; physician selection of, 15–17. *See also* Hospitals
Health Employers Data Information Set (HEDIS), 12
Health maintenance organizations (HMOs), patient satisfaction with, 116

Health plan providers: Customer Satisfaction for, 7–8; health care facilities and, 8–10
Hewlett-Packard, 56, 80
High structure, 346
"High-light/spot-light" meetings, 270–271, 331
Holiday cards, 207
Holy Cross Hospital (Chicago), call lights performance tracking at, 130,131; CEO Welcome Letter of, 69, 71–72; Customer interviews at, 184; Customer Satisfaction improvement at, 16; Customer Satisfaction ratings of, 17; Customer Satisfaction Reports of, 125, 126–127; high-light/spot-light meetings at, 270–271; ideation at, 34–35, 252, 253, 254; market share growth of, 11; patient care values of, 349; recognition, reward, and reinforcement at, 348–349, 350; service recovery at, 344–345, 347; valuing of Associates at, 350–351
Home alteration services, 209
Home visits, 323
Hospitals: Customer dissatisfaction in, case example, 170–176; Customer Satisfaction improvement in, 98–100; food service in, 94, 95, 97, 148, 318; healing environment in, 315, 319–321; hospitality services in, 94–97; importance of friendliness and sensitivity in, 93–97, 99; navigation in, 312–313; nursing staff behaviors in, 93; patient concern with physicians in, 95; patients' likelihood to recommend, factors in, 92–100; physician practice privileges in multiple, 5; physician referrals to, 5–6; priority index for improvement of, 98–100; room temperature in, 94, 95, 97
"Hospitals Forgetting to Query Customers in Quality Process," 236
Hotlines: Customer, 32, 309–310; DIG/JDI, 280, 297; patient, 74, 75
Housing for families, 324
Human Resources Executive, 2
Human Resources management, 350–351
Humility, 353
Hygiene, personal, 52–53
Hyper-allergenic materials, 243

I

Idea representatives, 277
Ideas: of adding value to services, 322–323; of Associates, 251–254, 264–274; barriers to, 265–267, 285; central clearinghouse of, 276, 277–278; for Customer "Wow!" experiences, 327; listening to Customers for, 232–236, 237–240, 242–244; maintaining the flow of, 267–274, 278, 351–352; managers' role in supporting, 262; plugging the black hole of, 285; reward system for, 266–267, 351–352; sources of, 264–265; strategies for generating, 264–274; system for processing, 75, 274–285; tracking, 288–289. *See also* Implementation of ideas
Ideation: analysis of, 252–254; compensation structure and, 267–268; establishing the BHAG for, 287; initiation and support of, 261, 264–274; maintaining, 267–274, 278, 351–352; performance bonus incentives for, 268–270, 271, 273–274; power of, 252, 253; staying power of, 254; tracking management of, 288–289; tracking return on investment in, 278. *See also* Implementation of ideas
Identification bracelets, 177
Implementation of ideas: manager support for, 261; system for, 75, 274–285
Implementation strategy, 294–296; highly controlled approach to, 294–296; rapid implementation approach to, 294–296,

345–346. *See also* Customer Satisfaction strategy
Impressions, first and last, 332–336
Incentives, Customer, 206
Inspirational quotes, 281
Insurance coverage, type of, and patient satisfaction, 116
Internal report card, 139
IBM, 53, 222
Interpersonal skills training, 241–245
Inventory on Customer Satisfaction Skills for Health Care Providers, 201
Irritations: compiling ambulatory care facilities list of, 316; continuum of care and, 136; dimensions of health care quality and, 316–318; observation of, 180; patients as tanks of, 136; removing, 314–321; value-added service and, 321–322. *See also* Complaints

J

Job swapping, 328–330
Joint Commission on Accreditation of Healthcare Organizations (JCAHO) standards, 317
Joint Commission on Hospital Accreditation, 1
Joking, 246
Journal of Ambulatory Care, 116
Just-Do-It-Groups (JDIs), 179; Communication Action Council and, 278–283; flow chart of, 276; Management Action Council and, 277–278; Physician Action Council and, 283–285; process of, 275, 276, 287; reporting topics and status of, 279–280; review of, 287; training for, 287–288
Just-in-time training, 291–292

K

Kaiser Permanente, 236
Kelleher, H., 231, 347
Key performance areas, Customer Satisfaction ratings break out by, 129–132
Key Result Areas (KRAs), 49–50, 82, 280
Kotulak, R., 249

L

Lab technician behavior, patient preferences for, 108, 109
Lab tests: efficiency of, in case example, 343–344; reliability of, 317
Last impressions, 332–336; dynamics of, 332–333; managing, 333–336
Leadership: disciplined, 353; uncommon, 340. *See also* Chief executive officers; Managers; Top executives
Leno, J., 225
Leonard, S., 222
Letters, complaint and compliment, 144–145; tracking, 144–145
Leveraging your Customer relationships, 209
Lighting, 319
Likelihood to recommend. *See* Recommend, likelihood to
"Listen Doctors" (Physician Insurers Association), 235, 249*n.*1
Listening to Customers: Associate responsibility for, 263; for comments, 176–177, 180, 207; in distribution chain, 211; for feedback, 145; for ideas, 232–236, 237–240, 242–244; multiple posts for, 211; training for, 78. *See also* Communication

M

Major U.S. Travel Service, 42
Mallardi, V., 85*n.*1
Malpractice claims, common causes of, 235
Managed care: criteria for contract awards by, 64; patent satisfaction with, 116

Management: high-structure, 346; short-sighted, 157–160; standardized system of, 353
Management Action Council (MAC), 275, 277–278; member selection and orientation for, 286–287; responsibilities of, 277–278, 285–286, 295
Management by objectives, 346
Management House, Inc., 57, 60, 75, 84, 201, 267, 275, 287, 332, 353
Management team, monthly meetings with, 30
Managers: as Customer Hotline staffers, 311–312; decision making of, 260–261; idea generation requirements for, 268; individual performance levels of, 331; needs evaluation for development of, 83–84; as new thinkers, 260; as role models, 262; roles and responsibilities of, 259–262; support of, for ideation, 266; as team coaches, 262; training and development of, 83–84, 353–354
Managing Quality Service (Martin), 198–199
Manners, 53–54
MANSYS System, 353
Market competition, 61–62
Market share: analysis of, 85; Customer share and, 58; loyal Customers and, 170
Marketing materials, 283
Marketing programs, Customer Satisfaction programs versus, 182
Marriott Hotels and Suites, 51, 56, 74, 184–185, 209
Marshall Fields Department Stores, 232–233
Martin, W., 198–199
Mayo Clinic, 229
McDonald's, 234–235, 329–330
MCI, 42
Mean scores, 118–120
Measurement. *See* Customer Satisfaction measurement
Medicaid reporting, 1
Medical practices: clustering, for account representatives, 304; Customer Satisfaction measurement for, 135; patients' likelihood to recommend, factors in, 107–109; priority index for improving, 109–112; size of, and patient satisfaction ratings, 116. *See also* Physician practices
Medical staff: company of, 320; negative and positive communication of, 226–229, 240–241, 246; patient relationship with, 107–109; training for, 84–85. *See also* Associates; Lab technician behaviors; Nursing staff behaviors
Medicare, patient satisfaction with, 116
Medication schedules, 242–243
Mentoring system, Customer Satisfaction, 217–218
Mergers, Associate-Customer satisfaction relationship and, 44
Merry Maids, 42
Mission, 349
Mobile Corporation, 223
Modern Health Care, 236
Moments of Truth, 169, 170–176, 315; testing departmental responsiveness to, 177–178
Monaghan, T., 210
Monitoring service, 211
Morgan, R. L., 161
Motorola, 212
Music, 318, 319
Mystery shoppers, 210

N

National databases, 120; mandates for, 11–12; participation in, 126–128
Natural sounds, 319
Navigation in facilities, 312–313, 333
Negative broadcasting, 161–164, 166–167

Negative communication, staff, 226–227, 228, 240–241, 246
Negotiation, of Customer contracts, 305–306
Negotiation power, of exceptional Customer Satisfaction, 13–14
New American Health Care organizations, 3; Associate ideas in, 251–252; components of, 337–339; Customer Hotlines in, 311–312; Customer Satisfaction in, 223–229; customer-focused, 341; hospital navigation systems in, 312; improved work systems, 341–344; performance review and rewards in, 48; powered-up Associates in, 340–341; recognition in, 49; staff retention and recruitment in, 79–80; values-driven, 339–340; vendor selection and, 151
New thinkers, 260
Newsletter Customer Satisfaction column, 73, 281–282
Newspapers, local, 282
Noise, 317–318, 319
Nordstrom's, 44
Nursing staff behaviors: patient preferences for, in emergency rooms, 102–103; patient preferences for, in hospitals, 93, 96–97, 99; patient preferences for, in medical practices, 107–109
Nuts: Southwest Airlines Crazy Recipe for Success (Kelleher), 231

O

Old National Bank, 157–160, 165
Olsen, K., 222
Olympics, 272–273, 347
Ombudsman, patient, 290–291
"One-time-stand," 3
On-site support, vendor, 149
Opel, J., 222
Operation Bandit, 264–265
Organizational culture: for Associate retention, 231–233; for exceptional Customer Satisfaction, 56–57; for ideation, 266; values-driven, 339–340
Organizational performance: CEO tips for sustaining, 344–355; Customer Satisfaction as driver of, 19–22. *See also* Associate performance; Customer Satisfaction improvement
Organizations: customer-focused, 341; improved work systems in, 341–344; powered-up Associates in, 340–341; primary components of, 337–339; values-driven, 339–340. *See also* New American Health Care organizations
Orientation, of council members, 286–287

P

Pacific Business Group on Health, 2
Pareto's 80/20 principle, 91–92
Parkside Associates, Inc., 44, 112, 137*n*.1
Partnership power, of exceptional Customer Satisfaction, 14–15
Pastoral care, 320
Patient advocacy, 75
Patient anxiousness, 28; methods to calm, 67–68; training for relief of, 78
Patient education, 205–206; materials for, 319–320; patient satisfaction and, 192–193
Patient hotline, 74, 75
Patient Ombudsman, 290–291
Patient preference card, 245
Patient satisfaction. *See* Customer Satisfaction
Patients: age and gender variables in, 112–116; constellation of, in the community, 207–209; inner life of, 183–185, 229; as irritation tanks, 136; as partners, 254–255; preferences of, in emergency room services, 100–103; preferences of, in hospital services, 92–100; preferences of, in medical practices, 107–109; preferences of,

patterns in, 106–107; as ultimate Customers, 7–8. *See also* Customer *headings*
Patron, 88–89
Pay-for-performance, 330–332
Peace and quiet, 317–318, 319
Peat Marwick, 190
Peer pressure, 271
Performance, as dimension of health care quality, 316
Performance improvement. *See* Associate performance; Customer Satisfaction improvement
Performance improvement checklist, 258
Performance review, 48
Performance standards, 51–54, 82–83
Personal appearance, uniform, 51–52
Personal hygiene, 52–53
Personal needs questions, 242–244
Pharmacies, on-site, 316
Philosophy: of "the Customer is always right," 221–225; of overserving Customers, 245–246; of putting the Customer first, 160
Physical plant, impressions of, 334. *See also* Health care facilities
Physician account management, 301–305
Physician account representatives: authority and accountability of, 304–305; selection of, 303–304; training for, 305
Physician Action Council (PAC), 283–286; member selection and orientation for, 286–287
Physician group ratings, 2
Physician Insurers Association, 235, 249*n*.1
Physician practices: Customer Satisfaction measurement for, 135–136; involving, in Customer Satisfaction initiatives, 84–85; patient likelihood to recommend, factors in, 107–109; priority index for improving, 109–112; size of, and patient satisfaction, 116; targeting, 301. *See also* Medical practices
Physician referrals, 5–6, 300–301
Physician satisfaction: costs of losing, 167; as Customer Satisfaction indicator, 145; management of, 300–301; measurement of, 22
Physician-patient relationship: importance of, in hospitals, 95; importance of, in medical practices, 107–109
Physicians: account representatives for, 303–304; as business people, 4–5; as Customers, 283, 301–302; grouping, by type of practice, 303; importance of, to patients in hospitals, 95; linking, to Customer Satisfaction initiative, 57–58, 283–285; as listeners and learners, 5–6; recruitment of, 15–17, 301; review of, 21–22, 300–301, 302–303; role of, in Customer Satisfaction improvement, 283–284; sharing Customer Satisfaction information with, 284; targeting, 301
Picker Institute, 120, 137*n*.1
Pink Flamingo awards, 258
Pizza Hut, 209
Policy, negative impact of invoking, 157–160
Politics, physician influence on, 284–285
Positive, happy, healthy attitudes, 264
Positive, happy, healthy communication, 227–229, 236–237, 240–241
Postdischarge surveys: mailed, 141–142; telephone, 142–143
Powered-up Associates, 295, 340–341, 345–346, 350. *See also* Associates; Empowerment
PPO Health Care Book of Providers (Sherman), 4
Preferred Provider Organization (PPO), patient satisfaction with, 116
Preferred providers, 8
Preoperative preparation room, comments observed in, 176–177

Preparedness, 334–335
Press, Ganey Associates, 118, 120, 137*n*.1; age and gender research of, 112–116; emergency room patient satisfaction study, 101–103; hospital patient satisfaction study, 92–100; medical practice patient satisfaction study, 107–109; national Customer Satisfaction database, 11, 16, 24, 128; national inpatient hospital Customer Satisfaction survey, 18
Preventative medicine, 205–206, 323–324
Priority index: creating, 118–120, 121; for improving emergency room Customer Satisfaction, 103–104; for improving hospital Customer Satisfaction, 98–100; for improving medical practice Customer Satisfaction, 109–112; sample, 120, 121; use of, to analyze improvement areas, 120, 122; use of, to research improvement areas, 122–123
Problem solving: assessment of ease of, 218; Associate responsibility for, 263; calendar for, 300; to control Customer defection, 61, 68, 164–166, 179, 180, 194–197, 219; to control staff negativity, 228, 246, 264; empowerment for, 56–57, 194–197, 218, 245–246; failure of, as reason for Customer defection, 161; patient and visitor participation in, 254–255; prioritizing, for each Customer, 299; for Service Excellence improvement, 247; skills in, value of, 199–200; timely, 165–166, 194–197; training for, 60, 68, 241–245. *See also* Do-It-Groups (DIGs); Just-Do-It Groups (JDIs)
Product and service extensions to health care, 208–209
Professionalism, 228
Profitability: Associate retention and, 229–233; Customer Satisfaction and, 41–42, 144, 201–204; ideation and, 252, 253; of one Customer, 167–168
Proof Rock Restaurant, 234–235
Protection of staff, 156
Providers, ways Customers select, 191–192
Publicity, Customer Satisfaction for, 17–18
Purpose, maintaining constancy of, 352

Q

Quality: cost and, 12, 64; dimensions of health care, 316–318; obsession with, 49–50; perceived, 318; service, 236–237
Quality improvement, 49, 185–186

R

R ranking, 118–120
Radiology tests, adding value to, 322–323
Radisson Hotel, 184
Rapid implementation, 294–296, 345–346
Ratings. *See* Customer Satisfaction ratings
Recognition, 48–49, 81–82, 348–349. *See also* Reward, recognition, and reinforcement
Recognition Action Council, 81–82
Recognition Action Guide, 267
Recommend, likelihood to, 105–106; emergency rooms, 100–103; hospitals, 92–100, 183; medical practices, 107–109; satisfaction survey questions' correlation to, 117–120, 119, 148
Recruitment: of Customers, 204–209; of physicians, 15–17, 301; of staff, 79–80
Reengineering: Customer Satisfaction initiative versus, 65–66; valuing Associates and, 350–351
Referrals, strategies for getting, 204–209
Registration process: first impressions and, 334; in-room, 324; speed of, 110, 111
Regression analysis, 143
Reif, R., 347

Reimbursement rates, Customer Satisfaction ratings and, 12–13
Reinforcement, 48–49, 81–82, 261–262. *See also* Reward, recognition, and reinforcement
Relationships: building, with Customers, 207–209; correlation of, with likelihood to recommend, 183; importance of, 183–185; leveraging Customer, 209
Reliability, as dimension of health care quality, 316–317
Remote clinics, 62
Repeat business, 105–106
Report cards of performance, Customer Satisfaction ratings as, 306–307
Reports: Customer Satisfaction reports: posting, in departments, 124–126, 127; sample, 125, 127; timeliness of, 150–151, 153; vendor flexibility in, 147. *See also* Customer Satisfaction measurement; Customer Satisfaction ratings
Retention, staff, 39–40, 45–46, 79–80, 229–233
Retirement homes, 205
Revenge, 156
Reward, recognition and reinforcement (3Rs), 48–49; for Associate retention, 232; departmental satisfaction statistics reporting and, 130; executive role in, 256–258, 348–349; for ideation and improvement, 266–270, 273–274, 351–352; linking, to Customer Satisfaction performance, 330–332; managers' role in, 261–262; organizational review of, 81–82; for service recovery innovation, 198, 204; varying, 351–352. *See also* Bonuses; Compensation
Right-to-satisfaction movement, 6–7, 14
Ritz-Carlton Hotels, 53, 211
Role models, managers as, 262
Rooms: design of, 320–321; healing elements in, 319–321; temperature of, 94, 95, 97; value-added, 324, 325. *See also* Waiting areas
Roykol, M., 163
Rural hospitals, market loss of, 61–62

S

St. Joseph's Hospital, 229
Satisfaction mirror, 43–44, 78–79, 230–231
Satisfaction Monitor, 22*n*.2
Satisfaction-Success Cycle, 8–10; Associate retention and, 229–233; quantification of, 42
Schlesinger, L., 42, 43, 229
Schneider, B., 42
Schulze, H., 211
Schwartz, J., 9, 17, 58, 251, 344
Screen savers, 282
Seafirst Bank, 160
Sears Corporation, 39–42, 229–230
Seibert, J., 3, 44, 116, 137*n*.2
Selection: for Associate service potential, 200–201, 202; of council members, 286; of physician account representatives, 303–304
Senior clubs, 206
Service and product extensions to health care, 208–209, 321–326. *See also* Value-added services
Service Excellence improvement plans, 246–248
Service potential, evaluation of Associate, 200–201, 202
Service quality: competitive advantage of, 236–237; as dimension of health care quality, 317; ideas for improving, 242–244. *See also* Complaints; Irritations; Value-added services
Service recovery, 164–166, 193–199, 219, 344–345. *See also* Complaints; Irritations; Problem solving
Service staff, seven essential traits of, 198–199

Service-profit-value chain. *See* Satisfaction-Success Cycle
Sherman, V. C., 4, 272
Shopping experiences, 221
Short-sighted management, 157–160
Signage, 312–313
Silver Cross Hospital (Joliet, Illinois), 36–37
Southwest Airlines (SWA), 56, 226, 230, 231–232, 236, 237, 347
Special needs: handling, 62–63; listening to, 38–39, 242–244. *See also* Customer needs and wants
Spot rewards, 331–332
Staff swapping, 328–330
Stage, being on, 228
Standardized management system, 353
Standards of Customer Satisfaction performance, 51–54, 82–83; in Adopt-a-Patient program, 292; conformance to, 317; Customer Satisfaction measures and, 129–132; high structure and, 346; for medical practices, 111–112; mentoring system and, 218
Stew Leonard's Dairy, 222
Strategy. *See* Customer Satisfaction strategy
Stream-of-consciousness log, 176–177
Stretch goals. *See* Big, Hairy, Audacious Goals
Strohmeyer, J., 116, 137*n.*2
Structure, high, 346
Success Cycle. *See* Satisfaction-Success Cycle
Suppliers, 186–187, 214
Support groups, 205
Survey return rates, 143–144
Surveys. *See* Associate Attitude and Opinion Surveys; Customer Satisfaction surveys
Sylvia, 225

T

Table tents, 73
Teen clubs, 206
Telemedicine, 62
Telephone calls, returning, 110, 111, 130
Telephone surveys, postdischarge, 142–143
Telephone systems: automated menu, 321–322; Customer-friendly, 336
Television remote reporting, 74, 75
Television viewing, charging for, 225, 226, 316
Temares, L., 182
Temporary assignments, 328–330
Terminations, natural-cause, 46
Terrorists, Customers as, 188–189
Testimonials, Customer, 280–281
Texas Medical Center, 229
3C Card-Complaints, Compliments, and Comments, 32, 69, 70, 75, 255, 313–314
Timeliness: of Customer Satisfaction data, 150–151, 153; defining, 213; of service recovery actions, 165–166, 194–197
Timing, 61
Tips: for Associates, for providing Customer Satisfaction, 125, 126, 281; for chief executive officers, for sustaining top performance, 344–355
Toilet tissue, 321
Tonight Show, 225
Top executives: active participation of, 259; communication of, 30, 68–69, 281–282; compensation for ideation for, 268; decision-making approaches of, and implementation strategy, 295–296; disciplined leadership of, 353; monthly meetings of, 30; role of, 256–259, 287; support of, for Customer Satisfaction management, 19, 21; sup-

port of, for ideation, 266, 287; valuing of Associates by, 350–351. *See also* Chief executive officer
Towels, 321
Training: for Adopt-a-Patient program, 291–292; on anxiety relief, 78; for Customer account representatives, 306; on Customer defection detection, 66–68; on Customer Satisfaction, 60, 197, 198, 337; on Do-It-Group/Just-Do-It-Group process, 287–288; in facility navigation, 312; on interpersonal skills, 241–245; investment in, 353–354; just-in-time, 291–292; on listening skills, 78; of medical staff, 84–85; needs evaluation for, 83–84; for physician account representatives, 305; on positive communication, 240–241; on problem solving, 199–200, 241–245; provided by Customer Satisfaction measurement vendors, 151; reference source for, 84; on service recovery, 197, 198; for standardized skills and behaviors, 83; work system improvement and, 341–342
Transportation services, 324
Travel services, 324
Trinity Hospital (Chicago), 9, 17, 47, 49, 58, 74, 196, 274, 344
Turnover, Associate, 45–46, 78–80, 229–230

U

Ubel, P., 226–227
Uncommon leadership, 340
Uniform standards, 51–54, 82–83. *See also* Standards of Customer Satisfaction performance
Uniforms, 51–52
University of Chicago Hospital, 229
University of Miami Colleague of Engineering, 182
University of Michigan, 39
University of Pennsylvania, 226
Unreasonable requests: "the Customer is always right" philosophy and, 221–225; hard choices and, 225–226; risks of responding to versus not responding to, 223–224
UPS, 56
USA Today, 182
User groups, vendor, 151

V

Value-added services, 208–209, 242–244, 321–326; application of, to every Customer encounter, 322–323; in general health care, 323–324; irritation removal and, 321–322; low cost of, 323, 325–326; in patient care, 323–324
Values-driven management, 339–340
Van, J., 249
Vendors. *See* Customer Satisfaction measurement vendors; Suppliers
Victory Scoreboard, 271–272, 278–280
Videos, testimonial, 280–281
Vision, 349
Visitors, as partners, 254–255

W

Waiting areas, 27–28, 68, 327
Waiting times, 26–29; communication with patient about, 122–123; as Customer defection point, 67; in emergency rooms, 27; in excess of fifteen minutes, 27, 28; excessive, 122–123; impact of reduced, 27, 28; in medical practices, 110, 111–112; observation of, 180; reducing, 122–123
Wannamaker, J., 221
Welcome letters and messages, 69, 71–72, 184–185, 335–336
Wellness services, 201–202, 205–206

Winners, 7–8
Women's health care centers, 321
Women's Services Center, 321
Work environment, 43, 45–46, 230–233
Work situations, interpretation of, in light of Customer Satisfaction standards, 260–261
Work systems: improving, 341–344; self-audit test of, 342
"Wow!" experiences, 326–327

X

Xerox Corporation, 42, 64, 188–191
X-ray staff, patient satisfaction and, 108, 109

Y

Youth: community involvement with, 205, 206; listening to, for ideas, 234–235

Z

Zero defections, 170
Zone of affection, 190
Zone of indifference, 189–190
Zone of defection, 188–189